Handbook of Systemic Autoimmune Diseases, Volume 17

The Lung in Autoimmune Diseases

Handbook of Systemic Autoimmune Diseases

Series Editor: F. Atzeni and P. Sarzi-Puttini

Volume 1 The Heart in Systemic Autoimmune Diseases
Edited by: Andrea Doria and Paolo Pauletto

Volume 2 Pulmonary Involvement in Systemic Autoimmune Diseases
Edited by: Athol U. Wells and Christopher P. Denton

Volume 3 Neurologic Involvement in Systemic Autoimmune Diseases
Edited by: Doruk Erkan and Steven R. Levine

Volume 4 Reproductive and Hormonal Aspects of Systemic Autoimmune Diseases
Edited by: Michael Lockshin and Ware Branch

Volume 5 The Skin in Systemic Autoimmune Diseases
Edited by: Piercarlo Sarzi-Puttini, Andrea Doria, Giampiero Girolomoni and Annegret Kuhn

Volume 6 Pediatrics in Systemic Autoimmune Diseases
Edited by: Rolando Cimaz and Thomas Lehman

Volume 7 The Kidney in Systemic Autoimmune Diseases
Edited by: Justin C. Mason and Charles D. Pusey

Volume 8 Digestive Involvement in Systemic Autoimmune Diseases
Edited by: Josep Font, Manuel Ramos-Casals and Juan Rodés

Volume 9 Endocrine Manifestations of Systemic Autoimmune Diseases
Edited by: Sara E. Walker and Luis J. Jara

Volume 10 Antiphospholipid Syndrome in Systemic Autoimmune Diseases
Edited by: Ricard Cervera, Joan Carles Reverter and Munther Khamashta

Volume 11 Pediatrics in Systemic Autoimmune Diseases, Second Edition
Edited by: Rolando Cimaz and Thomas Lehman

Volume 12 Antiphospholipid Syndrome in Systemic Autoimmune Diseases, Second Edition
Edited by: Ricard Cervera, Gerard Espinosa and Munther Khamashta

Volume 13 The Digestive Involvement in Systemic Autoimmune Diseases, Second Edition
Edited by: Manuel Ramos-Casals, Munther Khamashta, Pilar Brito-Zerón, Fabiola Atzeni and Joan Rodés Teixidor

Volume 14 The Heart in Systemic Autoimmune Diseases, Second Edition
Edited by: Fabiola Atzeni, Andrea Doria, Michael Nurmohamed and Paolo Pauletto

Volume 15 Surgery in Rheumatic and Muskuloskeletal Disease
Edited by: Fabiola Atzeni, Ignazio Francesco Masala, Daniel Aletaha, Marcus Lee and Xenofon Baraliakos

Volume 16 Infections in Systemic Autoimmune Diseases: Risk Factors and Management
Edited by: Fabiola Atzeni, James B. Galloway, Juan J. Gomez-Reino and Massimo Galli

Handbook of Systemic Autoimmune Diseases, Volume 17

The Lung in Autoimmune Diseases

Edited by

Fabiola Atzeni
Professor of Rheumatology, Rheumatology Unit,
University of Messina, Messina, Italy

José A. Gómez-Puerta
Rheumatology Department, Hospital Clínic, IDIBAPS,
University of Barcelona, Barcelona, Catalonia, Spain

Jacobo Sellares
Specialist in Respiratory Medicine, Interstitial Lung Diseases,
Hospital Clínic, IDIBAPS, University of Barcelona, Barcelona,
Catalonia, Spain

ELSEVIER

Elsevier
Radarweg 29, PO Box 211, 1000 AE Amsterdam, Netherlands
The Boulevard, Langford Lane, Kidlington, Oxford OX5 1GB, United Kingdom
50 Hampshire Street, 5th Floor, Cambridge, MA 02139, United States

Library of Congress Cataloging-in-Publication Data
A catalog record for this book is available from the Library of Congress

British Library Cataloguing-in-Publication Data
A catalogue record for this book is available from the British Library

ISBN: 978-0-323-91083-5
ISSN: 1571-5078

For information on all Elsevier publications visit our website at
https://www.elsevier.com/books-and-journals

Publisher: Stacy Masucci
Acquisitions Editor: Linda Versteeg-Buschman
Editorial Project Manager: Pat Gonzalez
Production Project Manager: Swapna Srinivasan
Cover designer: Christian J. Bilbow

Typeset by TNQ Technologies

The authors dedicate this book to their families.

Contents

Contributors xi

1. **Interstitial pneumonia with autoimmune features**
Anthony J. Esposito and Paul F. Dellaripa

Epidemiology 5
IPAF classification 6
Mechanisms of disease 10
Prognosis 12
Treatment considerations 13
Criticisms and potential shortcomings of the IPAF designation 14
Conclusions 16
Take home message 16
References 16

2. **Interstitial lung disease and rheumatoid arthritis**
Fabiola Atzeni, Cesare Siragusano and José A. Gómez-Puerta

Introduction 21
Risk factors and pathogenesis 21
Clinical manifestations 23
Diagnostic imaging 23
Different diagnostic methods 25
Therapy 26
Conclusions 33
Take-home messages 33
References 33

3. **Lung involvement in SLE**
Laurent Arnaud and Gerard Espinosa

Pleural involvement 41
Interstitial lung disease 42
Pulmonary arterial hypertension 45
Diffuse alveolar hemorrhage and pulmonary vasculitis 46
Acute lupus pneumonitis 46
Shrinking lung syndrome 48
References 50

4. Sjogren's syndrome and lung involvement
Ilektra Voulgareli, Vasiliki Koulouri, Alexandra Chroneou and Clio P. Mavragani

Introduction 55
Airway disease 56
Interstitial lung disease 58
Other pulmonary manifestations 65
References 66

5. Lung involvement in systemic sclerosis
Corrado Campochiaro, Cosimo Bruni, Sara Tomassetti, Lorenzo Dagna and Marco Matucci-Cerinic

Epidemiology 73
Pathogenesis 74
Clincal presentation 77
Diagnosis of ILD 78
Screening for ILD 86
ILD monitoring and progression 88
Prognosis 89
Treatment 90
COVID-19 and systemic sclerosis 94
Summary 95
Take-home messages 95
References 95

6. Inflammatory myopathy, mixed connective tissue disease, and antisynthetase syndrome
Albert Selva-O'Callaghan and Ernesto Trallero-Araguás

Introduction 105
The lung in inflammatory myopathies 105
The lung in mixed connective tissue disease 135
References 138

7. Lung involvement in ANCA-associated vasculitis
Sebastian Unizony and Andy Abril

Introduction 153
Pulmonary manifestations shared among all types of AAV 153
Pulmonary manifestations primarily seen in GPA and EGPA 158
Pulmonary manifestations primarily seen in GPA 159
Pulmonary manifestations primarily seen in EGPA 159
Treatment of lung involvement in ANCA-associated vasculitis 160
Conclusions 162
References 163

8. The lung in autoimmune diseases: sarcoidosis
Robert P. Baughman and Elyse E. Lower

Introduction 169
Lymphatic involvement 169
Parenchymal lung involvement 172
Pulmonary vascular involvement 174
Diagnosis of sarcoidosis 176
Treatment 178
Conclusion 182
Take home messages 182
References 182

9. COVID-19 and lung involvement
Jin-Seok You, Rosa Faner, Oriol Sibila and Jacobo Sellarés

Introduction 189
Epidemiology 190
Virology 191
Transmission 191
Pathogenesis 192
Clinical features 195
Laboratory findings 198
Imaging findings 198
Pathology findings 198
Diagnosis 200
Management 201
Conclusion 206
Take-home messages 206
References 207

Index 213

Contributors

Andy Abril, Division of Rheumatology, Mayo Clinic, Jacksonville, FL, United States

Laurent Arnaud, Department of Rheumatology, French National Reference Center for Autoimmune diseases (CRMR RESO), Strasbourg, France

Fabiola Atzeni, Rheumatology Unit, University of Messina, Messina, Italy

Robert P. Baughman, Department of Medicine, University of Cincinnati Medical Center, Cincinnati, OH, United States

Cosimo Bruni, Department of Experimental and Clinical Medicine, University of Florence, Florence, and Division of Rheumatology, AOUC, Florence, Italy

Corrado Campochiaro, Unit of Immunology, Rheumatology, Allergy and Rare diseases (UnIRAR), IRCCS San Raffaele Hospital, Milan, Italy; Vita-Salute San Raffaele University, Milan, Italy

Alexandra Chroneou, Department of Pulmonary Medicine, Sotiria Hospital, Athens, Greece

Lorenzo Dagna, Unit of Immunology, Rheumatology, Allergy and Rare diseases (UnIRAR), IRCCS San Raffaele Hospital, Milan, Italy; Vita-Salute San Raffaele University, Milan, Italy

Paul F. Dellaripa, Department of Medicine, Division of Rheumatology, Inflammation, and Immunity, Brigham and Women's Hospital, Harvard Medical School, Boston, MA, United States

Gerard Espinosa, Department of Autoimmune Diseases, Hospital Clinic, IDIBAPS, Universitat de Barcelona, Barcelona, Catalonia, Spain

Anthony J. Esposito, Department of Medicine, Division of Pulmonary and Critical Care Medicine, Northwestern University Feinberg School of Medicine, Chicago, IL, United States

Rosa Faner, Institut d'Investigacions Biomèdiques August Pi i Sunyer (IDIBAPS)-Centro de Investigación Biomedica en Red-Enfermedades Respiratorias (CIBERES), Madrid, Spain

José A. Gómez-Puerta, Rheumatology Department, Hospital Clínic, IDIBAPS, University of Barcelona, Barcelona, Catalonia, Spain

Vasiliki Koulouri, Department of Physiology, School of Medicine, National and Kapodistrian University of Athens, Athens, Greece

Elyse E. Lower, Department of Medicine, University of Cincinnati Medical Center, Cincinnati, OH, United States

Marco Matucci-Cerinic, Unit of Immunology, Rheumatology, Allergy and Rare diseases (UnIRAR), IRCCS San Raffaele Hospital, Milan, Italy; Department of Experimental and Clinical Medicine, University of Florence, Florence, and Division of Rheumatology, AOUC, Florence, Italy

Clio P. Mavragani, Department of Physiology, School of Medicine, National and Kapodistrian University of Athens, Athens, Greece

Jacobo Sellarés, Servei de Pneumologia, Institut Clínic Respiratori, Hospital Clínic, Barcelona, Spain

Albert Selva-O'Callaghan, Internal Medicine Department, Vall d'Hebron General Hospital, Barcelona, Spain

Oriol Sibila, Servei de Pneumologia, Institut Clínic Respiratori, Hospital Clínic, Barcelona, Spain

Cesare Siragusano, Rheumatology Unit, University of Messina, Messina, Italy

Sara Tomassetti, Department of Experimental and Clinical Medicine, University of Florence, and Division of Interventional Pneumology, AOUC, Florence, Italy

Ernesto Trallero-Araguás, Rheumatology Department, Vall d'Hebron General Hospital, Barcelona, Catalonia, Spain

Sebastian Unizony, Division of Rheumatology, Allergy and Immunology, The Edward A. Fox Chair in Medicine, Massachusetts General Hospital, Medicine Harvard Medical School, Boston, MA, United States

Ilektra Voulgareli, Department of Pulmonary Medicine, Sotiria Hospital, Athens, Greece

Jin-Seok You, Servei de Pneumologia, Institut Clínic Respiratori, Hospital Clínic, Barcelona, Spain

Chapter 1

Interstitial pneumonia with autoimmune features

Anthony J. Esposito[1] and Paul F. Dellaripa[2,*]
[1]*Department of Medicine, Division of Pulmonary and Critical Care Medicine, Northwestern University Feinberg School of Medicine, Chicago, IL, United States;* [2]*Department of Medicine, Division of Rheumatology, Inflammation, and Immunity, Brigham and Women's Hospital, Harvard Medical School, Boston, MA, United States*
[*]*Corresponding author at: pdellaripa@bwh.harvard.edu.*

Interstitial pneumonia with autoimmune features (IPAF) is a research classification proposed to describe individuals with idiopathic interstitial pneumonia (IIP) who have combinations of clinical, serologic, and/or thoracic morphologic features of a systemic autoimmune condition yet who fail to meet established criteria for an underlying connective tissue disease (CTD). Since its inception, several studies have retrospectively applied the classification criteria and have yielded significant heterogeneity across cohorts with regards to the characteristics of patients identified with IPAF, suggesting further refinement of the criteria is necessary. Nonetheless, those with IPAF seem to have an overall prognosis that is likely worse than those with defined CTD-associated interstitial lung disease (ILD) and better than those with idiopathic pulmonary fibrosis (IPF). The optimal treatment of IPAF is unknown though evidence is emerging for the use of antifibrotics for those with a progressive fibrosing phenotype. Further research is needed to elucidate which elements of the clinical, serologic, and morphologic domains confer the most prognostic information to a diagnosis of IPAF to help guide further development of the classification criteria and to facilitate clinical trial design in order to establish standardized treatment approaches.

The ILDs are a heterogenous collection of rare diffuse parenchymal lung disorders that are typified by varying combinations of fibrosis and inflammation and grouped by common clinical, radiologic, and histopathologic manifestations [1–5]. They are broadly characterized by those with or without an identifiable cause. The most commonly identifiable causes of ILD include CTD, sarcoidosis, occupational or environmental inhalational exposures, or drug- or radiation-induced lung injury. To be diagnosed with an IIP, of which IPF is the most common, exclusion of known causes of ILD is required [5].

The Lung in Autoimmune Diseases. https://doi.org/10.1016/B978-0-323-91083-5.00006-2

CTD is one of the most common causes of underlying ILD and is identified in up to 30% of new diagnoses [6]. Current guidelines recommend excluding a CTD not only because it is prevalent in ILD but also because it has important prognostic and therapeutic implications [3,5,7–9]. CTD-ILD, in general, has a more favorable prognosis than the IIPs [7,9]. Furthermore, management of CTD-ILD is often guided by treatment standards established for the underlying CTD [10,11], frequently employing immunosuppression which has been demonstrated to be harmful to individuals with IPF [12]. Despite the recommendation and clinical importance of identifying CTD, no standard approach to assess for one exists. If and how the evaluation for CTD is performed is clinician-dependent but typically involves assessing for extrathoracic features of CTD, testing for circulating autoantibodies, and integrating results from radiologic and/or histopathologic studies [13].

It has been estimated that 10%–20% of patients with IIP have subtle features suggestive of an autoimmune etiology without fulfillment of the American College of Rheumatology criteria for a CTD [8,14–18]. Interest in an intermediate phenotype between CTD-ILD and IIP resulted in multiple prior classifications. Undifferentiated CTD (UCTD)-associated ILD incorporated extrathoracic signs of autoimmunity (e.g., Raynaud's phenomenon, inflammatory arthritis, sicca symptoms, and proximal muscle weakness) with specific circulating autoantibodies in the presence of an interstitial pneumonia [8]. Diagnosis of UCTD-ILD was correlated with the presence of nonspecific interstitial pneumonia (NSIP)—the most common radiologic/histopathologic interstitial pneumonia in CTD [18]—but was not associated with a five-year survival advantage, faring worse than a CTD-ILD diagnosis [17]. Autoimmune-featured ILD combined extrathoracic symptoms with autoantibodies, but it failed in many aspects to differentiate CTD-ILD from IPF [17]. Finally, lung dominant-CTD integrated CTD-associated radiographic interstitial pneumonia patterns with autoantibodies, extrathoracic features of autoimmunity, and histopathologic findings [16]. These terminologies, while overlapping in many instances, fell short of capturing the diverse spectrum of phenotypes that can result when an autoimmune process is suspected of causing an ILD.

In 2015, the "European Respiratory Society/American Thoracic Society Task Force on Undifferentiated Forms of Connective Tissue Disease-associated Interstitial Lung Disease"—an international and multidisciplinary working group of experts from centers that had previously described suggestive forms of CTD-ILD—convened to establish consensus for the nomenclature and classification of patients with IIP and features of autoimmunity [19]. This task force published a research statement grounded in expert consensus that (1) designated the term "interstitial pneumonia with autoimmune features (IPAF)" to describe individuals with IIP who have combinations of clinical, serologic, and/or thoracic morphologic features of a systemic autoimmune condition yet who fail to meet established criteria for an underlying CTD (Figs. 1.1 and 1.2) proposed classification criteria for IPAF (Table 1.1) [19].

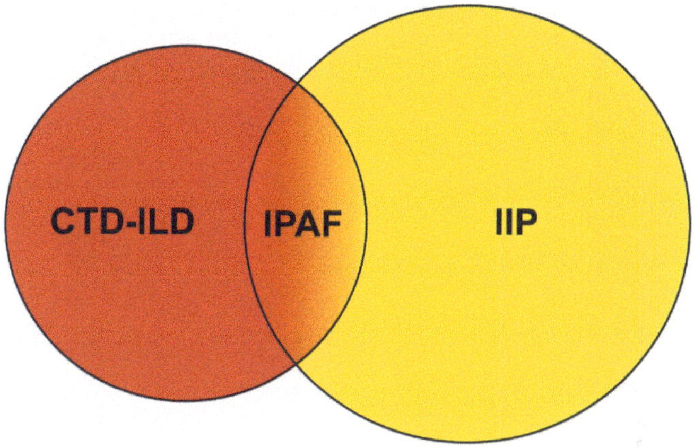

FIGURE 1.1 **Venn diagram displaying the relationship of interstitial pneumonia with autoimmune features (IPAF) to connective tissue disease (CTD)-associated interstitial lung disease (ILD) and idiopathic interstitial pneumonia (IIP).** IPAF is likely an intermediate phenotype with overlapping features of CTD-ILD and IIP.

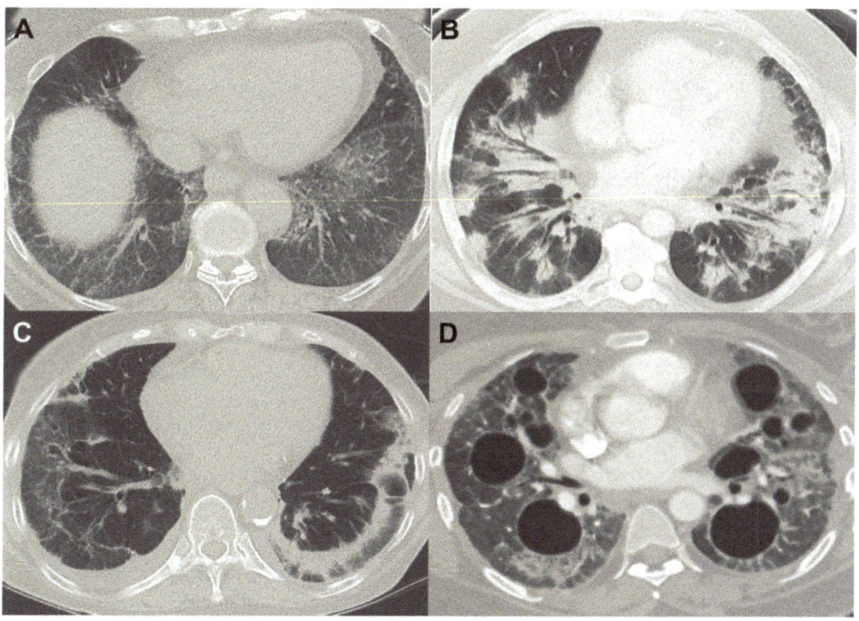

FIGURE 1.2 **Representative high-resolution computed tomography images of interstitial pneumonia patterns that can be associated with interstitial pneumonia with autoimmune features.** (A) Nonspecific interstitial pneumonia (NSIP). (B) Organizing Pneumonia (OP). (C) NSIP with OP overlap. (D) Lymphocytic Interstitial Pneumonia.

TABLE 1.1 Classification of interstitial pneumonia with autoimmune features.

1. Presence of an interstitial pneumonia as determined by HRCT or SLB
2. Exclusion of alternative etiologies
3. Does not meet criteria for a defined CTD
4. At least one feature from at least two of the following domains:
   A. Clinical domain
   B. Serologic domain
   C. Morphologic domain

A. Clinical domain
   1. Distal digital fissuring (i.e., "mechanic hands")
   2. Distal digital tip ulceration
   3. Inflammatory arthritis *or* polyarticular morning joint stiffness ≥60 min
   4. Palmar telangiectasia
   5. Raynaud's phenomenon
   6. Unexplained digital edema
   7. Unexplained fixed rash on digital extensor surfaces (Gottron sign)

B. Serologic domain
   1. ANA >1:320 titer (diffuse, speckled, homogeneous patterns) *or*
      a. ANA nucleolar pattern (any titer) *or*
      b. ANA centromere pattern (any titer)
   2. Rheumatoid factor ≥2× upper limit of normal
   3. Anti-CCP
   4. Anti-dsDNA
   5. Anti-Ro (SS-A)
   6. Anti-La (SS-B)
   7. Anti-ribonucleoprotein
   8. Anti-Smith
   9. Anti-topoisomerase (Scl-70)
   10. Anti-tRNA synthetase (e.g., Jo-1, PL-7, PL-12, EJ, OJ, KS, Zo, tRS)
   11. Anti-PM-Scl
   12. Anti-MDA-5

C. Morphologic domain
   1. Suggestive radiology patterns by HRCT:
      a. NSIP
      b. OP
      c. NSIP with OP overlap
      d. LIP
   2. Histopathology patterns or features by SLB:
      a. NSIP
      b. OP
      c. NSIP with OP overlap
      d. LIP
      e. Interstitial lymphoid aggregates with germinal centers
      f. Diffuse lymphoplasmacytic infiltration (with or without lymphoid follicles)

TABLE 1.1 Classification of interstitial pneumonia with autoimmune features.—cont'd

3. Multicompartment involvement (in addition to interstitial pneumonia): a. Unexplained pleural effusion or thickening b. Unexplained pericardial effusion or thickening c. Unexplained intrinsic airways disease (by PFT, imaging, or pathology)[a] d. Unexplained pulmonary vasculopathy

ANA, antinuclear antibody; *CTD*, connective tissue disease; *HRCT*, high-resolution computed tomography; *LIP*, lymphocytic interstitial pneumonia; *NSIP*, nonspecific interstitial pneumonia; *OP*, organizing pneumonia; *PFT*, pulmonary function testing; *SLB*, surgical lung biopsy.
[a]*Includes airflow obstruction, bronchiolitis, and bronchiectasis.*
Adapted with permission from reference Fischer A, Antoniou KM, Brown KK, Cadranel J, Corte TJ, du Bois RM, et al. An official European Respiratory Society/American Thoracic Society research statement: interstitial pneumonia with autoimmune features. Eur Respir J. 2015;46(4):976–87.

The statement cautions that the concepts proposed were not intended to guide clinical care but rather to serve as a platform for future, prospective research of this putative IIP subset. The term "connective tissue disease" was purposefully avoided in choosing the term IPAF as to not give the false impression that these patients have, or were destined to develop, a defined CTD.

Epidemiology

Since publication of these classification criteria, several retrospectively identified cohorts of patients with ILD who fulfill IPAF criteria have been described [20–26]. These single-center, observational studies are limited by the population examined, which was strongly influenced by the recruitment profile of each institution (i.e., referral bias); nevertheless, they provide insight into the prevalence and characteristics of patients with IPAF.

The prevalence of IPAF among those with ILD is estimated to be 7%–34% [20,21,26]. The mean age varies from 60 to 68 years [20,22–26], with some reporting a younger mean of about 55 years of age [21]. Patients with IPAF seem to have a balanced sex distribution although several studies have reported a skew toward females [21,23,25]. These patient characteristics notably differ from what has been observed for CTD-ILD, with a predominantly female and younger phenotype [9,18], and for patients with IPF who tend to be male and older [27]. Unlike CTD-ILD, smoking has been reported in about a third and as high as 55% of individuals with IPAF [20,21,26], which may be attributed to the greater percentage of cases with usual interstitial pneumonia (UIP) that meet IPAF criteria [26]. Published studies report that patients classified as IPAF who progress to a diagnosis of CTD-ILD exist but represent a minority (12% in one study) [24], suggesting that IPAF may truly be an intermediate phenotype between CTD-ILD and IIP (Fig. 1.1).

Interestingly, a significant proportion of patients previously diagnosed with IIP fulfilled a diagnosis of IPAF when the diagnostic criteria were retrospectively applied. In a series by Oldham et al. [26], 60% of patients with cryptogenic organizing pneumonia (OP), 30% with idiopathic NSIP, 25% with unclassifiable IIP, and 18% with IPF met criteria for IPAF. Those who were previously classified as UCTD-ILD met IPAF criteria in 91% of cases and accounted for 50% of IPAF diagnoses [26].

IPAF classification

To classify an IIP as IPAF, several a priori requirements must be fulfilled (Table 1.1) [19]:

1. Individuals must have evidence of interstitial pneumonia by high-resolution computed tomography (HRCT) imaging and/or by surgical lung biopsy (SLB).
2. Clinical evaluation must exclude known causes for interstitial pneumonia (e.g., exposure-related, sarcoidosis).
3. Criteria for a characterizable CTD cannot be satisfied.

For disease to be considered IPAF, the individual must meet all a priori requirements and have at least one feature from at least two of three central domains [19]:

A. Clinical domain (extrathoracic features)
B. Serologic domain (circulating autoantibodies)
C. Morphologic domain (pulmonary imaging, histopathologic, or physiologic features)

An illustrative case of a patient with IPAF is provided in Box 1.1.

Clinical domain

The clinical domain includes extrathoracic features suggestive of an underlying CTD. While these features are specific to various CTDs, they are not on their own sufficient to establish a diagnosis [19]. They include distal digital fissuring ("mechanic hands"), distal digital tip ulceration, inflammatory arthritis or polyarticular morning joint stiffness lasting greater than 60 minutes, palmar telangiectasia, Raynaud's phenomenon, unexplained digital edema, and unexplained fixed rash on the digital extensor surfaces (Gottron sign) (Table 1.1). Between 20% and 63% of patients with IPAF have at least

BOX 1.1 Case example: idiopathic pneumonia with autoimmune features (IPAF).

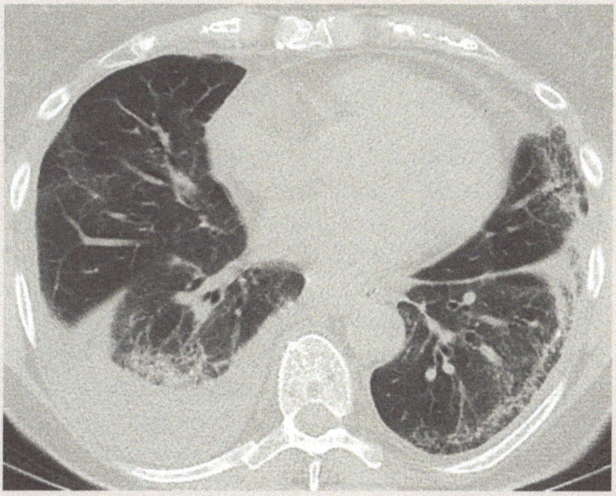

Case: A 70-year-old, previously healthy female presented with chronic cough and pleuritic chest pain. She did not have any significant occupational or environmental exposures. Exam revealed bibasilar crackles and diminished breath sounds at the right base. There were no extrathoracic features of autoimmune disease present, specifically no Raynaud's phenomenon, synovitis, distal digital fissuring, distal digital tip ulceration, palmar telangiectasia, digital edema, or rash. Chest radiograph revealed a large volume pleural effusion, which was sampled via thoracentesis. Pleural fluid analysis yielded a lymphocytic-predominant exudative effusion with negative cultures, including acid fast bacilli. Chest CT (displayed) revealed a large right sided pleural effusion and peripheral, basilar-predominant reticulations with subpleural sparing, consistent with NSIP. Serologic studies were notable for an ANA titer of 1:640 in a speckled pattern with positive anti-double stranded DNA and anti-Ro52 antibodies. She was HIV negative.

Discussion: This patient fulfills criteria for classification of IPAF. She meets all three a priori criteria in that (1) she has an interstitial pneumonia (i.e., NSIP), (2) she does not have obvious alternative etiologies, and (3) she does not meet criteria for a defined CTD. While she does not meet any criteria for the clinical domain, she meets several in the serologic and morphologic domains. Her ANA titer is > 1:320, and she has a circulating anti-Ro antibody. For the morphologic domain, she meets two of the subdomains: (1) she has CT evidence of NSIP, and (2) she has multicompartment involvement with an unexplained pleural effusion.

one clinical criterion, which is the least common criterion fulfilled for diagnosis. The most commonly reported are Raynaud's phenomenon (13%–74%), inflammatory arthritis or morning stiffness (5%–48%), mechanic hands (2%–29%), and Gottron sign (1%–18%) [20–26].

Serologic domain

In this domain, autoantibodies that are strongly associated with CTD and that are commonly assessed in the evaluation of an individual with presumed IIP are included; nonspecific markers of inflammation, such as erythrocyte sedimentation rate and C-reactive protein, are explicitly excluded (Table 1.1). For less-specific antibodies (i.e., antinuclear antibody [ANA] and rheumatoid factor [RF]), high titers are required to fulfill the domain's criteria with the exception of a nucleolar or centromere ANA-staining pattern which is sufficient at any titer [19]. The reason for this distinction is twofold: (1) weakly reactive ANA testing (specifically in diffuse, homogeneous, or speckled patterns) and low-level titers of RF are present in many nonrheumatic patients and not infrequently in "healthy" control populations, particularly the elderly [28,29], and (2) nucleolar and centromere-staining patterns of ANA are strongly associated with systemic sclerosis (SSc) but are not diagnostic for disease in solitude [28]. It should be noted that the current guidelines for ANA testing recommend indirect immunofluorescence [30], which allows for the reporting of both the titer and staining pattern. Enzyme-linked immunosorbent assay for ANA is discouraged, as it is less reliable, does not allow for assessment of a staining pattern, and can be falsely negative in a subset of patients with SSc [31]. Furthermore, antineutrophil cytoplasmic antibodies are also excluded from this domain due to their association with the vasculitides rather than the CTD-ILD spectra of disorders despite reports of positivity in those with IIP, particularly those with UIP [32].

More than 90% of patients with IPAF have at least one serologic criterion, which is the most commonly fulfilled for diagnosis. High-titer ANA is the most frequently observed (48%–82%). Other frequently reported autoantibodies include anti-tRNA synthetase (e.g., Jo-1, PL-7, PL-12, EJ, OJ, KS, ZO, and tRS), anti-Ro (SS-A), and high-titer RF [20–26].

Morphologic domain

The morphologic domain is divided into three subdomains: HRCT patterns, histopathologic features from SLB, and multicompartment thoracic features determined by imaging, histopathology, right heart catheterization, or pulmonary function testing. If any one of these three subdomains is present, the criteria for the morphologic domain are fulfilled [19].

The radiologic subdomain includes interstitial pneumonia patterns on HRCT that are commonly associated with CTD-ILD and whose presence should raise suspicion for an underlying autoimmune process. These are NSIP, OP, NSIP with OP, and lymphoid interstitial pneumonia (LIP) [19]. Representative examples of these HRCT patterns are provided in Fig. 1.2. It is important to note that a UIP pattern is also identified in some CTD-ILDs and is most commonly described in patients with rheumatoid arthritis (RA)-associated ILD [33]; however, UIP was excluded as a morphologic feature, as its presence is less specific for CTD compared to the other IIP patterns. Having a UIP pattern on HRCT does not exclude a diagnosis of IPAF, but one does not accrue "credit" toward the diagnosis as would be the case for NSIP, OP, or LIP patterns [19]. To be considered IPAF with a UIP HRCT pattern, a patient would need to fulfill criteria in both the clinical and serologic domains or have multicompartment thoracic involvement of disease, which would necessarily argue against a diagnosis of IPF. In several series, NSIP is the most common HRCT pattern reported (41%–57%) followed by NSIP with OP overlap [20–25]; however, a higher prevalence of the UIP pattern was found by Oldham et al. (55%) [26], which has been attributed to the recruitment profile of the study center.

The histopathologic subdomain requires evaluation of the lung parenchyma by SLB to identify patterns that are highly associated with the presence of a CTD. These include NSIP, OP, NSIP with OP, and LIP [19]. While these histopathologic patterns share nomenclature with the aforementioned radiologic patterns, the presence of one does not correlate with the other contrary to what has been described for UIP [34]; hence, this was the rationale to inform keeping the subdomains separate. The subdomain also includes secondary histopathologic features of interstitial lymphoid aggregates with germinal centers and diffuses lymphoplasmacytic infiltration with or without lymphoid follicles [19]. As with the radiologic subsection, UIP pattern on SLB was excluded due to its lack of association with an underlying CTD. Despite Oldham et al. describing UIP histopathology in 74% of surgical lung biopsies [26], the most common histopathologic pattern reported in IPAF patients is NSIP and is present in up to 59%. Interstitial lymphoid aggregates with germinal centers and diffuse lymphoplasmacytic infiltration are also frequently encountered, especially when UIP receives "credit" for the morphologic domain [20–26].

The last of the morphologic subdomains is the multicompartment designation. Disease in several concurrent thoracic compartments is often encountered in patients with CTDs but, as is the case with the other domains, is not diagnostic of any particular disease. This subdomain considers "unexplained" airway, vascular, pleural, or pericardial abnormalities as suggestive of underlying autoimmunity [19]. While these abnormalities can be evident on HRCT or histopathology, ancillary testing in the form of pulmonary function testing (airways), right heart catheterization (vascular; e.g., pulmonary arterial hypertension), and echocardiogram (pericardium) are often necessary for diagnosis. Outside of the interstitium, the most common thoracic compartment affected in IPAF is the vasculature (17%–30%) followed by the airways (9%–22%) [20–26].

Mechanisms of disease

IPAF represents an entity that has features between or incorporates elements of CTD-ILD and IIP (Fig. 1.1), particularly IPF [19]. Attempts to delineate mechanisms of disease in IPAF from those identified or postulated in CTD-ILD or IPF are a useful starting point to understand the pathogenesis of ILD in IPAF but may be limited by distinct features that may make IPAF a separate and unique entity. Given the heterogeneity within CTD-ILD (RA-ILD vs. SSc-associated ILD for example), elucidation of mechanism of disease in IPAF represents a particular challenge given the diversity of disease manifestations and the broad phenotypic classification inherent to the IPAF designation. Hence, caution must be taken to extrapolate how mechanisms of disease hypothesized in CTD-ILD and IPF apply to IPAF. This discussion will focus on immune dysregulation of specific immune T and B cells, the effects of immune mediators including cytokines and chemokines, and genetic mechanisms that may play a role in promoting ILD and pulmonary fibrosis. Special attention is given to how these mechanisms may affect clinical outcomes and prognosis, as they are applied with the limited data available from described IPAF cohorts.

Role of the immune system

Immune response to injury of the lung epithelium—potentially due to environmental exposures like cigarette smoking, pollution, or aspiration—leads to a homeostatic repair response in normal circumstances; however, in pathologic environments, repetitive injury activates fibrotic pathways marked by differentiation of myofibroblasts as part of the wound healing process [35]. Both the innate and adaptive immune system play a role in this process. Macrophages are a critical aspect of the innate immune systems and play an important role in the development of fibrosis in the lung via numerous mechanisms [36]. Macrophages can differentiate into profibrotic or proinflammatory forms leading to the secretion of cytokines which include but are not limited to interleukin (IL)-1B, IL-6, IL-8, IL-10, transforming growth factor (TGF)-beta, vascular endothelial growth factor, and platelet-derived growth factor in addition to numerous chemokines including chemokine ligand (CXCL) 9, CXCL10, and CXCL12 [37,38]. Specifically, IL-6 is a proinflammatory cytokine that can stimulate fibroblasts, lead to differentiation into myofibroblasts, and promote the production of extracellular matrix, leading to fibrosis [39]. Increased IL-6 activity noted in early SSc-ILD has led to utilization of IL-6 antagonists in its treatment [40,41]. Neutrophils, another important part of the innate immune system, also play a role in the development of fibrosis via modulation of extracellular matrix turnover and the excretion of neutrophil extracellular traps [42,43].

Adaptive immune responses have also been postulated to participate in both profibrotic and antifibrotic processes via T helper cell Th1, Th2, Th17, and T regulatory cells. Specifically, T cell profiles that exhibit an increased Th2 response have been noted in IPF and SSc-ILD, and Th17 cells may play an important role in RA-ILD and IPF [44,45]. B cell activation, as evidenced by the presence of B cell laden lymphoid follicles in lung tissue as noted in RA-ILD and other CTD-ILDs [46], is also part of the morphologic criteria in the IPAF designation; however, characterization of specific T and B cell populations that have been identified in IPF or CTD-ILD, like SSc-, RA-, or Sjogren's-associated ILD, have not been studied in a similar fashion in IPAF, limiting their application. Theoretically, these pathways and histopathologic phenotypes may be expressed in varying degrees in IPAF and thus reflect the diversity of immune responses and phenotypes noted in patients with IPAF.

While understanding of mechanisms of disease is slowly emerging in SSc-ILD and IPF and to a lesser extent in RA-ILD, there has been a paucity of investigation in ILD related to IPAF. One recent study compared IPAF patients with IPF and CTD-ILD and identified significantly increased serum levels of the chemokines CXCL9, CXCL10, and CXCL1 in CTD-ILD and IPAF compared to IPF [47]. More specifically, IPAF levels were intermediate between IPF and CTD-ILD.

Circulating autoantibodies are an important part of the classification criteria for IPAF though the role that autoantibody formation plays in the pathogenesis of ILD, especially CTD-ILD and IPAF, is unclear. With regards to lung and synovial pathology in RA and perhaps IPF, the role of anti-citrullinated protein antibodies (anti-CCP) and protein conformational changes that result in the face of antigenic exposure is an area of active investigation [48]. Other autoantibodies such as anti-topoisomerase (Scl-70) have been postulated to interact and promote fibrosis via CD4+ T cells in patients with SSc-ILD [49]. Furthermore, anti-melanoma differentiation-associated protein 5 (MDA5) and the Th/To and ribonucleoprotein autoantibody confer a higher risk for ILD and worse prognosis, though the role of these antibodies in the formation of inflammatory and fibrotic changes in the lung is unknown.

Genetics

Several lines of evidence point to an important role for genetics in the development of ILD and particularly IPAF. Telomeres represent distal elements of chromosomes that maintain their integrity. Loss of function of telomere maintenance enzymes or telomere destabilization can compromise the ability to effectively heal after alveolar epithelial injury in the lung [50]. Shortened leukocyte telomere length (LTL) and mutations in telomere maintenance genes (*TERT, TERC*, and *RTEL1* among others) have been described in a variety of ILDs including IPF, hypersensitivity pneumonitis, and RA-ILD [51]; their presence can be associated with lung fibrosis and worse outcomes [52]. Studies investigating telomere abnormalities in IPAF in a large observational cohort comparing IPAF and CTD-ILD with IPF have demonstrated that LTLs are longer in CTD-ILD and IPAF compared to IPF and that LTL less than the 10th percentile among IPAF patients is associated with worsened decline in lung function compared to LTL greater than 10th percentile [53].

In addition to telomere abnormalities, variants in the mucin 5B gene (*MUC5B*) have been associated with disease severity in IPF and other ILDs such as RA-ILD [54,55]. In RA-ILD, the *MUC5B* promoter variant portends a worse prognosis associated with a UIP pattern [55], which is of interest as UIP is not part of the morphologic domain in IPAF. IPAF patients have been noted to have a higher frequency of *MUC5B* allele representation and this appeared to confer a worse transplant-free survival [53].

Prognosis

Although several studies have examined overall survival in patients with IPAF compared to other ILDs, the findings are often conflicting and are limited to retrospective, single-center designs. Oldham et al. identified 144 patients previously classified as having IIP or UCTD-ILD who met IPAF criteria from their ILD registry at the University of Chicago [26]. They found that patients with IPAF had worse survival than those with CTD-ILD and marginally better survival than those with IPF though not statistically significant. When stratified by presence of UIP on HRCT or SLB, those with a non-UIP pattern had similar survival to CTD-ILD and those with a UIP pattern had similar survival to those with IPF. Both age and diffusion capacities of the lung for carbon monoxide were significant predictors of mortality in multivariate analyses. Interestingly, presence of the clinical domain was associated with a decrease in the risk of mortality by about a half while the serologic and morphologic domains were associated with a nonsignificant increase in morality risk. Nonetheless, the presence of multicompartment features was associated with a greater than twofold increase in mortality risk. A major criticism of this study is the high proportion of patients with UIP (55% by HRCT and 74% of those who had SLB) who met IPAF criteria, which was explained by the referral pattern of the university; 30% previously had a diagnosis of IPF. This may be the reason these authors found older age and a higher percentage of smokers in those with IPAF than what had previously been reported for UCTD-ILD.

Ahmad et al. identified 57 patients with IPAF from the Claude Bernard Lyon University in France [20]. They also found that the probability of survival in IPAF patients was no different than those with IPF over a median follow-up of 16 months. Contrasting the results of Oldham et al. [26], the authors did not find a difference when patients with IPAF were stratified by NSIP or UIP HRCT pattern [20]. A history of smoking was the only variable associated with higher mortality. A similar study from a rheumatology clinic at the University of Colorado found stable lung function and no deaths in 56 predominantly female, never smokers with IPAF who were observed for a mean of 285 weeks [21]. It is important to note that all but one of the patients in this study were receiving immunosuppressive treatments, most commonly in the form of corticosteroids (82%). These studies illustrate the variability in outcomes data and suggest that at least some of this variability may be explained by the recruitment characteristics of the cohorts examined.

Lim et al. in a South Korean cohort reported IPAF survival that was worse than CTD-ILD but better than IPF [23]; however, no significant difference was observed between patients with IPAF and a UIP pattern compared to IPF though the UIP-IPAF group tended to survive a longer duration. They also investigated acute exacerbations of ILD with a definition that was extrapolated from the IPF literature [56]. While the proportion of patients with IPAF having an acute ILD exacerbation was lower (26%) than that for CTD-ILD (33%) and IPF (35%) and was significantly different one, three, and five years after cohort enrollment, time to first exacerbation was no different between the IPAF and IPF groups while those with CTD-ILD had a significantly longer duration to first exacerbation compared to the IPF group [23]. As has been shown to be a strong risk factor for mortality in IPF [56], acute exacerbation of ILD was a significant risk factor for mortality from IPAF in multivariate analyses [23].

In a large study from China, 177 patients with IPAF were identified from 1429 patients with previously diagnosed ILD [22]. Patients with IPAF were found to have significantly worse survival compared to those without IPAF. In subgroup analyses, patients with IPAF were found to have similar survival to those with UCTD-ILD and dramatically better survival than the IPF group. Predictors of poor survival in multivariate analyses were age, smoking history, anti-ribonucleoprotein positivity, and OP pattern on HRCT.

These studies suggest that patients with IPAF have an intermediate prognosis that is worse than those with CTD-ILD but likely better than those with IPF. Those with IPAF and a UIP pattern may have worse outcomes. Solid conclusions cannot be drawn from the available studies due to the differences in the cohorts studied and methodology used. The only available prospective study of IPAF patients did not report survival data [57]; therefore, rigorous, prospective data from multiple centers are needed to better define the prognostic significance of the IPAF designation.

Treatment considerations

Treatment standards for patients with IPAF have not been established, as prospective clinical trials are lacking. Current practice is guided by expert opinion and by outcome observations from retrospective studies. In general, treatment of IPAF is directed by the overall impression of the lung morphology, namely whether it conforms to a predominately inflammatory or fibrotic phenotype.

Patients with predominantly inflammatory lung disease usually present with ground glass opacities on HRCT (such as in cellular NSIP) and lymphoplasmocytic infiltration of lung tissue with or without lymphoid follicles on histopathology. Treatment strategies for these patients consist primarily of corticosteroids usually in combination with a second agent: mycophenolate mofetil, azathioprine, a calcineurin inhibitor, and in some cases a JAK inhibitor are all considerations. In more severe cases, B cell depletion with rituximab or cyclophosphamide are options [22,26,58].

Patients with predominantly fibrotic lung disease usually present with reticulations, honeycombing, and/or traction bronchiectasis on HRCT and interstitial collagen deposition on histopathology. There is some evidence from clinical trials supporting the use of antifibrotics (pirfenidone or nintedanib) in these patients [59−61]; however, IPAF was neither specifically investigated in subgroup analyses nor did it represent a significant number of patients recruited to those trials. Of note, if UIP is evident despite its exclusion from the IPAF designation, adding antifibrotic therapy in the event of progressive disease is reasonable given that UIP likely portends a worse prognosis. Nonetheless, some patients with IPAF will have evidence of both inflammation and fibrosis. Consideration for both forms of therapy (immunosuppression plus antifibrotics) in these cases may be reasonable though prospective data for this strategy are still lacking.

A general treatment approach to IPAF involves the use of corticosteroids in combination with either azathioprine or mycophenolate mofetil in mild to moderate cases with consideration for addition of rituximab or cyclophosphamide in more severe cases. Lung transplant evaluation, pneumocystis prophylaxis, pulmonary rehabilitation, oxygen supplementation, and immunization are also essential components of the treatment plan as with any other IIP.

Criticisms and potential shortcomings of the IPAF designation

The IPAF designation is predicated on the presence of a group of features within the clinical domain, the serologic domain, and the morphologic domain [19]. It was developed by and agreed upon through a consensus process by a group of experienced clinicians as a framework to understand hard-to-classify patients with ILD. The designation was meant to serve as a launching pad for further investigation and refinement as our understanding of this disease entity evolves over time.

Each of these domains raises questions moving forward about which criteria are most appropriate for the IPAF designation or whether some criteria will be recategorized into a more defined CTD. For clinical criteria, while some features appear to be nonspecific and generalizable clinically (such as adult-onset Raynaud's phenomenon, inflammatory arthritis, and perhaps digital edema), other clinical features may be more clearly linked to known phenotypes. For example, distal digital fissures are most closely associated with the antisynthetase syndrome or can sometimes be seen in the anti-MDA5 syndrome [62], while Gottron sign is closely linked phenotypically with dermatomyositis [63]. As such, these features in future iterations of the IPAF schema may be removed. Similarly, a group of clinical features that are not included in the IPAF designation yet are associated with a variety of CTDs—for example, abnormalities seen with nailfold capillary microscopy or esophageal dysmotility—but are not necessarily specific for a defined CTD may in the future be included in the IPAF criteria. The limited attention paid to diagnostic testing for Sjogren's syndrome in the criteria that may in the future include salivary gland imaging, function, and biopsy may shift patients otherwise designated as IPAF into Sjogren's-associated ILD. The designation of "arthritis" is also fraught with some degree of diagnostic ambiguity, as the evaluation for this criterion is dependent on the level of expertise of the clinician performing the examination. The use of ancillary radiologic and ultrasonic imaging may affect the accuracy of this particular physical finding.

The serologic domain also presents significant classification challenges. While ANA testing is an important marker of autoimmunity, it is associated with a high degree of false positivity [28,29], and quality concerns with test performance related to the type of assay utilized remain an issue [30]. Findings such as cytoplasmic staining, which can be seen with ANA testing and is often associated with an "ANA negative" result, can be associated with the antisynthetase syndrome yet may not be reported or incorporated into the evaluation of a patient with ILD where an autoimmune phenotype is being considered [64]. Other antibodies like anti-MDA5, Ro, K52, and Th/To may ultimately be linked to identifiable phenotypes and thus be removed from the IPAF designation entirely.

Regarding the morphologic domain, most cases are adjudicated by HRCT, and while the correlation between a UIP pattern on HRCT and histopathologic findings is established [34], NSIP and other IIP patterns within the IPAF domain show less correlation between HRCT and histopathologic findings. The concept of multicompartmentalism, often considered supportive of a systemic process and included in the IPAF criteria, is controversial in that it can be challenging to link what may appear to be disparate lung findings to an underlying autoimmune process. However, such findings may, in reality, be related to other etiologies or a different diagnosis altogether. In summary, these challenges highlight the need for continued engagement of multidisciplinary groups of clinicians and investigators to help improve our understanding of and enhance our ability to classify patients with IPAF.

Conclusions

The IPAF designation is an important research classification established to provide consensus for the nomenclature and classification of patients with IIP and features of autoimmunity. Initial single-center studies of retrospectively identified patients with IPAF have demonstrated significant heterogeneity between cohorts, suggesting that further refinement of the criteria is needed. Nonetheless, patients with IPAF seem to have an overall prognosis that is likely worse than those with defined CTD-ILD and better than those with IPF. Both the pathophysiology and treatment of IPAF have yet to be defined. Further research is needed to elucidate which elements of the clinical, serologic, and morphologic domains confer the most prognostic information to a diagnosis of IPAF to help guide further development of the classification criteria and to facilitate clinical trial design in order to establish standardized treatment approaches.

Take home message

- IPAF is a designation that encompasses features of autoimmunity based on clinical, serologic, and morphologic features.
- Morbidity and mortality can be significant and in most studies suggest an intermediate survival between IPF and ILD related to CTD.
- Treatment options are tailored to the degree of inflammation and fibrosis with each specific patient and may involve both types of therapy.
- The IPAF designation continues to undergo refinement and will likely evolve as our understanding of the genetic, immunologic, and clinical features of IIPs in general improves.

References

[1] American Thoracic Society, European Respiratory Society. American Thoracic Society/European Respiratory Society international multidisciplinary consensus classification of the idiopathic interstitial pneumonias. This joint statement of the American Thoracic Society (ATS), and the European Respiratory Society (ERS) was adopted by the ATS board of directors, June 2001 and by the ERS executive committee, June 2001. Am J Respir Crit Care Med 2002;165(2):277–304.

[2] Crouser ED, Maier LA, Wilson KC, Bonham CA, Morgenthau AS, Patterson KC, et al. Diagnosis and detection of sarcoidosis. An official American Thoracic Society clinical practice guideline. Am J Respir Crit Care Med 2020;201(8):e26–51.

[3] Raghu G, Collard HR, Egan JJ, Martinez FJ, Behr J, Brown KK, et al. An official ATS/ERS/JRS/alat statement: idiopathic pulmonary fibrosis: evidence-based guidelines for diagnosis and management. Am J Respir Crit Care Med 2011;183(6):788–824.

[4] Raghu G, Remy-Jardin M, Myers JL, Richeldi L, Ryerson CJ, Lederer DJ, et al. Diagnosis of idiopathic pulmonary fibrosis. An official ATS/ERS/JRS/alat clinical practice guideline. Am J Respir Crit Care Med 2018;198(5):e44–68.

[5] Travis WD, Costabel U, Hansell DM, King Jr TE, Lynch DA, Nicholson AG, et al. An official american thoracic society/european respiratory society statement: update of the international multidisciplinary classification of the idiopathic interstitial pneumonias. Am J Respir Crit Care Med 2013;188(6):733–48.

[6] Lee CT, Oldham JM. Interstitial pneumonia with autoimmune features: overview of proposed criteria and recent cohort characterization. Clin Pulm Med 2017;24(5):191–6.

[7] Park JH, Kim DS, Park IN, Jang SJ, Kitaichi M, Nicholson AG, et al. Prognosis of fibrotic interstitial pneumonia: idiopathic versus collagen vascular disease-related subtypes. Am J Respir Crit Care Med 2007;175(7):705–11.

[8] Corte TJ, Copley SJ, Desai SR, Zappala CJ, Hansell DM, Nicholson AG, et al. Significance of connective tissue disease features in idiopathic interstitial pneumonia. Eur Respir J 2012;39(3):661–8.

[9] Cottin V. Significance of connective tissue diseases features in pulmonary fibrosis. Eur Respir Rev 2013;22(129):273–80.

[10] Mathai SC, Danoff SK. Management of interstitial lung disease associated with connective tissue disease. BMJ 2016;352:h6819.

[11] Vij R, Strek ME. Diagnosis and treatment of connective tissue disease-associated interstitial lung disease. Chest 2013;143(3):814–24.

[12] Idiopathic Pulmonary Fibrosis Clinical Research N, Raghu G, Anstrom KJ, King Jr TE, Lasky JA, Martinez FJ. Prednisone, azathioprine, and n-acetylcysteine for pulmonary fibrosis. N Engl J Med 2012;366(21):1968–77.

[13] Fischer A, Lee JS, Cottin V. Interstitial lung disease evaluation: detecting connective tissue disease. Respiration 2015;90(3):177–84.

[14] Cottin V. Interstitial lung disease: are we missing formes frustes of connective tissue disease? Eur Respir J 2006;28(5):893–6.

[15] Fischer A, West SG, Swigris JJ, Brown KK, du Bois RM. Connective tissue disease-associated interstitial lung disease: a call for clarification. Chest 2010;138(2):251–6.

[16] Omote N, Taniguchi H, Kondoh Y, Watanabe N, Sakamoto K, Kimura T, et al. Lung-dominant connective tissue disease: clinical, radiologic, and histologic features. Chest 2015;148(6):1438–46.

[17] Vij R, Noth I, Strek ME. Autoimmune-featured interstitial lung disease: a distinct entity. Chest 2011;140(5):1292–9.

[18] Kinder BW, Collard HR, Koth L, Daikh DI, Wolters PJ, Elicker B, et al. Idiopathic nonspecific interstitial pneumonia: lung manifestation of undifferentiated connective tissue disease? Am J Respir Crit Care Med 2007;176(7):691–7.

[19] Fischer A, Antoniou KM, Brown KK, Cadranel J, Corte TJ, du Bois RM, et al. An official European Respiratory Society/American Thoracic Society research statement: interstitial pneumonia with autoimmune features. Eur Respir J 2015;46(4):976–87.

[20] Ahmad K, Barba T, Gamondes D, Ginoux M, Khouatra C, Spagnolo P, et al. Interstitial pneumonia with autoimmune features: clinical, radiologic, and histological characteristics and outcome in a series of 57 patients. Respir Med 2017;123:56–62.

[21] Chartrand S, Swigris JJ, Stanchev L, Lee JS, Brown KK, Fischer A. Clinical features and natural history of interstitial pneumonia with autoimmune features: a single center experience. Respir Med 2016;119:150–4.

[22] Dai J, Wang L, Yan X, Li H, Zhou K, He J, et al. Clinical features, risk factors, and outcomes of patients with interstitial pneumonia with autoimmune features: a population-based study. Clin Rheumatol 2018;37(8):2125–32.

[23] Lim JU, Gil BM, Kang HS, Oh J, Kim YH, Kwon SS. Interstitial pneumonia with autoimmune features show better survival and less exacerbations compared to idiopathic pulmonary fibrosis. BMC Pulm Med 2019;19(1):120.

[24] Ito Y, Arita M, Kumagai S, Takei R, Noyama M, Tokioka F, et al. Serological and morphological prognostic factors in patients with interstitial pneumonia with autoimmune features. BMC Pulm Med 2017;17(1):111.

[25] Yoshimura K, Kono M, Enomoto Y, Nishimoto K, Oyama Y, Yasui H, et al. Distinctive characteristics and prognostic significance of interstitial pneumonia with autoimmune features in patients with chronic fibrosing interstitial pneumonia. Respir Med 2018;137:167–75.

[26] Oldham JM, Adegunsoye A, Valenzi E, Lee C, Witt L, Chen L, et al. Characterisation of patients with interstitial pneumonia with autoimmune features. Eur Respir J 2016;47(6):1767–75.

[27] Raghu G, Chen SY, Hou Q, Yeh WS, Collard HR. Incidence and prevalence of idiopathic pulmonary fibrosis in us adults 18–64 years old. Eur Respir J 2016;48(1):179–86.

[28] Reveille JD, Solomon DH, American College of Rheumatology Ad Hoc Committee of Immunologic Testing Guidelines. Evidence-based guidelines for the use of immunologic tests: anticentromere, scl-70, and nucleolar antibodies. Arthritis Rheum 2003;49(3):399–412.

[29] Ruffatti A, Rossi L, Calligaro A, Del Ross T, Lagni M, Marson P, et al. Autoantibodies of systemic rheumatic diseases in the healthy elderly. Gerontology 1990;36(2):104–11.

[30] Solomon DH, Kavanaugh AJ, Schur PH, American College of Rheumatology Ad Hoc Committee on Immunologic Testing Guidelines. Evidence-based guidelines for the use of immunologic tests: antinuclear antibody testing. Arthritis Rheum 2002;47(4):434–44.

[31] Shanmugam VK, Swistowski DR, Saddic N, Wang H, Steen VD. Comparison of indirect immunofluorescence and multiplex antinuclear antibody screening in systemic sclerosis. Clin Rheumatol 2011;30(10):1363–8.

[32] Ando M, Miyazaki E, Ishii T, Mukai Y, Yamasue M, Fujisaki H, et al. Incidence of myeloperoxidase anti-neutrophil cytoplasmic antibody positivity and microscopic polyangitis in the course of idiopathic pulmonary fibrosis. Respir Med 2013;107(4):608–15.

[33] Esposito AJ, Chu SG, Madan R, Doyle TJ, Dellaripa PF. Thoracic manifestations of rheumatoid arthritis. Clin Chest Med 2019;40(3):545–60.

[34] Hunninghake GW, Zimmerman MB, Schwartz DA, King Jr TE, Lynch J, Hegele R, et al. Utility of a lung biopsy for the diagnosis of idiopathic pulmonary fibrosis. Am J Respir Crit Care Med 2001;164(2):193–6.

[35] Thannickal VJ, Toews GB, White ES, Lynch 3rd JP, Martinez FJ. Mechanisms of pulmonary fibrosis. Annu Rev Med 2004;55:395–417.

[36] Joshi N, Watanabe S, Verma R, Jablonski RP, Chen CI, Cheresh P, et al. A spatially restricted fibrotic niche in pulmonary fibrosis is sustained by M-CSF/M-CSFR signalling in monocyte-derived alveolar macrophages. Eur Respir J 2020;55(1).

[37] Barratt SL, Blythe T, Jarrett C, Ourradi K, Shelley-Fraser G, Day MJ, et al. Differential expression of VEGF-A_{xxx} isoforms is critical for development of pulmonary fibrosis. Am J Respir Crit Care Med 2017;196(4):479–93.

[38] Desai O, Winkler J, Minasyan M, Herzog EL. The role of immune and inflammatory cells in idiopathic pulmonary fibrosis. Front Med 2018;5:43.

[39] Fielding CA, Jones GW, McLoughlin RM, McLeod L, Hammond VJ, Uceda J, et al. Interleukin-6 signaling drives fibrosis in unresolved inflammation. Immunity 2014;40(1):40–50.

[40] De Lauretis A, Sestini P, Pantelidis P, Hoyles R, Hansell DM, Goh NS, et al. Serum interleukin 6 is predictive of early functional decline and mortality in interstitial lung disease associated with systemic sclerosis. J Rheumatol 2013;40(4):435–46.

[41] Khanna D, Lin CJF, Furst DE, Goldin J, Kim G, Kuwana M, et al. Tocilizumab in systemic sclerosis: a randomised, double-blind, placebo-controlled, phase 3 trial. Lancet Respir Med 2020;8(10):963–74.

[42] Chrysanthopoulou A, Mitroulis I, Apostolidou E, Arelaki S, Mikroulis D, Konstantinidis T, et al. Neutrophil extracellular traps promote differentiation and function of fibroblasts. J Pathol 2014;233(3):294–307.

[43] Martinod K, Witsch T, Erpenbeck L, Savchenko A, Hayashi H, Cherpokova D, et al. Peptidylarginine deiminase 4 promotes age-related organ fibrosis. J Exp Med 2017;214(2):439–58.

[44] Saito A, Okazaki H, Sugawara I, Yamamoto K, Takizawa H. Potential action of il-4 and il-13 as fibrogenic factors on lung fibroblasts in vitro. Int Arch Allergy Immunol 2003;132(2):168–76.

[45] Zhang J, Wang D, Wang L, Wang S, Roden AC, Zhao H, et al. Profibrotic effect of il-17a and elevated il-17ra in idiopathic pulmonary fibrosis and rheumatoid arthritis-associated lung disease support a direct role for il-17a/il-17ra in human fibrotic interstitial lung disease. Am J Physiol Lung Cell Mol Physiol 2019;316(3):L487–97.

[46] Wang D, Zhang J, Lau J, Wang S, Taneja V, Matteson EL, et al. Mechanisms of lung disease development in rheumatoid arthritis. Nat Rev Rheumatol 2019;15(10):581–96.

[47] Kameda M, Otsuka M, Chiba H, Kuronuma K, Hasegawa T, Takahashi H, et al. CXCL9, CXCL10, and CXCL11; biomarkers of pulmonary inflammation associated with autoimmunity in patients with collagen vascular diseases-associated interstitial lung disease and interstitial pneumonia with autoimmune features. PLoS One 2020;15(11):e0241719.

[48] Solomon JJ, Matson S, Kelmenson LB, Chung JH, Hobbs SB, Rosas IO, et al. Iga antibodies directed against citrullinated protein antigens are elevated in patients with idiopathic pulmonary fibrosis. Chest 2020;157(6):1513–21.

[49] Fava A, Cimbro R, Wigley FM, Liu QR, Rosen A, Boin F. Frequency of circulating topoisomerase-i-specific CD4 t cells predicts presence and progression of interstitial lung disease in scleroderma. Arthritis Res Ther 2016;18(1):99.

[50] Naikawadi RP, Disayabutr S, Mallavia B, Donne ML, Green G, La JL, et al. Telomere dysfunction in alveolar epithelial cells causes lung remodeling and fibrosis. JCI Insight 2016;1(14):e86704.

[51] Newton CA, Batra K, Torrealba J, Kozlitina J, Glazer CS, Aravena C, et al. Telomere-related lung fibrosis is diagnostically heterogeneous but uniformly progressive. Eur Respir J 2016;48(6):1710–20.

[52] Courtwright AM, El-Chemaly S. Telomeres in interstitial lung disease: the short and the long of it. Ann Am Thorac Soc 2019;16(2):175–81.

[53] Newton CA, Oldham JM, Ley B, Anand V, Adegunsoye A, Liu G, et al. Telomere length and genetic variant associations with interstitial lung disease progression and survival. Eur Respir J 2019;53(4).

[54] Seibold MA, Wise AL, Speer MC, Steele MP, Brown KK, Loyd JE, et al. A common muc5b promoter polymorphism and pulmonary fibrosis. N Engl J Med 2011;364(16):1503–12.

[55] Juge PA, Lee JS, Ebstein E, Furukawa H, Dobrinskikh E, Gazal S, et al. Muc5b promoter variant and rheumatoid arthritis with interstitial lung disease. N Engl J Med 2018;379(23):2209–19.

[56] Collard HR, Ryerson CJ, Corte TJ, Jenkins G, Kondoh Y, Lederer DJ, et al. Acute exacerbation of idiopathic pulmonary fibrosis. An international working group report. Am J Respir Crit Care Med 2016;194(3):265–75.

[57] Sambataro G, Sambataro D, Torrisi SE, Vancheri A, Colaci M, Pavone M, et al. Clinical, serological and radiological features of a prospective cohort of interstitial pneumonia with autoimmune features (IPAF) patients. Respir Med 2019;150:154–60.

[58] Kim HC, Lee JH, Chae EJ, Song JS, Song JW. Long-term clinical course and outcome of interstitial pneumonia with autoimmune features. Respirology 2020;25(6):636–43.

[59] Distler O, Highland KB, Gahlemann M, Azuma A, Fischer A, Mayes MD, et al. Nintedanib for systemic sclerosis-associated interstitial lung disease. N Engl J Med 2019;380(26):2518–28.

[60] Flaherty KR, Wells AU, Cottin V, Devaraj A, Walsh SLF, Inoue Y, et al. Nintedanib in progressive fibrosing interstitial lung diseases. N Engl J Med 2019;381(18):1718–27.

[61] Maher TM, Corte TJ, Fischer A, Kreuter M, Lederer DJ, Molina-Molina M, et al. Pirfenidone in patients with unclassifiable progressive fibrosing interstitial lung disease: design of a double-blind, randomised, placebo-controlled phase ii trial. BMJ Open Respir Res 2018;5(1):e000289.

[62] Solomon J, Swigris JJ, Brown KK. Myositis-related interstitial lung disease and antisynthetase syndrome. J Bras Pneumol 2011;37(1):100–9.

[63] Cao H, Xia Q, Pan M, Zhao X, Li X, Shi R, et al. Gottron papules and gottron sign with ulceration: a distinctive cutaneous feature in a subset of patients with classic dermatomyositis and clinically amyopathic dermatomyositis. J Rheumatol 2016;43(9):1735–42.

[64] Aggarwal R, Dhillon N, Fertig N, Koontz D, Qi Z, Oddis CV. A negative antinuclear antibody does not indicate autoantibody negativity in myositis: role of anticytoplasmic antibody as a screening test for antisynthetase syndrome. J Rheumatol 2017;44(2):223–9.

Chapter 2

Interstitial lung disease and rheumatoid arthritis

Fabiola Atzeni,[1] Cesare Siragusano[1] and José A. Gómez-Puerta[2,*]
[1]*Rheumatology Unit, University of Messina, Messina, Italy;* [2]*Rheumatology Department, Hospital Clínic, IDIBAPS, University of Barcelona, Barcelona, Catalonia, Spain*
[*]*Corresponding author at: jagomez@clinic.cat.*

Introduction

Interstitial lung disease (ILD) is an extra-articular manifestation of rheumatoid arthritis (RA), first reported by Ellman and Ball in 1948 [1]. The prevalence and incidence of ILD associated with RA (RA-ILD) are unknown, ranging from 1% to 58% depending on the method used [2–5]. Population studies performed in the United States suggest that the cumulative incidence of clinically manifest RA-ILD (defined by the presence of abnormalities on high-resolution computed tomography [HRCT] and abnormal lung function tests) is 5% at 10 years [6], 6.3% at 15 years [7], and 6.8% at 30 years [2]. Another US study that examined death certificates of patients with RA reported a clinically relevant incidence of ILD in 6.8% of women and 9.8% of men [3]. Patients with RA undergoing screening, regardless of the presence of symptoms, often have radiologic abnormalities on HRCT, referred to as subclinical ILD and/or interstitial lung abnormalities, with prevalence ranging from 19% to 57% [5,8]. It has been shown that these radiographic features progress in ~50% of cases [4]. However, there is currently a lack of tools capable of predicting the individual risk of progression to clinically manifest RA-ILD.

Risk factors and pathogenesis

There are several risk factors associated with the development of ILD in RA patients, but the most frequent are advanced age [7,9,10], male gender [5,8,9], cigarette smoking [5,8,11] and positivity for rheumatoid factor (FR) or for antibodies anticyclic citrullinated peptide (anti-CCP) [5,11,12]. In particular,

The Lung in Autoimmune Diseases. https://doi.org/10.1016/B978-0-323-91083-5.00010-4

cigarette smoking appears to be associated with both an increased risk of developing RA [13] and a greater risk of developing RA-ILD [12,13].

A recent study reported a higher prevalence of anticarbamylated antibodies specificities in patients with RA-associated ILD than in patients without ILD. All anticarbamylated antibodies conferred a higher risk for ILD, after adjusting for confounders factors including smoking and disease duration [14].

The development of RA-ILD has also been associated with disease activity, but this association is still unclear [7,9]. Recently, a study evaluating as a risk factor for RA-ILD the polymorphism in the region of the promoter of the 5b mucin gene (a gene that encodes for mucin) [15], showed this to be associated with an increased risk of idiopathic pulmonary fibrosis (IPF) [16], ILD [17], and chronic obstructive pulmonary disease [18].

The MUC5B promoter variant (rs35705950) alters host's mucosa defenses, resulting in lung injuries from inhaled substances, inflammation, and fibrosis, but particularly increasing by three times the risk of ILD in patients with RA, with the usual interstitial pneumonia (UIP) subtype [14]. No other gene is so strongly associated with the development of RA-ILD [19].

Other factors have been linked to the development of ILD in patients with RA, such as some alleles of the major histocompatibility complex, including HLA-B54, HLA-DQB1*0601, HLA-B40, and HLA-DR4 [20].

Literature data also demonstrates that serum biomarkers such as IL-33, IL-18, MMP-7, PARC, and SPD at a high titers promote the development of ILD in patients with RA [12,21].

Risk factors and pathogenesis pathway of RA-ILD is summarized in Fig. 2.1.

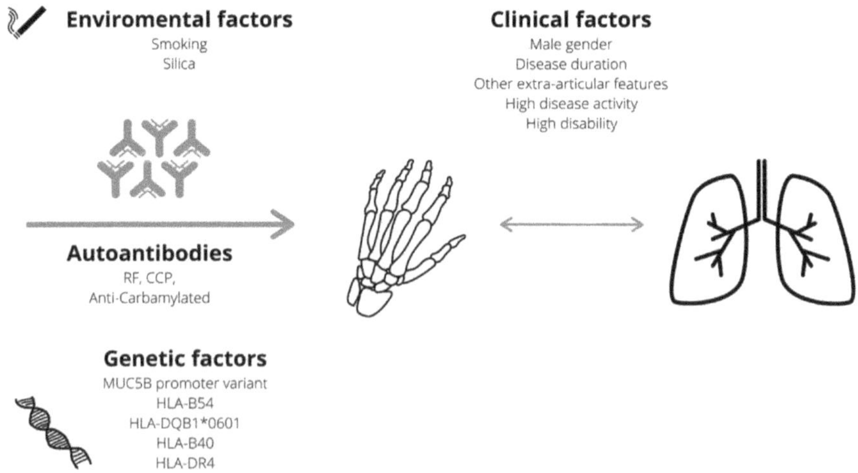

FIGURE 2.1 Risk factors and pathogenic pathway for RA-associated ILD.

Clinical manifestations

Clinical manifestations of RA-ILD are similar to those of idiopathic interstitial pneumonia, although patients with RA-ILD can remain asymptomatic despite significant radiographic changes. The most common presenting symptoms include nonproductive cough, tachypnea, and exertional dyspnea, which in patients with arthritis pain can be masked by limited mobility. The physical examination highlights inspiratory crackles at the lung bases [22]. Pleural rubbing can be occasionally heard, and cyanosis, edema, and signs of pulmonary hypertension (PH) may be observed in an advanced stage of disease. In particular, PH should be suspected in the presence of typical symptoms or arterial oxygen desaturation induced by exercise, which is disproportionate to the severity of the pulmonary involvement. Clubbing occurs less frequently than in IPF [23]. The relationship between the onset of joint disease and the onset of ILD is variable. One study showed a median of 4.9 years from RA diagnosis to ILD diagnosis [24], but lung disease can also precede joint manifestations [25].

Diagnostic imaging

Chest X-rays show poor sensitivity and specificity for ILD. In fact, in a prospective study of asymptomatic patients with early disease, chest radiography showed ILD features in only 6% of patients [5]. Alterations observable on chest X-ray range from bibasal ground glass opacities to lattice and nodular frameworks, as well as to a honeycomb pattern. In advanced stage of disease, enlargement of the central pulmonary arteries and attenuation of the peripheral vessels may suggest PH.

HRCT is the primary method for ILD diagnosis. In fact, compared to chest radiographs, HRCT can detect minimal structural changes in lung tissue in the early stages of disease [26]. HRCT can replace lung biopsy since topographic images correlate with histopathological changes [27,28].

The predominant HRCT pattern of RA-ILD is UIP (Fig. 2.2), followed by nonspecific interstitial pneumonia (NSIP) (Fig. 2.3). Other patterns are less frequent, including organized pneumonia (OP) (Fig. 2.4), obliterative bronchiolitis, acute interstitial pneumonia with diffuse alveolar damage, desquamating interstitial pneumonia, and lymphocytic interstitial pneumonia [29,30].

The UIP pattern on HRCT is characterized by heterogeneous honeycombs, reticulations, and architectural distortions at both the bases and periphery of the lungs. Typical NSIP's features on HRCT are bilateral ground glass opacity and minimal or no architectural distortion or honeycomb distortion [23,31]. NSIP is more common in connective tissue disease (CTD)-associated ILDs, while UIP is more common in RA-ILD [25,32]. The UIP pattern observed in patients with RA is very similar to that observed in patients with IPF [28,33]. However, straight edges, exuberant honeycomb pattern, and involvement of the superior lobe are significantly more common in the RA-UIP pattern [34], which has a worse prognosis than the non-UIP pattern of RA-ILD [28,33].

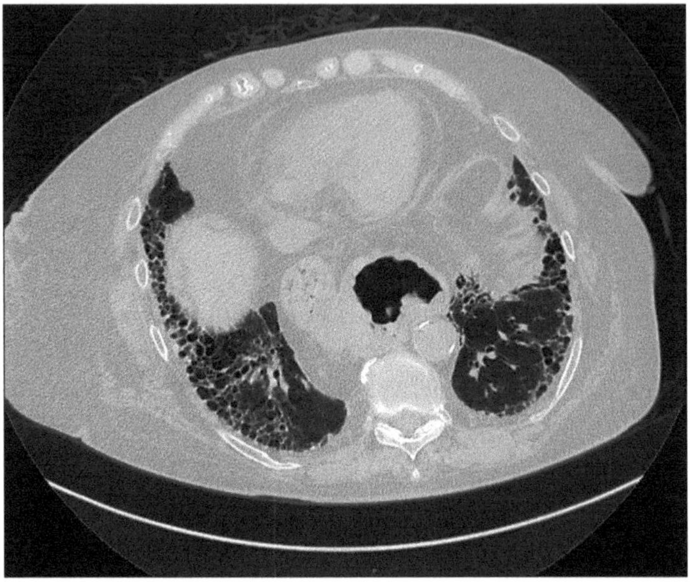

FIGURE 2.2 **Usual interstitial pneumonia.** High-resolution computed tomography scan revealing cystic images of honeycombing in subpleural locations associated with reticular opacities and traction bronchiectasis. *Images courtesy of Dr. Marcelo Sanchez, Radiology Department, Hospital Clinic, Barcelona.*

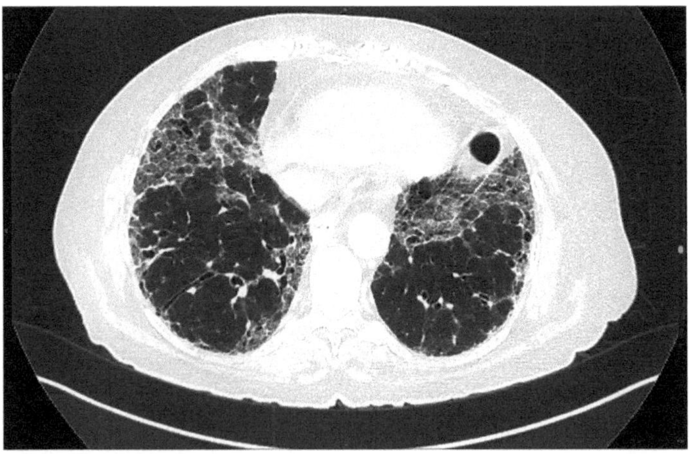

FIGURE 2.3 **Non-specific interstitial pneumonia.** High-resolution computed tomography scan showing ground glass opacities associated with traction bronchiectasis and bronchioloectasia without honeycombing. *Images courtesy of Dr. Marcelo Sanchez, Radiology Department, Hospital Clinic, Barcelona.*

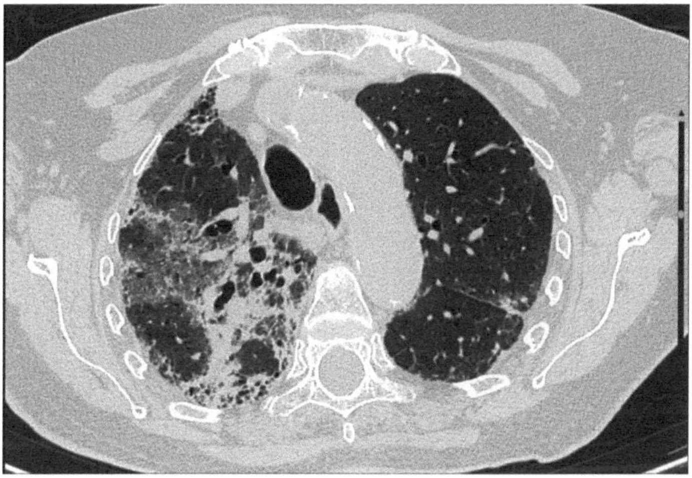

FIGURE 2.4 **Organizing pneumonia.** High-resolution computed tomography scan revealing an upper lobe consolidation with irregular bronchial dilatations in a perilobular distribution with reverse halo sign. *Images courtesy of Dr. Marcelo Sanchez, Radiology Department, Hospital Clinic, Barcelona.*

As well as the idiopathic UIP associated with IPF, the clinical course of UIP associated with RA is quite variable and can be characterized by "acute exacerbations." These exacerbations are defined as a clinically significant lung function worsening, and/or as the onset of dyspnea typically lasting less than one month, accompanied by new diffuse pulmonary infiltrates on chest X-ray or HRCT, and in the absence of heart failure and fluid overload [35]. There are no studies comparing the prevalence of these acute exacerbations in CTD-ILDs, but patients with UIP pattern appear to be at increased risk of developing this complication regardless of the disease [36]. In a retrospective study involving 51 patients with RA-ILD, acute exacerbation occurred in 22% of patients (11 out of 51) during a median follow-up period of 8.5 years, with a mortality rate of 64% (7 out of 11 patients) [37]. As expected, patients who experienced acute exacerbation had a significantly worse outcome than the others ($P = .001$).

Different diagnostic methods

The high prevalence of subclinical ILD on HRCT images in RA patients demonstrates that screening procedures based on clinical signs and symptoms have a low sensitivity in detecting ILD [5,38]. To overcome this limit, an algorithm has been developed to detect Velcro crackles using an electronic stethoscope. Out of 137 RA patients undergoing HRCT, the recorded Velcro crackles showed a sensitivity of 93.2% and a specificity of 76.9% for the detection of ILD, far exceeding clinical signs, chest radiography, and lung function tests [39].

Although several studies have shown that pulmonary function tests (PFTs) are useful for the early diagnosis of ILD, they are actually more suitable for assessing disease progression. In patients with RA-ILD, PFTs can reveal a restrictive ventilatory defect characterized by a reduced diffusion capacity of the lungs for carbon monoxide (DLCO) even in the absence of symptoms. In a study of patients with RA at onset, 33% had a DLCO <80% compared to what expected, but only 14% had symptoms [5]. DLCO is sensitive for detecting the presence of ILD, while the respiratory pulmonary volumes are more useful to evaluate the extent of the disease [26,40]. As in IPF, clinically relevant changes over time include a 10% decrease in forced vital capacity (FVC) or a 15% decrease in DLCO over a time span of 6–12 months [40].

Recently, lung ultrasound was introduced as a safe and readily available tool to detect ILD [41,42]. Ultrasound signs, such as multiple B lines, pleural line irregularity, or pleural nodules, may be indicative of interstitial disease [43].

Broncho alveolar lavage (BAL) fluid reports of RA-ILD patients are often altered but not specific, although it has been observed that an increase in the number of neutrophils is more frequent in patients with UIP, while an increase in lymphocytes is more frequent in patients with NSIP or organizing pneumonia [44]. However, alterations in the cellular components of BAL fluid are not helpful in predicting the clinical course of the disease or the response to treatment. Therefore, BAL is not performed regularly for the diagnosis of these patients. However, in patients with acute onset RA and/or rapid progression of respiratory symptoms and X-ray changes, BAL is useful for excluding neoplastic processes and infections [40].

Therapy

The therapeutic approach to patients with RA-ILD represents a clinical challenge as no randomized controlled clinical trials (RCTs) have been published so far. Several disease-modifying antirheumatic drugs (DMARDs), such as methotrexate (MTX), leflunomide (LEF), antitumor necrosis factor alpha (anti-TNF-α), tocilizumab (TCZ), and less frequently rituximab (RTX) and abatacept (ABA), have been reported as inducing or promoting the progression of RA-ILD [45,46]. The majority of the studies suggest that DMARDs do not cause RA-ILD. However, it is uncertain whether they contribute to the onset of drug-induced lung disease/pneumonia, and whether some DMARDs are more effective for treating RA-ILD compared to others. For this reason, the recent American College of Rheumatology/European League Against Rheumatism (ACR/EULAR) guidelines for RA management have not proposed specific recommendations for the treatment of patients with RA-ILD [47,48]. The differential effect of DMARDs and targeted therapies over joint involvement and RA-associated ILD is summarized in Table 2.1.

TABLE 2.1 Therapeutic effects of DMARDs and targeted therapies over articular involvement and ILD in RA.

Conventional DMARD		
DMARD	**Joint involvement**	**ILD**
AZA	+/−	+[a]
CYC	+/−	+[a]
LEF	+	+/−
MMF	−	+[a]
MTX	+	+/−
Targeted therapies and antifibrotic		
Therapy	**Joint involvement**	**ILD**
Antifibrotic	−	+[b]
ABA	+	+
JAKi	+	+/−
RTX	+	+
TNFi	+	+/−
TCZ	+	+/−

Abbreviations: *AZA*, azathioprine; *ABA*, Abatacept; *CYC*, Cyclophosphamide; *LEF*, Leflunomide; *JAKi*, Jak inhibitors; *MMF*, mycophenolate mofetil; *MTX*, Methotrexate; *RTX*, Rituximab; *TNFi*, Tumor necrosis factors inhibitors; *TCZ*, Tocilizumab. +, Demonstrated benefit; −, no benefit; +/−, not benefit proven yet.
[a]*More benefit in NSIP forms.*
[b]*More benefit in UIP forms.*

Glucocorticoids

Glucocorticoids (GCs) are no longer considered as first-line therapy for the treatment of patients with RA-ILD. However, they can be considered in cases of severe flare-up or when a rapid action of drugs on the disease is desired. GCs are no longer used for the treatment of fibrotic forms of lung disease, since they have shown to cause a worsening of the clinical picture in IPF [40]. The inflammatory subtypes of RA-ILD, in particular NSIP and OP can benefit from the use of steroids [49]. The treatment with GCs includes the use of 0.5−1 mg/kg/die of prednisone, or in case of severe disease, an intravenous bolus of 1 g/day of methylprednisolone is recommended. GCs should be administered under close monitoring and careful management of side effects, particularly pneumonia or other opportunistic infections. It has been shown that GCs in elderly subjects with RA are associated with a four times greater risk of serious infections [50,51]. Prophylaxis for *Pneumocystis* pneumonia should be considered in RA-ILD patients who are going to be treated with GCs, although threshold doses and duration of GCs treatment to set prophylaxis in RA-ILD are not yet well established [52]. GCs-induced osteoporosis represents another adverse event that requires careful screening and follow-up, since RA itself represents a risk factor for osteoporosis [51]. In fact, GCs therapy is responsible for the most frequent form of secondary osteoporosis [53].

Conventional disease-modifying antirheumatic drugs

Methotrexate

MTX is recommended as first-line therapy for the treatment of RA patients, as it decreases disease activity and progression, disability, and mortality [54]. However, the association between MTX and the onset or exacerbation of ILD in patients with RA has also been reported [37].

The "lung complications" associated with MTX fall into two categories: infectious and noninfectious complications. Infectious complications are caused by the immunosuppressive action of the drug, while the noninfectious include an acute event called "MTX-induced pneumonia" (MTXip), which is a rare acute inflammatory lung complication, observed in 1% of RA patients starting MTX [55], and with onset within the first year of therapy [56].

HRCT changes include bilateral ground glass alterations. The treatment is based on the immediate suspension of MTX, possibly associated with a short course of GCs to improve symptoms. If MTXip is not recognized and MTX suspended, this drug can prove fatal in 20% of cases.

Over the years, several articles in literature have associated the use of MTX with fibrosing ILD (fILD). The hypothesis that MTX could cause fILD probably arose for two main reasons. First, the inability to discriminate between the different forms of lung "toxicity" that MTX can induce. MTX can actually cause one type of ILD, but this uncommon pharmacological reaction is an inflammatory pneumonia and not a truly fibrotic progressive ILD. In addition, infectious insults can also leave some degree of static fibrotic damage after resolution. It may therefore be suspected that patients have developed fILD, but in fact they do not suffer from it.

Secondly, several patients with RA receive MTX as the only therapy. Fibrotic ILD as an intrinsic manifestation of the disease has an incidence of 4%–7% in patients with RA [9]. Therefore, it is not reasonable to suspect that fILD may be due to the use of MTX.

To assess the correlation between MTX and ILD, Conway carried out a meta-analysis of 22 randomized controlled double-blind studies (RCTs), including 8584 patients with RA [57] divided into two groups based on whether they took MTX. The results of this study showed that the use of MTX was associated with an increased risk of respiratory infections, but the risk of ILD was lower than previously reported. In conclusion, MTX may not be responsible for ILD, and in addition it may play an important role in the treatment of RA-ILD being an effective treatment on joint manifestations. Additionally, a recent observational study of 2701 RA patients found no association between MTX and ILD, rather suggesting that MTX may delay the onset of ILD [58].

Leflunomide

LEF is a drug used to effectively treat RA, but an observational study involving 5054 patients with RA reported that 61 patients under LEF treatment developed ILD, and others showed a worsening of the same [59]. A recent meta-analysis reported that patients treated with LEF do not present an increased risk of respiratory adverse events, even showing a decrease in noninfectious respiratory adverse events. The results of this study support the safety of LEF in RA patients and regarding the possible risk of ILD [60].

Mycophenolate mofetil

Most of the data on mycophenolate mofetil (MMF) comes from observational studies on CTD-ILD, particularly on systemic sclerosis (SSc), which has been demonstrated to have the ability to stabilize the disease [61,62]. It has also been demonstrated that MMF has a higher safety profile than cyclophosphamide (CYC) per os in SSc-ILD [63]. A small study involving 10 CTD-ILD patients reported that MMF is associated with an improvement of symptoms, imaging features, respiratory function tests, and CO diffusion capacity [64]. However, these studies are limited by the small size of the sample, and further larger controlled studies are therefore needed to provide more reliable results. MMF is relatively ineffective on the typical joint manifestations of RA, and it must be associated with another DMARD to control joint disease activity [65].

Cyclophosphamide

CYC has been used to treat various types of ILD, and studies have shown its ability to stabilize the pulmonary function in case of fibrosis [66]. A recent Cochrane systematic review on CYC for the treatment of CTD-ILD, which included four trials for a total of 495 patients, showed that CYC led to a small improvement of FVC, but not of DLCO, and that there was no difference between CYC and MMF [67]. Due to the toxicity of CYC, it is recommended to administer it only to those who have a rapidly progressive or resistant lung disease. Finally, for the same reason, although this drug is effective on the articular component, its use must be limited to serious or resistant inflammation both at the lung and joint level.

Azathioprine

There are no controlled studies on the use of azathioprine (AZA) in RA-ILD, but following the results of the PANTHER-IPF study, the enthusiasm for its use in any form of ILD is scarce. Based on IPF data, the association of GCs with AZA was thought to be able to improve survival, but the results of the 2012 PANTHER-IPF study abruptly modified this therapeutic approach [68]. This study ended early due to increased rates of mortality and hospitalization for lung infections in the GCs + AZA and N-acetylcysteine arm compared to placebo [69]. However, in a 2016 retrospective cohort study on CTD-ILD involving 54 patients, AZA showed to be able to stabilize the lung function over time, with an incidence of adverse events overlapping with the group under MMF [70]. AZA can be used in patients with poor or mild joint involvement that does not justify the use of biological DMARDs, or with contraindications to the administration of other drugs.

Biological disease-modifying antirheumatic drugs

Tumor necrosis factor inhibitors

Although several cases of ILD onset or ILD exacerbation have been reported after the use of tumor necrosis factor inhibitors (TNFi), data on the effects of TNFi on ILD are controversial [71,72]. In retrospective cohort studies of the British Society for Rheumatology Biologics Register (BSRBR), the use of TNFi in patients with RA-ILD was not associated with a higher risk of death than patients treated with DMARDs [73], but a better survival was observed with the use of RTX compared to that of TNFi (hazard ratio 0.53%, 95%, CI 0.26−1.10) [74]. Data from a large US administrative claims database showed no significant differences between patients with RA-ILD using TNFi compared to those treated with TCZ, RTX and ABA [75]. Nonetheless, there have been fewer respiratory events in patients treated with ABA than in those treated with TNFi [75].

Tocilizumab

TCZ is a monoclonal antibody directed toward the interleukin-6 receptor (IL-6R) approved for the treatment of RA. A retrospective study of 28 patients with RA-ILD treated with TCZ showed a stabilization of the lung disease and an acceptable safety profile [76]. In particular, 28 patients with RA-ILD were identified (women/men 18/10, average age 61.6 years), treated with TCZ and subject to an average follow-up of 30 months. At the end of the follow-up, it was observed that FVC remained stable in 14 (56%) patients, improved in 5 (20%), and worsened in 6 (24%). DLCO remained stable in 14 (56%) patients, improved in 5 (20%), and worsened in 6 (24%), although in three patients DLCO and FVC showed an opposite trend. HRCT remained stable in most (25) cases, worsened in two patients with an UIP pattern, and improved in only one case with a pattern of NSIP.

By contrast, early RCTs and case reports suggested the association between the onset of ILD and therapy with TCZ [77]. In addition, a recent meta-analysis which included observational studies in patients with RA suggested a possible association between the use of TCZ and the worsening of RA-ILD [78].

Abatacept

ABA is the only drug currently approved to treat RA that targets the co-stimulatory signal required for full T-cell activation. An open label study of 63 RA-ILD patients in Spain showed that most patients had an effect on symptoms, stabilization of PFTs, and a significant improvement was observed in 20%–25% of patients [79].

An extended real-world clinical study with a bigger cohort of RA-ILD patients (N = 263) also reported stabilization of FVC, DLCO, dyspnea scale, and chest HRCT in addition to improvement in RA activity in patients with ABA treatment. An additional GC-sparing effect was seen in patients with combined therapy (ABA + MTX) [80].

A recent meta-analysis including nine observational studies reported that patients who received ABA versus. TNFi had significant lower ILD worsening rates with an important reduction of relative risk of deterioration after 24 months of follow-up in comparison with TNFi and DMARDs [81]. An open label phase 2 study is currently enrolling patients to study the safety of abatacept in patients with RA-ILD [82].

Rituximab

RTX is an anti-CD20 chimeric monoclonal antibody causing depletion of B lymphocytes, which has been proven effective in treating CTD-ILDs. Studies have shown that a therapy with RTX stabilizes or improves lung function in patients with systemic SSc-ILD or dermatomyositis-ILD [83,84]. RTX was also used to treat severe and progressive CTD-ILDs [85]. A 10-year observational study involving patients with RA and ILD, reported that RTX is safe and stops ILD progression [86]. A study carried out by the BSRBR for RA (BSRBR-RA), compared the results of RA-ILD patients treated with RTX (n = 43) with those treated with TNFi (n = 309), showing lower mortality in the arm under RTX therapy than in the arm under TNFi [74]. RTX has proven effective on joint involvement, so that it can also be considered in patients with simultaneous lung and joint involvement. Moreover, in some patients it may also be used in conjunction with MMF.

Janus kinase inhibitors

Janus kinase inhibitors (JAKi) also known as JAK inhibitors or jakinibs, are a type of medication that functions by inhibiting the activity of one or more of the Janus kinase family of enzymes (JAK1, JAK2, JAK3, TYK2), thereby interfering with the JAK-STAT signaling pathway. To date, data on the safety of JAKi on lungs are inconclusive. In the RCTs and postmarketing studies of tofacitinib and baricitinib, the number of patients with RA-ILD was quite limited, so no conclusions can be drawn [87]. An open label study involving 18 patients with amyopathic dermatomyositis-associated ILD, showed an improvement in pulmonary function and survival in the group treated with tofacitinib compared to controls [88]. The phase IV RCT comparing the effectiveness of tofacitinib and MTX in RA-ILD (PULMORA) has not yet started recruiting [89].

Antifibrotic drugs

Nintedanib is a drug that works by blocking several tyrosine-kinase enzymes, and it is approved by the US Food and Drugs Administration (FDA) for IPF, SSc-ILD and ILD with chronic progressive fibrosis, which may also include RA-ILD. Nintedanib was shown to be effective in progressive fibrotic ILD in a randomized double-blind phase 3 placebo-controlled study (INBUILD study) involving 663 patients [90]. The study included 89 (13%) patients with RA-ILD. Patients treated with nintedanib showed a slower FVC reduction than placebo at 52 weeks, with a benefit similar to that observed in IPF (INPULSIS study) [91]. Among patients with CTD-ILD, the benefit was more evident in the UIP subtype than other subtypes, although no improvement was observed compared to placebo, but the extent of the clinical benefit is still unknown. Finally, nintedanib may be considered in patients with RA-ILD, but gastrointestinal side effects may limit its use. Pirfenidone is an antifibrotic drug with anti-inflammatory properties, which in RCTs has shown effectiveness on IPF, in particular by improving lung function and reducing mortality [92]. It has been approved by the FDA for the treatment of mild or moderate IPF and "unclassifiable ILD," which may include interstitial pneumonia with autoimmune features) and RA-ILD, as it showed a slower FVC reduction than placebo [93]. The onset of rash and gastrointestinal side effects, such as nausea, limits its use. A phase 2 open label study of SSc-ILD patients has shown the tolerability of pirfenidone, even in those taking MMF at the same time [94]. The treatment of RA-ILD with pirfenidone is currently under study in a phase 2 clinical study (TRAIL1) [95]. As well as nintedanib, pirfenidone can be considered in patients with RA-ILD, although the extent of the clinical benefit is not yet clear and side effects are frequent. In conclusion, although data are limited and studies have not yet been carried out, this drug can be used to treat fibrotic subtypes of RA-ILD such as UIP.

Lung transplantation

Lung transplantation can be considered in patients with terminal RA-ILD who do not respond to therapy. Data on lung transplant results in RA-ILD patients are limited. A retrospective study of 10 patients with RA-ILD versus 53 patients with IPF who underwent lung transplantation, showed that the one-year survival was comparable between the two groups (67% vs. 69%, respectively). The study also found a significant improvement in the quality of life related to respiratory symptoms [96]. The decision of lung transplantation in RA-ILD must be carefully evaluated due to the comorbidities involving patients with RA, such as osteoporosis and cardiovascular diseases.

Conclusions

Lung involvement in patients with RA is relatively frequent, and in recent years there has been a growing interest in RA-related ILD. Although several important gaps around its optimal treatment still exist, in recent years, there has been enormous progress in the definition of RA-ILD subtypes, risk factors involved in its development, and in the pathogenesis and management of this complication.

Take-home messages

- ILD is an extra-articular manifestation of RA.
- There are several risk factors associated with the development of ILD in RA patients, but the most frequent are advanced age, male gender, cigarette smoking and positivity for rheumatoid factor or for antibodies anti-CCP.
- Clinical manifestations of RA-ILD are similar to those of idiopathic interstitial pneumonia, although patients with RA-ILD can remain asymptomatic.
- HRCTis the primary method for ILD diagnosis.
- Several conventional and biological disease-modifying antirheumatic drugs have been reported as inducing or promoting the progression of RA-ILD. The majority of the studies suggest that DMARDs do not cause RA-ILD.
- JAK inhibitors, antifibrotic drugs, and lung transplant have also been used with a controversial results.

References

[1] Ellman P, Ball RE. "Rheumatoid disease" with joint and pulmonary manifestations. Br Med J 1948;2:816–20. https://doi.org/10.1136/bmj.2.4583.816.

[2] Turesson C, O'Fallon WM, Crowson CS, Gabriel SE, Matteson EL. Extra-articular disease manifestations in rheumatoid arthritis: incidence trends and risk factors over 46 years. Ann Rheum Dis 2003;62:722–7. https://doi.org/10.1136/ard.62.8.722.

[3] Olson AL, Swigris JJ, Sprunger DB, Fischer A, Fernandez-Perez ER, Solomon J, et al. Rheumatoid arthritis-interstitial lung disease-associated mortality. Am J Respir Crit Care Med 2011;183:372–8. https://doi.org/10.1164/rccm.201004-0622OC.

[4] Gochuico BR, Avila NA, Chow CK, Novero LJ, Wu HP, Ren P, et al. Progressive preclinical interstitial lung disease in rheumatoid arthritis. Arch Intern Med 2008;168:159–66. https://doi.org/10.1001/archinternmed.2007.59.

[5] Gabbay E, Tarala R, Will R, Carroll G, Adler B, Cameron D, et al. Interstitial lung disease in recent onset rheumatoid arthritis. Am J Respir Crit Care Med 1997;156:528–35. https://doi.org/10.1164/ajrccm.156.2.9609016.

[6] Myasoedova E, Crowson CS, Turesson C, Gabriel SE, Matteson EL. Incidence of extra-articular rheumatoid arthritis in olmsted county, Minnesota, in 1995–2007 versus

1985–1994: a population-based study. J Rheumatol 2011;38:983–9. https://doi.org/10.3899/jrheum.101133.

[7] Koduri G, Norton S, Young A, Cox N, Davies P, Devlin J, et al. Interstitial lung disease has a poor prognosis in rheumatoid arthritis: results from an inception cohort. Rheumatology 2010;49:1483–9. https://doi.org/10.1093/rheumatology/keq035.

[8] Saag KG, Kolluri S, Koehnke RK, Georgou TA, Rachow JW, Hunninghake GW, et al. Rheumatoid arthritis lung disease: determinants of radiographic and physiologic abnormalities. Arthritis Rheum 1996;39:1711–9. https://doi.org/10.1002/art.1780391014.

[9] Bongartz T, Nannini C, Medina-Velasquez YF, Achenbach SJ, Crowson CS, Ryu JH, et al. Incidence and mortality of interstitial lung disease in rheumatoid arthritis - a population-based study. Arthritis Rheum 2010;62:1583–91. https://doi.org/10.1002/art.27405.

[10] Mori S, Koga Y, Sugimoto M. Different risk factors between interstitial lung disease and airway disease in rheumatoid arthritis. Respir Med 2012;106:1591–9. https://doi.org/10.1016/j.rmed.2012.07.006.

[11] Kelly CA, Saravanan V, Nisar M, Arthanari S, Woodhead FA, Price-Forbes AN, et al. Rheumatoid arthritis-related interstitial lung disease: associations, prognostic factors and physiological and radiological characteristics-a large multicentre UK study. Rheumatology 2014;53:1676–82. https://doi.org/10.1093/rheumatology/keu165.

[12] Doyle TJ, Patel AS, Hatabu H, Nishino M, Wu G, Osorio JC, et al. Detection of rheumatoid arthritis-interstitial lung disease is enhanced by serum biomarkers. Am J Respir Crit Care Med 2015;191:1403–12. https://doi.org/10.1164/rccm.201411-1950OC.

[13] Saag KG, Cerhan JR, Kolluri S, Ohashi K, Hunninghake GW, Schwartz DA. Cigarette smoking and rheumatoid arthritis severity. Ann Rheum Dis 1997;56:463–9. https://doi.org/10.1136/ard.56.8.463.

[14] Castellanos-Moreira R, Rodríguez-García SC, Gomara MJ, Ruiz-Esquide V, Cuervo A, Casafont-Solé I, et al. Anti-carbamylated proteins antibody repertoire in rheumatoid arthritis: evidence of a new autoantibody linked to interstitial lung disease. Ann Rheum Dis 2020;79:587–94. https://doi.org/10.1136/annrheumdis-2019-216709.

[15] Juge P-A, Lee JS, Ebstein E, Furukawa H, Dobrinskikh E, Gazal S, et al. MUC5B promoter variant and rheumatoid arthritis with interstitial lung disease. N Engl J Med 2018;379:2209–19. https://doi.org/10.1056/nejmoa1801562.

[16] Seibold MA, Wise AL, Speer MC, Steele MP, Brown KK, Loyd JE, et al. A common MUC5B promoter polymorphism and pulmonary fibrosis. N Engl J Med 2011;364:1503–12. https://doi.org/10.1056/nejmoa1013660.

[17] Hunninghake GM, Hatabu H, Okajima Y, Gao W, Dupuis J, Latourelle JC, et al. MUC5B promoter polymorphism and interstitial lung abnormalities. N Engl J Med 2013;368:2192–200. https://doi.org/10.1056/nejmoa1216076.

[18] Kesimer M, Ford AA, Ceppe A, Radicioni G, Cao R, Davis CW, et al. Airway mucin concentration as a marker of chronic bronchitis. N Engl J Med 2017;377:911–22. https://doi.org/10.1056/nejmoa1701632.

[19] Wang D, Zhang J, Lau J, Wang S, Taneja V, Matteson EL, et al. Mechanisms of lung disease development in rheumatoid arthritis. Nat Rev Rheumatol 2019;15:581–96. https://doi.org/10.1038/s41584-019-0275-x.

[20] Sugiyama Y, Kano S, Ohno S, Maeda H, Kitamura S. Diffuse panbronchiolitis and rheumatoid arthritis: a possible correlation with HLA-B54. Intern Med 1994;33:612–4. https://doi.org/10.2169/internalmedicine.33.612.

[21] Matsuo T, Hashimoto M, Ito I, Kubo T, Uozumi R, Furu M, et al. Interleukin-18 is associated with the presence of interstitial lung disease in rheumatoid arthritis: a cross-sectional

study. Scand J Rheumatol 2019;48:87–94. https://doi.org/10.1080/03009742.2018.1477989.

[22] Shaw M, Collins BF, Ho LA, Raghu G. Rheumatoid arthritis-associated lung disease. Eur Respir Rev 2015;24. https://doi.org/10.1183/09059180.00008014.

[23] Rajasekaran BA, Shovlin D, Lord P, Kelly CA. Interstitial lung disease in patients with rheumatoid arthritis: a comparison with cryptogenic fibrosing alveolitis. Rheumatology 2001;40:1022–5. https://doi.org/10.1093/rheumatology/40.9.1022.

[24] Zamora-Legoff JA, Krause ML, Crowson CS, Ryu JH, Matteson EL. Patterns of interstitial lung disease and mortality in rheumatoid arthritis. Rheumatology 2017;56:344–50. https://doi.org/10.1093/rheumatology/kew391.

[25] Lee HK, Kim DS, Yoo B, Seo JB, Rho JY, Colby Tv, et al. Histopathologic pattern and clinical features of rheumatoid arthritis-associated interstitial lung disease. Chest 2005;127:2019–27. https://doi.org/10.1378/chest.127.6.2019.

[26] Dawson JK, Fewins HE, Desmond J, Lynch MP, Graham DR. Fibrosing alveolitis in patients with rheumatoid arthritis as assessed by high resolution computed tomography, chest radiography, and pulmonary function tests. Thorax 2001;56:622–7. https://doi.org/10.1136/thorax.56.8.622.

[27] Assayag D, Elicker BM, Urbania TH, Colby Tv, Kang BH, Ryu JH, et al. Rheumatoid arthritis-associated interstitial lung disease: radiologic identification of usual interstitial pneumonia pattern. Radiology 2014;270:583–8. https://doi.org/10.1148/radiol.13130187.

[28] Solomon JJ, Ryu JH, Tazelaar HD, Myers JL, Tuder R, Cool CD, et al. Fibrosing interstitial pneumonia predicts survival in patients with rheumatoid arthritis-associated interstitial lung disease (RA-ILD). Respir Med 2013;107:1247–52. https://doi.org/10.1016/j.rmed.2013.05.002.

[29] Ascherman DP. Interstitial lung disease in rheumatoid arthritis. Curr Rheumatol Rep 2010;12:363–9. https://doi.org/10.1007/s11926-010-0116-z.

[30] Kim EJ, Elicker BM, Maldonado F, Webb WR, Ryu JH, van Uden JH, et al. Usual interstitial pneumonia in rheumatoid arthritis-associated interstitial lung disease. Eur Respir J 2010;35:1322–8. https://doi.org/10.1183/09031936.00092309.

[31] Katzenstein ALA, Mukhopadhyay S, Myers JL. Diagnosis of usual interstitial pneumonia and distinction from other fibrosing interstitial lung diseases. Hum Pathol 2008;39:1275–94. https://doi.org/10.1016/j.humpath.2008.05.009.

[32] Doyle TJ, Dellaripa PF. Lung manifestations in the rheumatic diseases. Chest 2017;152:1283–95. https://doi.org/10.1016/j.chest.2017.05.015.

[33] Jacob J, Hirani N, van Moorsel CHM, Rajagopalan S, Murchison JT, van Es HW, et al. Predicting outcomes in rheumatoid arthritis related interstitial lung disease. Eur Respir J 2019;53. https://doi.org/10.1183/13993003.00869-2018.

[34] Chung JH, Cox CW, Montner SM, Adegunsoye A, Oldham JM, Husain AN, et al. CT features of the usual interstitial pneumonia pattern: differentiating connective tissue disease-associated interstitial lung disease from idiopathic pulmonary fibrosis. Am J Roentgenol 2018;210:307–13. https://doi.org/10.2214/AJR.17.18384.

[35] Collard HR, Ryerson CJ, Corte TJ, Jenkins G, Kondoh Y, Lederer DJ, et al. Acute exacerbation of idiopathic pulmonary fibrosis an international working group report. Am J Respir Crit Care Med 2016;194:265–75. https://doi.org/10.1164/rccm.201604-0801CI.

[36] Spagnolo P, Wuyts W. Acute exacerbations of interstitial lung disease: lessons from idiopathic pulmonary fibrosis. Curr Opin Pulm Med 2017;23:411–7. https://doi.org/10.1097/MCP.0000000000000405.

[37] Hozumi H, Nakamura Y, Johkoh T, Sumikawa H, Colby Tv, Kono M, et al. Acute exacerbation in rheumatoid arthritis-associated interstitial lung disease: a retrospective case control study. BMJ Open 2013;3. https://doi.org/10.1136/bmjopen-2013-003132.

[38] Salaffi F, Carotti M, di Carlo M, Tardella M, Giovagnoni A, Adamek M. High-resolution computed tomography of the lung in patients with rheumatoid arthritis: prevalence of interstitial lung disease involvement and determinants of abnormalities. Medicine 2019;98. https://doi.org/10.1097/MD.0000000000017088.

[39] Manfredi A, Cassone G, Cerri S, Venerito V, Fedele AL, Trevisani M, et al. Diagnostic accuracy of a velcro sound detector (VECTOR) for interstitial lung disease in rheumatoid arthritis patients: the InSPIRAtE validation study (INterStitial pneumonia in rheumatoid ArThritis with an electronic device). BMC Pulm Med 2019;19. https://doi.org/10.1186/s12890-019-0875-x.

[40] Wells AU, Hirani N. Interstitial lung disease guideline: the British Thoracic Society in collaboration with the Thoracic Society of Australia and New Zealand and the Irish Thoracic Society. Thorax 2008;63. https://doi.org/10.1136/thx.2008.101691.

[41] Caiulo VA, Gargani L, Caiulo S, Fisicaro A, Moramarco F, Latini G, et al. Lung ultrasound in bronchiolitis: comparison with chest X-ray. Eur J Pediatr 2011;170:1427–33. https://doi.org/10.1007/s00431-011-1461-2.

[42] Wohlgenannt S, Gehmacher O, Gehmacher U, Kopf A, Mathis G. Sonographische befunde bei interstitiellen lungenerkrankungen. Ultraschall der Med 2001;22:27–31. https://doi.org/10.1055/s-2001-11252.

[43] Sperandeo M, Varriale A, Sperandeo G, Filabozzi P, Piattelli ML, Carnevale V, et al. Transthoracic ultrasound in the evaluation of pulmonary fibrosis: our experience. Ultrasound Med Biol 2009;35:723–9. https://doi.org/10.1016/j.ultrasmedbio.2008.10.009.

[44] Garcia JGN, Parhami N, Killam D, Keogh BA. Bronchoalveolar lavage fluid evaluation in rheumatoid arthritis. Am Rev Respir Dis 1986;133:450–4. https://doi.org/10.1164/arrd.1986.133.3.450.

[45] Rojas-Serrano J, Herrera-Bringas D, Pérez-Román DI, Pérez-Dorame R, Mateos-Toledo H, Mejía M. Rheumatoid arthritis-related interstitial lung disease (RA-ILD): methotrexate and the severity of lung disease are associated to prognosis. Clin Rheumatol 2017;36:1493–500. https://doi.org/10.1007/s10067-017-3707-5.

[46] Wada T, Akiyama Y, Yokota K, Sato K, Funakubo Y, Mimura T. A case of rheumatoid arthritis complicated with deteriorated interstitial pneumonia after the administration of abatacept. Jpn J Clin Immunol 2012;35:433–8. https://doi.org/10.2177/jsci.35.433.

[47] Chatzidionysiou K, Emamikia S, Nam J, Ramiro S, Smolen J, van der Heijde D, et al. Efficacy of glucocorticoids, conventional and targeted synthetic disease-modifying antirheumatic drugs: a systematic literature review informing the 2016 update of the EULAR recommendations for the management of rheumatoid arthritis. Ann Rheum Dis 2017;76:1102–7. https://doi.org/10.1136/annrheumdis-2016-210711.

[48] Singh JA, Saag KG, Bridges SL, Akl EA, Bannuru RR, Sullivan MC, et al. 2015 American College of Rheumatology guideline for the treatment of rheumatoid arthritis. Arthritis Care Res 2016;68:1–25. https://doi.org/10.1002/acr.22783.

[49] Kim EJ, Collard HR, King TE. Rheumatoid arthritis-associated interstitial lung disease: the relevance of histopathologic and radiographic pattern. Chest 2009;136:1397–405. https://doi.org/10.1378/chest.09-0444.

[50] Dixon WG, Abrahamowicz M, Beauchamp ME, Ray DW, Bernatsky S, Suissa S, et al. Immediate and delayed impact of oral glucocorticoid therapy on risk of serious infection in

older patients with rheumatoid arthritis: a nested case-control analysis. Ann Rheum Dis 2012;71:1128–33. https://doi.org/10.1136/annrheumdis-2011-200702.
[51] Laan RFJM, Buijs WCAM, Verbeek ALM, Draad MP, Corstens FHM, van de Putte LBA, et al. Bone mineral density in patients with recent onset rheumatoid arthritis: influence of disease activity and functional capacity. Ann Rheum Dis 1993;52:21–6. https://doi.org/10.1136/ard.52.1.21.
[52] Yukawa K, Nagamoto Y, Watanabe H, Funaki M, Iwahashi M, Yamana J, et al. Risk factors for pneumocystis jirovecii pneumonia in patients with rheumatoid arthritis and a prophylactic indication of trimethoprim/sulfamethoxazole. J Clin Rheumatol 2018;24:355–60. https://doi.org/10.1097/RHU.0000000000000731.
[53] Canalis E, Mazziotti G, Giustina A, Bilezikian JP. Glucocorticoid-induced osteoporosis: pathophysiology and therapy. Osteoporos Int 2007;18:1319–28. https://doi.org/10.1007/s00198-007-0394-0.
[54] Smolen JS, Landewé R, Breedveld FC, Buch M, Burmester G, Dougados M, et al. EULAR recommendations for the management of rheumatoid arthritis with synthetic and biological disease-modifying antirheumatic drugs: 2013 update. Ann Rheum Dis 2014;73:492–509. https://doi.org/10.1136/annrheumdis-2013-204573.
[55] Sathi N, Chikura B, Kaushik Vv, Wiswell R, Dawson JK. How common is methotrexate pneumonitis? A large prospective study investigates. Clin Rheumatol 2012;31:79–83. https://doi.org/10.1007/s10067-011-1758-6.
[56] Saravanan V, Kelly CA. Reducing the risk of methotrexate pneumonitis in rheumatoid arthritis. Rheumatology 2004;43:143–7. https://doi.org/10.1093/rheumatology/keg466.
[57] Conway R, Low C, Coughlan RJ, O'Donnell MJ, Carey JJ. Methotrexate and lung disease in rheumatoid arthritis: a meta-analysis of randomized controlled trials. Arthritis Rheumatol 2014;66:803–12. https://doi.org/10.1002/art.38322.
[58] Kiely P, Busby AD, Nikiphorou E, Sullivan K, Walsh DA, Creamer P, et al. Is incident rheumatoid arthritis interstitial lung disease associated with methotrexate treatment? Results from a multivariate analysis in the ERAS and ERAN inception cohorts. BMJ Open 2019;9. https://doi.org/10.1136/bmjopen-2018-028466.
[59] Sawada T, Inokuma S, Sato T, Otsuka T, Saeki Y, Takeuchi T, et al. Leflunomide-induced interstitial lung disease: prevalence and risk factors in Japanese patients with rheumatoid arthritis. Rheumatology 2009;48:1069–72. https://doi.org/10.1093/rheumatology/kep052.
[60] Conway R, Low C, Coughlan RJ, O'Donnell MJ, Carey JJ. Leflunomide use and risk of lung disease in rheumatoid arthritis: a systematic literature review and metaanalysis of randomized controlled trials. J Rheumatol 2016;43:855–60. https://doi.org/10.3899/jrheum.150674.
[61] Tzouvelekis A, Galanopoulos N, Bouros E, Kolios G, Zacharis G, Ntolios P, et al. Effect and safety of mycophenolate mofetil or sodium in systemic sclerosis-associated interstitial lung disease: a meta-analysis. Pulm Med 2012;2012. https://doi.org/10.1155/2012/143637.
[62] Fischer A, Brown KK, du Bois RM, Frankel SK, Cosgrove GP, Fernandez-Perez ER, et al. Mycophenolate mofetil improves lung function in connective tissue disease-associated interstitial lung disease. J Rheumatol 2013;40:640–6. https://doi.org/10.3899/jrheum.121043.
[63] Tashkin DP, Roth MD, Clements PJ, Furst DE, Khanna D, Kleerup EC, et al. Mycophenolate mofetil versus oral cyclophosphamide in scleroderma-related interstitial lung disease (SLS II): a randomised controlled, double-blind, parallel group trial. Lancet Respir Med 2016;4:708–19. https://doi.org/10.1016/S2213-2600(16)30152-7.

[64] Saketkoo LA, Espinoza LR. Experience of mycophenolate mofetil in 10 patients with autoimmune-related interstitial lung disease demonstrates promising effects. Am J Med Sci 2009;337:329–35. https://doi.org/10.1097/MAJ.0b013e31818d094b.

[65] Kelly C, Saravanan V. Treatment strategies for a rheumatoid arthritis patient with interstitial lung disease. Expet Opin Pharmacother 2008;9:3221–30. https://doi.org/10.1517/14656560802591430.

[66] Schupp JC, Köhler T, Müller-Quernheim J. Usefulness of cyclophosphamide pulse therapy in interstitial lung diseases. Respiration 2016;91:296–301. https://doi.org/10.1159/000445031.

[67] Barnes H, Holland AE, Westall GP, Goh NSL, Glaspole IN. Cyclophosphamide for connective tissue disease-associated interstitial lung disease. Cochrane Database Syst Rev 2018;2018. https://doi.org/10.1002/14651858.CD010908.pub2.

[68] Raghu G, Depaso WJ, Cain K, Hammar SP, Wetzel CE, Dreis DF, et al. Azathioprine combined with prednisone in the treatment of idiopathic pulmonary fibrosis: a prospective double-blind, randomized, placebo-controlled clinical trial. Am Rev Respir Dis 1991;144:291–6. https://doi.org/10.1164/ajrccm/144.2.291.

[69] Idiopathic Pulmonary Fibrosis Clinical Research Network, Raghu G, Anstrom KJ, King Jr TE, Lasky JA, Martinez FJ. Prednisone, azathioprine, and N -acetylcysteine for pulmonary fibrosis. N Engl J Med 2012;366:1968–77. https://doi.org/10.1056/nejmoa1113354.

[70] Oldham JM, Lee C, Valenzi E, Witt LJ, Adegunsoye A, Hsu S, et al. Azathioprine response in patients with fibrotic connective tissue disease-associated interstitial lung disease. Respir Med 2016;121:117–22. https://doi.org/10.1016/j.rmed.2016.11.007.

[71] Perez-Alvarez R, Perez-de-Lis M, Diaz-Lagares C, Pego-Reigosa JM, Retamozo S, Bove A, et al. Interstitial lung disease induced or exacerbated by TNF-targeted therapies: analysis of 122 cases. Semin Arthritis Rheum 2011;41:256–64. https://doi.org/10.1016/j.semarthrit.2010.11.002.

[72] Nakashita T, Ando K, Kaneko N, Takahashi K, Motojima S. Potential risk of TNF inhibitors on the progression of interstitial lung disease in patients with rheumatoid arthritis. BMJ Open 2014;4. https://doi.org/10.1136/bmjopen-2014-005615.

[73] Dixon WG, Hyrich KL, Watson KD, Lunt M, Symmons DPM. Influence of anti-TNF therapy on mortality in patients with rheumatoid arthritis-associated interstitial lung disease: results from the British Society for Rheumatology Biologics Register. Ann Rheum Dis 2010;69:1086–91. https://doi.org/10.1136/ard.2009.120626.

[74] Druce KL, Iqbal K, Watson KD, Symmons DPM, Hyrich KL, Kelly C. Mortality in patients with interstitial lung disease treated with rituximab or TNFi as a first biologic. RMD Open 2017;3. https://doi.org/10.1136/rmdopen-2017-000473.

[75] Kang EH, Jin Y, Desai RJ, Liu J, Sparks JA, Kim SC. Risk of exacerbation of pulmonary comorbidities in patients with rheumatoid arthritis after initiation of abatacept versus TNF inhibitors: a cohort study. Semin Arthritis Rheum 2020;50:401–8. https://doi.org/10.1016/j.semarthrit.2019.11.010.

[76] Manfredi A, Cassone G, Furini F, Gremese E, Venerito V, Atzeni F, et al. Tocilizumab therapy in rheumatoid arthritis with interstitial lung disease: a multicentre retrospective study. Intern Med J 2020;50:1085–90. https://doi.org/10.1111/imj.14670.

[77] Jani M, Hirani N, Matteson EL, Dixon WG. The safety of biologic therapies in RA-associated interstitial lung disease. Nat Rev Rheumatol 2014;10:284–94. https://doi.org/10.1038/nrrheum.2013.197.

[78] Roubille C, Haraoui B. Interstitial lung diseases induced or exacerbated by DMARDS and biologic agents in rheumatoid arthritis: a systematic literature review. Semin Arthritis Rheum 2014;43:613–26. https://doi.org/10.1016/j.semarthrit.2013.09.005.

[79] Fernández-Díaz C, Loricera J, Castañeda S, López-Mejías R, Ojeda-García C, Olivé A, et al. Abatacept in patients with rheumatoid arthritis and interstitial lung disease: a national multicenter study of 63 patients. Semin Arthritis Rheum 2018;48:22–7. https://doi.org/10.1016/j.semarthrit.2017.12.012.

[80] Fernández-Díaz C, Atienza-Mateo B, Castañeda S, Melero-Gonzalez RB, Ortiz-SanJuan F, Loricera J, et al. Abatacept in monotherapy vs combined in interstitial lung disease of rheumatoid arthritis—multicentre study of 263 Caucasian patients. Rheumatology 2021. https://doi.org/10.1093/rheumatology/keab317.

[81] Vicente-Rabaneda EF, Atienza-Mateo B, Blanco R, Cavagna L, Ancochea J, Castañeda S, et al. Efficacy and safety of abatacept in interstitial lung disease of rheumatoid arthritis: a systematic literature review. Autoimmun Rev 2021;20. https://doi.org/10.1016/j.autrev.2021.102830.

[82] APRIL (AbatacePt in rheumatoid arthritis-ILD) (APRIL). ClinicalTrialsGov. Identifier: NCT03084419; n.d.

[83] Bosello SL, de Luca G, Rucco M, Berardi G, Falcione M, Danza FM, et al. Long-term efficacy of B cell depletion therapy on lung and skin involvement in diffuse systemic sclerosis. Semin Arthritis Rheum 2015;44:428–36. https://doi.org/10.1016/j.semarthrit.2014.09.002.

[84] Doyle TJ, Dhillon N, Madan R, Cabral F, Fletcher EA, Koontz DC, et al. Rituximab in the treatment of interstitial lung disease associated with antisynthetase syndrome: a multicenter retrospective case review. J Rheumatol 2018;45:841–50. https://doi.org/10.3899/jrheum.170541.

[85] Keir GJ, Maher TM, Hansell DM, Denton CP, Ong VH, Singh S, et al. Severe interstitial lung disease in connective tissue disease: rituximab as rescue therapy. Eur Respir J 2012;40:641–8. https://doi.org/10.1183/09031936.00163911.

[86] Md Yusof MY, Kabia A, Darby M, Lettieri G, Beirne P, Vital EM, et al. Effect of rituximab on the progression of rheumatoid arthritis-related interstitial lung disease: 10 years' experience at a single centre. Rheumatology 2017;56:1348–57. https://doi.org/10.1093/rheumatology/kex072.

[87] Harigai M. Growing evidence of the safety of JAK inhibitors in patients with rheumatoid arthritis. Rheumatology 2019;58:i34–42. https://doi.org/10.1093/rheumatology/key287.

[88] Chen Z, Wang X, Ye S. Tofacitinib in amyopathic dermatomyositis–associated interstitial lung disease. N Engl J Med 2019;381:291–3. https://doi.org/10.1056/nejmc1900045.

[89] Effects of tofacitinib vs methotrexate on rheumatoid arthritis interstitial lung disease (PULMORA). ClinicalTrialsGov. Identifier: NCT04311567; n.d.

[90] Flaherty KR, Wells AU, Cottin V, Devaraj A, Walsh SLF, Inoue Y, et al. Nintedanib in progressive fibrosing interstitial lung diseases. N Engl J Med 2019;381:1718–27. https://doi.org/10.1056/nejmoa1908681.

[91] Richeldi L, du Bois RM, Raghu G, Azuma A, Brown KK, Costabel U, et al. Efficacy and safety of nintedanib in idiopathic pulmonary fibrosis. N Engl J Med 2014;370:2071–82. https://doi.org/10.1056/nejmoa1402584.

[92] Noble PW, Albera C, Bradford WZ, Costabel U, Bois RMD, Fagan EA, et al. Pirfenidone for idiopathic pulmonary fibrosis: analysis of pooled data from three multinational phase 3 trials. Eur Respir J 2016;47:243–53. https://doi.org/10.1183/13993003.00026-2015.

[93] Maher TM, Corte TJ, Fischer A, Kreuter M, Lederer DJ, Molina-Molina M, et al. Pirfenidone in patients with unclassifiable progressive fibrosing interstitial lung disease: a double-blind, randomised, placebo-controlled, phase 2 trial. Lancet Respir Med 2020;8:147–57. https://doi.org/10.1016/S2213-2600(19)30341-8.

[94] Khanna D, Albera C, Fischer A, Khalidi N, Raghu G, Chung L, et al. An open-label, phase II study of the safety and tolerability of pirfenidone in patients with scleroderma-associated interstitial lung disease: the LOTUSS trial. J Rheumatol 2016;43:1672–9. https://doi.org/10.3899/jrheum.151322.

[95] Phase ll study of pirfenidone in patients with RAILD (TRAIL1). ClinicalTrialsGov. Identifier: NCT02808871; n.d.

[96] Yazdani A, Singer LG, Strand V, Gelber AC, Williams L, Mittoo S. Survival and quality of life in rheumatoid arthritis-associated interstitial lung disease after lung transplantation. J Heart Lung Transplant 2014;33:514–20. https://doi.org/10.1016/j.healun.2014.01.858.

Chapter 3

Lung involvement in SLE

Laurent Arnaud[1,*] and Gerard Espinosa[2]
[1]*Department of Rheumatology, French National Reference Center for Autoimmune diseases (CRMR RESO), Strasbourg, France;* [2]*Department of Autoimmune Diseases, Hospital Clinic, IDIBAPS, Universitat de Barcelona, Barcelona, Catalonia, Spain*
[*]*Corresponding author at: laurent.arnaud@chru-strasbourg.fr.*

Pulmonary manifestations of systemic lupus erythematosus (SLE) are quite diverse in their nature and frequency. While pleural involvement is relatively common (20%–40% of patients), other manifestations such as those involving the lung parenchyma (lupus pneumonitis, interstitial lung disease [ILD]), the diaphragm (shrinking lung syndrome [SLS]), or the lung vasculature (pulmonary arterial hypertension [PAH] and pulmonary vasculitis) are infrequent, with the exception of pulmonary embolism which is largely associated with the antiphospholipid syndrome. Also, the risk of lung infection is increased, due to the disease itself, but mostly to the use of immunosuppressive treatments. Most SLE patients with lung involvement will present with a combination of chest pain, cough, and dyspnea, but others may be asymptomatic. Diagnosis of SLE-associated lung involvement is typically made with thoracic imaging such as chest X-ray or nowadays more commonly with high-resolution computed chest tomography (HRCT), pulmonary function tests, echocardiography, lung scintigraphy, or transthoracic ultrasound of the lung [1].

Pleural involvement

Pleural involvement is the most common lung manifestation of SLE, observed as the presenting symptom in 5%–20% of patients [2] and in 20%–40% during the course of the disease [3]. It is also a common manifestation in drug-induced lupus [4]. Pleuritis is accompanied with pericarditis in about 20% of cases and most patients have active SLE in other organs [5]. Patients can present with pleuritic chest pain, which may occur with or without pleural effusion, but some patients may be asymptomatic with pleural involvement being found incidentally on thoracic imaging. Effusions are usually bilateral but may be unilateral. The causes of pleural effusion in SLE patients included

The Lung in Autoimmune Diseases. https://doi.org/10.1016/B978-0-323-91083-5.00001-3

lupus pleurisy in a majority of cases, as well as infectious pleural effusion with or without associated pneumonia, pulmonary embolism, congestive heart failure, and less commonly malignancy. Pleural aspiration can be useful to rule out differential diagnoses, especially if an infection is suspected. Pleural fluid analysis typically shows an exsudate with increased lactate dehydrogenase and leukocytes. Pleural fluid ANA titers ≥1:160 [6,7] as well as the occasional presence of LE cells in the pleural fluid have been demonstrated in some cases. Serum CRP levels are typically increased in lupus pleuritic [7]. Pleural biopsies are uncommonly performed, as these show aspecific lymphocytic and plasma cell infiltration, fibrosis, and fibrinous pleuritic, and are mainly used to rule out a differential diagnosis when needed. The mainstay treatment of pleurisy in SLE is corticosteroids [5]. Immunosuppressive agents can be indicated in case of refractory or relapsing pleural involvement, or when there is a concurrent flare in another organ. Of note, belimumab did not show any significant effect over pleurisy in the combined analysis of its two phase III pivotal trials (BLISS-52 and BLISS-76) [8].

Interstitial lung disease

The exact prevalence of SLE-associated ILD is not completely known. In three international registries that have included a large number of SLE patients, the prevalence of ILD ranges from 0.4% in the LUMINA (for Lupus in Minorities: Nature vs. Nurture) cohort [9] to 1.4% in the GLADEL (Latin American Group for the Study of Lupus) cohort [10], and 2% in the RELESSER (Spanish Rheumatology Society SLE Registry) cohort [3]. Recently, two studies from Sweden and Taiwan reported that the incidence rates of ILD in patients with incident SLE compared with the general population were 3.1 per 1000 years and 120 per 10^5 years, respectively [11,12]. Results of a recent systematic review of the literature and meta-analysis indicated that late-onset SLE patients, defined as ≥50 years of age, are more likely than early-onset patients to develop pulmonary manifestations. In fact, older-onset SLE patients had a nearly threefold increased odds of ILD, similar to age trends in idiopathic ILD [13].

From the clinical point of view, SLE patients with ILD may present with chest pain, nonproductive cough, and dyspnea resulting in decreased exercise tolerance. However, it is important to keep in mind that the majority of them are asymptomatic with no respiratory symptoms at the time of ILD diagnosis [14]. Of note, 55% of patients exhibited basilar crackles. Conversely, clubbing and peripheral cyanosis, which are characteristic of idiopathic pulmonary fibrosis, are rarely found in SLE-ILD. In a recent series of 55 SLE patients with ILD, the chronic form was the commonest present in 35 (63.6%) patients, whereas the remaining presented by subacute and acute ILD [15]. In the largest series of SLE patients with associated ILD including 379 Chinese patients, acute ILD with rapidly progressive deterioration within one month presented in only 1.1% of them and subacute ILD with progressive deterioration within three months in only 10.8%, respectively. The remaining presented with chronic ILD [16]. Considering the presentation form, ILD in SLE may develop following a flare of acute lupus pneumonitis (ALP). Those patients who survived the acute episode developed residual infiltrates with abnormal pulmonary function. On the other hand, in most SLE patients, ILD followed a slow and a more insidious clinical course [17]. In general, up to 50% of patients are diagnosed with ILD and SLE concomitantly.

Some risk factors have been associated with the development of SLE-ILD such as longstanding disease, older age, a history of ALP, anti-U1RNP antibodies, and overlapping clinical features with scleroderma such as Raynaud's phenomenon and sclerodactyly [18,19].

From the histopathological and radiographic point of view, the most common form of SLE-ILD is the nonspecific interstitial pneumonia (NSIP), but other forms have also been described such as organizing pneumonia, lymphocytic interstitial pneumonia, follicular bronchitis, and usual interstitial pneumonia [19,20]. Given the low prevalence of SLE-ILD, screening with lung function test of all patients with SLE is not recommended. Diagnosis of SLE-associated ILD should be based on a compatible clinical picture or the finding of basilar crackles on the pulmonary auscultation. It is imperative to perform an imaging study with chest radiography and HRCT (Fig. 3.1). In addition, lung function tests may show a restrictive pattern of disease and a decrease in diffusing capacity for carbon monoxide (DLCO) [21]. The following step should be to exclude other potential causes of ILD such as concomitant overlap disorders. In this sense, it is important to rule out the coexistence of rheumatoid arthritis by measuring rheumatoid factor, antisynthetase syndrome by measuring serum muscle enzymes and an extended myositis panel, and systemic sclerosis by measuring specific autoantibodies such as antitopoisomerase, anticentromere, and anti-RNA polymerase autoantibodies if the clinical suspicion is high. At this point, the role of

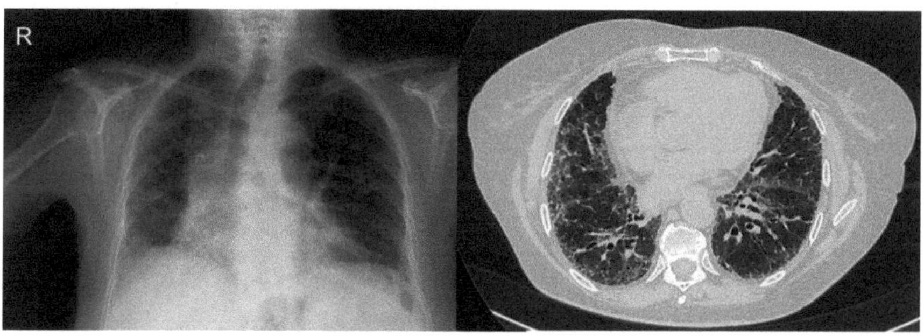

FIGURE 3.1 Interstitial lung disease (ILD) associated with systemic lupus erythematosus. Chest X-ray (left) showing ILD with peripheral distribution. HRCT (right) showing an ILD with a pattern of usual interstitial pneumonia.

pulmonologist may be very important to rule out other nonautoimmune causes of ILD such as hypersensitivity pneumonitis or ILD associated to environmental exposure or drugs. Interestingly, in the majority of patients, anti-dsDNA antibody titer or complement levels do not associate with the development of ILD [16]. Bronchoalveolar lavage (BAL) or transbronchial lung biopsy may be useful to evaluate for alternative causes such as hypersensitivity pneumonitis or associated infection or neoplasm. Histological studies have reported the presence of lymphocytic and mononuclear interstitial and peribronchiolar infiltrates in biopsies taken from those with SLE-related NSIP [22].

In terms of treatment, there is a lack of clinical trials assessing the efficacy of immunosuppressive agents for the ILD in the context of SLE, a lack of data about the potential role of new antifibrotic therapies and finally, a lack of biomarkers to assess from the pathogenic point of view, the therapeutic response to all these treatments. Therefore, recommendations are predominantly based on case reports, small case series, physician expertise, and mainly by applying findings from studies of ILD in other autoimmune diseases. In this sense, the combination of glucocorticoids (GCs) and intravenous cyclophosphamide (IVCYC) or mycophenolate mofetil (MMF) may be the first line therapy. Considering GC, it is important to take into account the last EULAR recommendations for the management of SLE patients to avoid the adverse events associated with high doses of steroids. Pulses of intravenous methylprednisolone (125–500 mg per day, for 1–3 days) provide immediate therapeutic effect and enable the use of lower starting dose of oral GC (0.5 mg/kg/day) [23]. It is important to remember that as maintenance dose, prednisone should be minimized to less than 7.5 mg/day (or equivalent). Owing its better safety profile, MMF could be considered before IVCYC [24]. It is important to highlight that there are no head-to-head studies assessing the efficacy of these immunosuppressive therapies. Therefore, in some milder cases, azathioprine, methotrexate, or tacrolimus may be also considered or as treatment to maintain long-term control of the disease.

Anecdotal reports of the efficacy of rituximab in severe or refractory cases of SLE-ILD have been described [25,26]. Unfortunately, in a recent review of the efficacy and safety of rituximab in the treatment of connective tissue disease-related ILD, there is no specific data for SLE patients [27]. Recently, a patient with ILD associated to SLE and scleroderma overlap who was successfully treated with belimumab has been reported [28]. Unfortunately, in the randomized controlled trials of belimumab, no data of pulmonary manifestations were described in detail. In a survey among SLE experts, the preferred treatment algorithm for the ILD was the induction with GC and MMF or CYC, then rituximab or intravenous immunoglobulin (IVIG), and maintenance followed with azathioprine or MMF [29].

Considering antifibrotic therapy, nintedanib has been approved by the Food and Drug Administration and European Medicaments Agency for the treatment of idiopathic pulmonary fibrosis and chronic fibrosing ILDs with a progressive phenotype and for reducing the rate of decline in forced vital capacity (FVC) in patients with ILD associated with systemic sclerosis [30]. Moreover, in the randomized, placebo-controlled INBUILD trial, conducted in 663 subjects with non-IPF chronic fibrosing ILDs that had progressed within the previous two years despite management in clinical practice, nintedanib slowed the rate of decline in FVC over 52 weeks by 57% versus placebo [31]. Approximately one-quarter (25.6%) of the patients in this trial had autoimmune disease-related ILDs. The most common diagnosis was rheumatoid arthritis followed by systemic sclerosis. Ten patients in the nintedanib group had "other" autoimmune disease, but the authors did not describe them in detail. Although the INBUILD trial was not powered to study individual ILDs, subgroup analyses suggested that there was no heterogeneity in the rate of FVC decline across subgroups by ILD diagnosis. The adverse events associated with nintedanib were predominantly gastrointestinal events, particularly diarrhea [32]. The other antifibrotic agent is pirfenidone. The results of RELIEF study suggest that pirfenidone might attenuate disease progression as measured by decline in FVC in patients with non-IPF progressive fibrotic ILDs [33]. From 127 patients, 37 had ILD associated to autoimmune disease. Unfortunately, none of them presented with SLE. In the light of these results and in addition to conventional immunosuppressive and/or biologic therapy, in some SLE patient with ILD antifibrotic treatment may be considered, mainly in those with progressive fibrotic ILD phenotype.

Pulmonary arterial hypertension

PAH is a chronic and progressive disease leading to right heart failure and ultimately death if untreated. The exact prevalence of PAH in SLE is unknown with the broad range of 1%–43% being reported depending on the cohort [34], although this is likely to reflect both referral and screening biases, as well as the inclusion of patients with PH among those with PAH. The majority of PAH cases occur within the first five years following SLE diagnosis [35]. Symptoms of PAH in SLE are nonspecific and not different from those observed with other causes of pulmonary hypertension (PH), and include breathlessness, fatigue, chest pain, edema, and exertional syncope. There are a number of possible underlying causes which may result in PH during SLE, including left ventricular dysfunction, chronic thromboembolic disease, or less commonly in SLE parenchymal lung disease. In a meta-analysis of 31 studies, the prevalence of PH in aPL-positive SLE individuals was 12.3% versus 7.3% in those without aPL (OR: 2.28 [95% CI, 1.65 to 3.15]). Also, systemic hypertension has been shown to be an independent predictor of PAH occurrence among SLE patients [35]. In the multicenter Chinese SLE Treatment and Research group (CSTAR) registry, serositis and antiribonucleoprotein (RNP) antibody positivity were independent predictors of PAH. While risk prediction of mortality based on 6-min walking distance (6MWD), World Health Organization (WHO) functional class, right atrial pressure (RAP), cardiac index (CI), and brain natriuretic peptides (BNP or NT-proBNP) is well studied in iPAH and SSc-PAH, data are largely lacking in SLE. In a meta-analysis, the pooled 1-, 3-, and 5-year survival rates for PAH in SLE were 88% (95% CI, 0.80–0.93), 81% (95% CI, 0.67–0.90), and 68% (95% CI, 0.52–0.80), respectively [36]. Pharmacological treatments for PAH typically include a combination of endothelin receptor antagonists, soluble guanylate cyclase stimulators, phosphodiesterase-5 inhibitors (PDE-5i), as well as prostacyclin analogs and lung transplantation in more severe cases. In the context of SLE, those drugs are typically associated with corticosteroids and immunosuppressive therapy. The use of anticoagulation in patients without chronic thromboembolic disease remains controversial.

Diffuse alveolar hemorrhage and pulmonary vasculitis

Diffuse alveolar hemorrhage (DAH) is a rare but life-threatening complication of SLE, which originates from the pulmonary microcirculation, including the alveolar capillaries, arterioles, and venules. DAH may occur in the context of pulmonary vasculitis [37], but also with coagulopathy, decompensated heart failure and infection [37]. Also DAH can occur in SLE in relation with another condition such as diffuse alveolar damage, inhalation, or cytotoxic drug therapy. Among immune-meditated causes of DAH, ANCA-associated vasculitis and SLE are the most common causes. The most common clinical manifestations are dyspnea, cough, fever, and less commonly hemoptysis and anemia along with pulmonary infiltrates on thoracic imaging. Many patients with pulmonary vasculitis will also present with extrapulmonary manifestations suggesting a systemic flare of the disease. In the majority of cases of DAH associated with SLE, lupus nephritis is also present, and 80% of these cases occur in young female patients with known SLE [38]. Early bronchoscopy with BAL is generally required to confirm the diagnosis of DAH and exclude infection. Transbronchial biopsy is rarely used in identifying the cause of DAH, but Direct IF examination typically shows immunoglobulin and complement deposits in the alveolar interstitium and intra-alveolar blood vessels [38] as well as the occasional presence of pulmonary vasculitis. Therapeutic management typically includes oxygen, transfusion support when appropriate, and glucocorticoids in conjunction with immunosuppressive agents. Prompt diagnosis and intensive treatment of pulmonary vasculitis is essential to improve early mortality and long-term outcomes [39].

Acute lupus pneumonitis

ALP is a life-threatening and uncommon manifestation of SLE that requires prompt diagnosis and treatment. In terms of prevalence, it affects around 2%

of SLE patients [20]. In the GLADEL cohort [10], lupus pneumonitis was the second pulmonary manifestation present in 2.3% of patients and it was associated with nonischemic heart disease (OR 2.48; 95%CI: 1.20–5.13). In the RELESSER cohort, 118 (3.6%) patients presented with ALP after 5.4 years from the SLE diagnosis, had worse survival rate (78.6% vs. 95.6%; $P < .01$), and 26% of them who survived developed pulmonary fibrosis [3].

Clinically, ALP presents in the context of a systemic flare of SLE in addition to fever, dyspnea, cough with or without hemoptysis, hypoxemia, and pleuritic chest pain [21]. Onset is acute but nonspecific making a clinical challenge to differentiate from infection, alveolar hemorrhage, or organizing pneumonia. In some cases, ALP may also be the initial presenting symptom of SLE. Wan et al. described the main clinical characteristics of five patients who presented with lupus pneumonitis during the initial SLE manifestation representing 0.007% of 633 SLE patients in their center [40]. All of them were female and had concomitantly other clinical features of SLE such as malar rash, arthritis, oral ulcers, and hematological involvement.

Patients are frequently hypoxemic with bibasilar crackles on examination. The diagnosis is based on the presence of a suggestive clinical picture and data from imaging techniques, immunological features, and in some cases BAL or lung biopsy. Chest radiographs show unilateral or bilateral infiltrates predominantly in the lower lung fields. Associated pleural effusions may be present in up to 50%. Computed tomography (CT) angiography may be needed to exclude pulmonary embolism and HRCT show ground glass opacities with patchy consolidations uni- or bilaterally. However, all this radiographical findings are nonspecific. High levels of anti-dsDNA antibodies and hypocomplementemia are frequently found in this context. Some authors have proposed the association of ALP with anti-SSA/Ro antibodies positivity [41]. BAL is useful to rule out alternative causes such as alveolar hemorrhage and infection. Characteristically, there is an increase in cellularity at the expense of activated polymorphonuclear cells. Lung biopsy should be limited to cases of uncertain diagnosis for the exclusion of alternative etiologies or in those patients who fail to respond to immunosuppressive therapy. Histological data are also nonspecific including alveolar wall damage, inflammatory cell infiltration, edema, hemorrhage, and hyaline membranes without evidence of vasculitis or hemorrhage [42].

Data suggest a high mortality of up to 40%–50% in ALP despite adequate treatment [40,43]. The cell-type present in BAL has been associated with prognosis. Thus, the predominance of lymphocytes in BAL is associated with a more favorable course, whereas the predominance of eosinophils or neutrophils is associated with a higher rate of mortality [44].

As in ILD associated with SLE, treatment recommendations of ALP are based on clinical experience and case reports. It is important to keep in mind that until infection is ruled out, broad-spectrum antibiotic coverage is mandatory. GC combined with immunosuppressant agents are the cornerstone of the treatment of ALP. If ALP is considered as a severe manifestation of SLE, according to the most recent British Society for Rheumatology guideline for the management of SLE in adults, initial pulses of intravenous methylprednisolone (500 mg per day, for 1–3 days) followed by prednisone ≤0.5 mg/kg/day combined with IVCYC or MMF would be the initial treatment [45]. In the retrospective series of five patients with ALP as presenting manifestation of SLE, all of them received GC and four patients were treated with IVCYC, in three of them in combination with IVIg [40]. Given that differential diagnosis often includes infection, and as infection can commonly co-exist with ALP, IVIg represents a useful option as it does not increase the high risk of immunosuppression associated with GC, IVCYC, and MMF [46]. In refractory cases, plasma exchange [47] and rituximab may be an option [48,49].

Shrinking lung syndrome

SLS was described for the first time in 1965 by Hoffbrand and Beck [50]. They described two SLE patients with unexplained breathlessness and raised sluggish diaphragms. The actual prevalence is unknown because the method and criteria used for diagnosis vary between different studies. In the RELESSER cohort, SLS was present in 0.8% of patients [3] and in the GLADEL cohort in 1.6% of them [10].

In a recent review of 164 cases published between 1964 and 2014 in the English and French literature, diagnosis of SLS was made at the time of SLE diagnosis in 9.5% of them. In the remaining cases, SLS was discovered after SLE with a mean delay between diagnosis of SLE and occurrence of SLS of 66.7 months [51]. The median age of the patients at SLS diagnosis was 32 years old (range 11–69) with a female predominance (6.1/1). From the clinical point of view, respiratory symptoms were present in 100% of cases, in form of dyspnea (100%), pleuritic chest pain (80%), and coughing (17%). Of note, extra-thoracic manifestations of SLE included arthralgia (89%), cutaneous involvement (52%), glomerulonephritis (49%), fever (42%), pericardial effusion (19%), alopecia (18%), and neurological involvement (20%). Thoracic imaging (chest X-ray or CT scan) was reported in 139 cases and was abnormal in 98% of them. The most frequent finding was elevated hemidiaphragm with reduced lung volume (96%), uni- or bilaterally (Fig. 3.2). Basal atelectasis due to poor chest expansion was reported in 34% of 139 cases. Pleural effusions and pleural thickening were less frequent, present in 14% and 11%, respectively. Respiratory function showed a restrictive pattern in all cases without obstructive defects with a reduced FVC (52% of theoretical measurement), reduced mean total lung capacity (52%), reduced mean DLCO (49%), but with normal mean DLCO corrected by vital capacity (95%). Maximal inspiratory and expiratory pressures were decreased in 78% and 81%

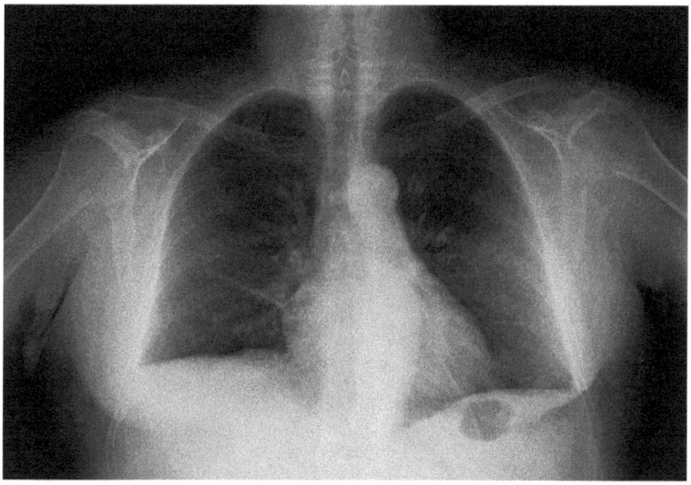

FIGURE 3.2 Chest X-ray showing a bilateral elevation hemidiaphragm with reduced lung volume in an SLE patient with shrinking lung syndrome.

of cases. Among 12 phrenic nerve stimulations, 9 were normal and 3 showed mild signs of neuropathy [51].

There are no diagnostic criteria for SLS. Diagnosis is based on the combination of suggestive clinical picture such as progressive exertional dyspnea that characteristically is worse when supine, pleuritic chest pain, and reducing lung volumes. Physical examination may reveal decreased breath sounds at the bases sometimes with associated crackles. The radiographic imaging in SLS is not specific and the main utility of HRCT in SLS is ruling out parenchymal, interstitial, or vascular lung disease.

The pathophysiology of SLS is unknown. In the majority of patients, tests for diaphragmatic muscle strength or phrenic nerve function are normal. The results of respiratory function and maximal inspiratory and expiratory pressures suggest that may exist a restriction in chest wall expansion, but the mechanism behind this is unknown. Failure of surfactant production resulting in microatelectasis, phrenic neuropathy, pleural inflammation, diaphragm adhesions and fibrosis, steroid induced myopathy, and pain have all been postulated to play a role in pathogenesis [52,53].

Because the cause of the SLS is not known, we do not have appropriate treatments that are based only on case reports and clinician experience. In general, therapeutic approach of SLS is based on antiinflammatory agents. The GCs are the first line of the former with or without immunosuppressive agents. Concerning GC dosing, think on pulses of methylprednisolone (125–500 mg/day for 3 days) followed by prednisone (0.5 mg/kg/day) or equivalent in a decreasing schedule. As immunosuppressants, azathioprine, MMF, methotrexate, or IVCYC have been used [51]. However, there are no trials that have compared the efficacy between them, and choice is usually guided by other factors such as physician expertise, extrapulmonary manifestations, or SLS severity. Most recently, biological therapy has been used successfully with rituximab [54] and belimumab [55]. In addition to antiinflammatory therapy, other treatments should be considered. Among them, bronchodilators such as theophylline and β-agonist therapies may improve diaphragmatic strength and noninvasive positive pressure ventilation at night may also be beneficial. Long-term prognosis is generally good with clinical response within weeks after starting treatment [56]. A recent literature review of 155 SLE patients with SLS revealed clinical improvement in 94% of them, functional improvement in 77% and radiological improvement in 57% after treatment [51].

References

[1] Moazedi-Fuerst FC, Kielhauser S, Brickmann K, Tripolt N, Meilinger M, Lufti A, Graninger W. Sonographic assessment of interstitial lung disease in patients with rheumatoid arthritis, systemic sclerosis and systemic lupus erythematosus. Clin Exp Rheumatol 2015;33:S87–91.

[2] Torre O, Harari S. Pleural and pulmonary involvement in systemic lupus erythematosus. Presse Med 2011;40:e19–29.

[3] Narvaez J, Borrell H, Sanchez-Alonso F, Rua-Figueroa I, Lopez-Longo FJ, Galindo-Izquierdo M, Calvo-Alen J, Fernandez-Nebro A, Olive A, Andreu JL, Martinez-Taboada V, Nolla JM, Pego-Reigosa JM, Group RS. Primary respiratory disease in patients with systemic lupus erythematosus: data from the Spanish rheumatology society lupus registry (RELESSER) cohort. Arthritis Res Ther 2018;20:280.

[4] Arnaud L, Mertz P, Gavand PE, Martin T, Chasset F, Tebacher-Alt M, Lambert A, Muller C, Sibilia J, Lebrun-Vignes B, Salem JE. Drug-induced systemic lupus: revisiting the ever-changing spectrum of the disease using the WHO pharmacovigilance database. Ann Rheum Dis 2019;78:504–8.

[5] Palavutitotai N, Buppajarntham T, Katchamart W. Etiologies and outcomes of pleural effusions in patients with systemic lupus erythematosus. J Clin Rheumatol 2014;20:418–21.

[6] Toworakul C, Kasitanon N, Sukitawut W, Wichinun R, Louthrenoo W. Usefulness of pleural effusion antinuclear antibodies in the diagnosis of lupus pleuritis. Lupus 2011;20:1042–6.

[7] Choi BY, Yoon MJ, Shin K, Lee YJ, Song YW. Characteristics of pleural effusions in systemic lupus erythematosus: differential diagnosis of lupus pleuritis. Lupus 2015;24:321–6.

[8] Manzi S, Sanchez-Guerrero J, Merrill JT, Furie R, Gladman D, Navarra SV, Ginzler EM, D'Cruz DP, Doria A, Cooper S, Zhong ZJ, Hough D, Freimuth W, Petri MA, Bliss, Groups B-S. Effects of belimumab, a B lymphocyte stimulator-specific inhibitor, on disease activity across multiple organ domains in patients with systemic lupus erythematosus: combined results from two phase III trials. Ann Rheum Dis 2012;71:1833–8.

[9] Bertoli AM, Vilá LM, Apte M, Fessler BJ, Bastian HM, Reveille JD, et al. Systemic lupus erythematosus in a multiethnic US Cohort LUMINA XLVIII: factors predictive of pulmonary damage. Lupus 2007;16:410–7.

[10] Haye Salinas MJ, Caeiro F, Saurit V, Alvarellos A, Wojdyla D, Scherbarth HR, et al. Pleuropulmonary involvement in patients with systemic lupus erythematosus from a Latin American inception cohort (GLADEL). Lupus 2017;26:1368–77.

[11] Forbess LJ, Rossides M, Weisman MH, Simard JF. New-onset non-infectious pulmonary manifestations among patients with systemic lupus erythematosus in Sweden. Arthritis Res Ther 2019;21:48.
[12] Ng KG, Chen DY, Lin CH, Chao WC, Chen YM, Chen YH, et al. Risk of interstitial lung disease in patients with newly diagnosed systemic autoimmune rheumatic disease: a nationwide, population-based cohort study. Semin Arthritis Rheum 2020;50:840–5.
[13] Medlin JL, Hansen KE, McCoy SS, Bartels CM. Pulmonary manifestations in late versus early systemic lupus erythematosus: a systematic review and meta-analysis. Semin Arthritis Rheum 2018;48:198–204.
[14] Toyoda Y, Koyama K, Kawano H, Nishimura H, Kagawa K, Morizumi S, et al. Clinical features of interstitial pneumonia associated with systemic lupus erythematosus. Respir Invest 2019;57:435–43.
[15] Enomoto N, Egashira R, Tabata R, Hashisako M, Kitani M, Waseda Y, et al. Analysis of systemic lupus erythematosus-related interstitial pneumonia: a retrospective multicentre study. Sci Rep 2019;9:7355.
[16] Lian F, Zhou J, Wang Y, Cui W, Chen D, Li H, et al. Clinical features and independent predictors of interstitial lung disease in systemic lupus erythematosus. Int J Clin Exp Med 2016;9:4233–42.
[17] Weinrib L, Sharma P, Quismorio FP. A long-term study of interstitial lung disease in systemic lupus erythematosus. Semin Arthritis Rheum 1990;20:48–56.
[18] Lopez-Velazquez M, Highland KB. Pulmonary manifestations of systemic lupus erythematosus and Sjögrens's síndrome. Curr Opin Rheumatol 2018;30:449–64.
[19] Mathai SC, Danoff SK. Management of interstitial lung disease associated with connective tissue disease. Br Med J 2016;352:h6819.
[20] Amarnani R, Yeoh SA, Denneny MK, Wincup C. Lupus and the Lungs: the assessment and management of pulmonary manifestations of systemic lupus erythematosus. Front Med 2021;7:610257.
[21] Hannah JR, D'Cruz DP. Pulmonary complications of systemic lupus erythematosus. Semin Respir Crit Care Med 2019;40:227–34.
[22] Vivero M, Padera RF. Histopathology of lung disease in the connective tissue diseases. Rheum Dis Clin N Am 2015;41:197–211.
[23] Fanouriakis A, Kostopoulou M, Alunno A, Aringer M, Bajema I, Boletis JN, et al. Update of the EULAR recommendations for the management of systemic lupus erythematosus. Ann Rheum Dis 2019;78:736–45.
[24] Cassone G, Sebastiani M, Vacchi C, Erre GL, Salvarani C, Manfredi A. Efficacy and safety of mycophenolate mofetil in the treatment of rheumatic disease-related interstitial lung disease: a narrative review. Drugs Context 2021;10. 2020-2028-8.
[25] Reynolds JA, Toescu V, Yee CS, Prabu A, Situnayake D, Gordon C. Effects of rituximab on resistant SLE disease including lung involvement. Lupus 2009;18:67–73.
[26] Lim SW, Gillis D, Smith W, Hissaria P, Greville H, Peh CA. Rituxumab use in systemic lupus erythematosus pneumonitis and a review of current reports. Intern Med J 2006;36:260–2.
[27] Vacchi C, Manfredi A, Cassone G, Erre GL, Salvarani C, Sebastiani M. Efficacy and safety of rituximab in the treatment of connective tissue disease-related interstitial lung disease. Drugs Context 2021;10. 2020-2028-7.
[28] Gorthi R, Attoti Y, Atluri R, Mwangi JK. Belimumab in the treatment of interstitial lung disease associated with systemic lupus erythematosus. Am J Respir Crit Care Med 2020;201:A6643.

[29] Muangchan C, van Vollenhoven R, Bernatsky SR, Douglas Smith C, Hudson M, Inanç M, et al. Treatment algorithms in systemic lupus erythematosus. Arthritis Care Res 2015;67:1237–45.

[30] Distler O, Highland KB, Gahlemann M, Azuma A, Fischer A, Mayes MD, et al. Nintedanib for systemic sclerosis-associated interstitial lung disease. N Engl J Med 2019;380:2518–28.

[31] Flaherty KR, WellS AU, Cottin V, Devaraj A, Walsh SLF, Inoue Y, et al. Nintedanib in progressive fibrosing interstitial lung diseases. N Engl J Med 2019;381:1718–27.

[32] K Brown K, Martinez FJ, Walsh SL, Thannickal VJ, Prasse A, Schlenker-Herceg R, et al. The natural history of progressive fibrosing interstitial lung diseases. Eur Respir J 2020;55:2000085.

[33] Beher J, Prasse A, Kreuter M, Johow J, Rabe KF, Bonella F, et al. Pirfenidone in patients with progressive fibrotic interstitial lung diseases other than idiopathic pulmonary fibrosis (RELIEF): a double-blind, randomised, placebo-controlled, phase 2b trial. Lancet Resp Med 2021;9:476–86.

[34] Arnaud L, Agard C, Haroche J, Cacoub P, Piette JC, Amoura Z. Pulmonary arterial hypertension in systemic lupus erythematosus. Rev Med Interne 2011;32:689–97.

[35] Chen HA, Hsu TC, Yang SC, Weng CT, Wu CH, Sun CY, Lin CY. Incidence and survival impact of pulmonary arterial hypertension among patients with systemic lupus erythematosus: a nationwide cohort study. Arthritis Res Ther 2019;21:82.

[36] Qian J, Wang Y, Huang C, Yang X, Zhao J, Wang Q, Tian Z, Li M, Zeng X. Survival and prognostic factors of systemic lupus erythematosus-associated pulmonary arterial hypertension: a PRISMA-compliant systematic review and meta-analysis. Autoimmun Rev 2016;15:250–7.

[37] Bhushan A, Choi D, Maresh G, Deodhar A. Risk factors and outcomes of immune and nonimmune causes of diffuse alveolar hemorrhage: a tertiary-care academic single-center experience. Rheumatol Int 2021. https://doi.org/10.1007/s00296-021-04842-2.

[38] Park MS. Diffuse alveolar hemorrhage. Tuberc Respir Dis 2013;74:151–62.

[39] Casian A, Jayne D. Current modalities in the diagnosis of pulmonary vasculitis. Expert Opin Med Diagn 2012;6:499–516.

[40] Wan SA, Teh CL, Jobli AT. Lupus pneumonitis as the initial presentation of systemic lupus erythematosus: case series from a single institution. Lupus 2018;25:1485–90.

[41] Tselios K, UrowitZ MB. Cardiovascular and pulmonary manifestations of systemic lupus erythematosus. Curr Rheumatol Rev 2017;13:206–18.

[42] Mira-Avendano IC, Abril A. Pulmonary manifestations of Sjögren syndrome, systemic lupus erythematosus, and mixed connective tissue disease. Rheum Dis Clin N Am 2015;41:263–77.

[43] Alamoudi OSB, Attar SM. Pulmonary manifestations in systemic lupus erythematosus: association with disease activity. Respirology 2015;20:474–80.

[44] Aguilera-Pickens G, Abud-Mendoza C. Pulmonary manifestations in systemic lupus erythematosus: pleural involvement, acute pneumonitis, chronic interstitial lung disease and diffuse alveolar hemorrhage. Reumatol Clínica 2018;14:294–300.

[45] Gordon C, Amissah-Arthur MB, Gayed M, Brown S, Bruce IN, D'Cruz D, et al. The British Society for Rheumatology guideline for the management of systemic lupus erythematosus in adults. Rheumatology 2018;57:e1–45.

[46] Martinez T, García-Robledo J, Plata I, Urbano MJ, Posso-Osorio I, Rios-Serna LJ, et al. Mechanisms of action and historical facts on the use of intravenous immunoglobulins in systemic lupus erythematosus. Autoimmun Rev 2019;18:279–86.

[47] Kronbichler A, Brezina B, Quintana LF, Jayne DR. Efficacy of plasma exchange and immunoadsorption in systemic lupus erythematosus and antiphospholipid syndrome: a systematic review. Autoimmun Rev 2016;15:38–49.

[48] Cobo-Ibáñez T, Loza-Santamaria E, Pego-Reigosa JM, Olive Marques A, Rúa-Figueroa I, Fernández-Nebro A, et al. Efficacy and safety of rituximab in the treatment of non-renal systemic lupus erythematosus: a systematic review. Semin Arthritis Rheum 2014;44:175–85.

[49] Robles-Perez A, Dorca J, Castellví I, Nolla JM, Molina-Molina M, Narváez J. Rituximab effect in severe progressive connective tissue disease-related lung disease: preliminary data. Rheumatol Int 2020;40:719–26.

[50] Hoffbrand BI, Beck ER. "Unexplained" dyspnoea and shrinking lungs in systemic lupus erythematosus. Br Med J 1965;1:1273–7.

[51] Duron L, Cohen-Aubart F, Diot E, Borié R, Abad S, Richez C, et al. Shrinking lung syndrome associated with systemic lupus erythematosus: a multicenter collaborative study of 15 new cases and a review of the 155 cases in the literature focusing on treatment response and long-term outcomes. Autoimmun Rev 2016;15:994–1000.

[52] Henderson LA, Loring SH, Gill RR, Liao KP, Ishizawar R, Kim S, et al. Shrinking lung syndrome as a manifestation of pleuritis: a new model based on pulmonary physiological studies. J Rheumatol 2013;40:273–81.

[53] Nemec M, Pradella M, Jahn K, Tamm M, Walker UA. Magnetic resonance imaging-confirmed pleuritis in systemic lupus erythematosus-associated shrinking lung syndrome. Arthritis Rheum 2015;67:1880.

[54] Goswami RP, Mondal S, Lahiri D, Basu K, Das S S, Ghosh P, et al. Shrinking lung syndrome in systemic lupus erythematosus successfully treated with rituximab. QJM 2016;109:617–8.

[55] Reyes F, Lazaro D. Systemic lupus erythematosus complicated by shrinking lung syndrome treated with belimumab: a case report. Chest 2016;150:300A.

[56] Smyth H, Flood R, Kane D, Donnelly S, Mullan RH. Shrinking lung syndrome and systemic lupus erythematosus: a case series and literature review. QJM 2018;111:839–43.

Chapter 4

Sjogren's syndrome and lung involvement

Ilektra Voulgareli,[1,#] Vasiliki Koulouri,[2,#] Alexandra Chroneou[1] and Clio P. Mavragani[2,*]
[1]*Department of Pulmonary Medicine, Sotiria Hospital, Athens, Greece;* [2]*Department of Physiology, School of Medicine, National and Kapodistrian University of Athens, Athens, Greece*
[*]*Corresponding author at: kmauragan@med.uoa.gr.*

Introduction

Sjogren's syndrome (SS) is a systemic autoimmune rheumatic disease (SARD) primarily affecting lachrymal and salivary glands, leading to dry eyes and dry mouth, respectively. It is one of the most common SARDs, with a predilection for the female sex, and is designated as primary SS (pSS) when no other concomitant autoimmune disease is present. Apart from exocrine gland involvement, systemic manifestations in the setting of pSS often occur [1]. For instance, pulmonary involvement in pSS can be both the result of exocrine and extraglandular dysfunction manifested as airway, parenchymal, pleural, and vascular disease and/or combination of the above; among them, airway and interstitial lung disease (ILD) are the most commonly observed [2]. Lung disease can be a serious complication as these patients present with higher mortality rates and lower quality of life. Prevalence rates of pulmonary insult in SS patients display a wide range from 9% to 79%, depending on the definitions and methods employed for the description of lung involvement, though most studies report a prevalence rate of 9%–20% [3–13]. Imaging abnormalities are also detected in up to 65% of asymptomatic SS patients [12], highlighting the importance of careful evaluation, monitoring, and potential treatment of pulmonary involvement in SS patients.

In this chapter, we will discuss the major different types of respiratory involvement in pSS, as depicted in Fig. 4.1.

[#] Equally contributed.

The Lung in Autoimmune Diseases. https://doi.org/10.1016/B978-0-323-91083-5.00008-6

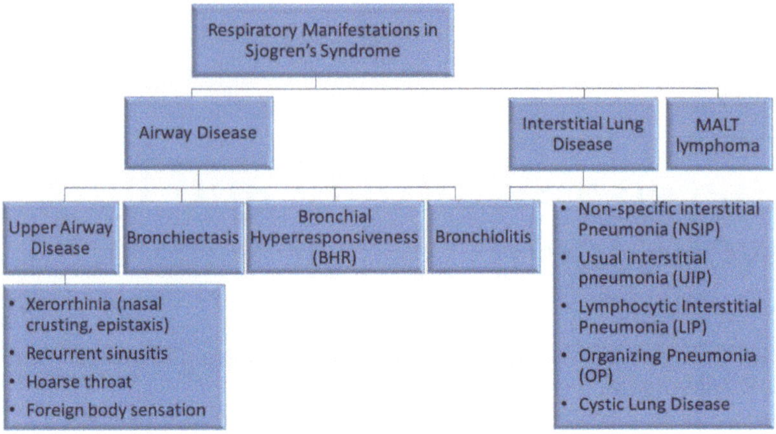

FIGURE 4.1 Major types of respiratory involvement in Sjogren's syndrome.

Airway disease

Overview

As an autoimmune exocrinopathy, pSS is characterized by glandular lymphocytic infiltration and impaired function which can also affect airway epithelial lining [14]. Upper airway involvement, resulting from reduced mucus secretion, commonly presents as persistent nasal crusting and irritation, epistaxis, recurrent sinusitis, throat hoarseness, and foreign body sensation [15,16]. Dry cough is a very common symptom among pSS patients and can be attributed to both upper airway and tracheobronchial desiccation (xerotrachea/xerobronchitis), ineffective mucous clearance, airway inflammation, and hyperresponsiveness [17,18]. Since dry cough can be the primary and/or initial manifestation, as seen in up to 50% of pSS patients, a misdiagnosis of asthma or bronchitis is frequently made [15]. Lower airway pathology includes bronchiectasis, bronchiolitis, and bronchial hyperresponsiveness (BHR) and is mainly manifested as chronic cough, shortness of breath, recurrent lower respiratory infections, and rarely hemoptysis (associated with bronchiectasis) [19]. Small airway disease is the most common pulmonary SS complication among symptomatic patients [20], typically affecting peripheral bronchioles with $\leq$2 mm internal diameter. Interestingly, chronic obstructive pulmonary disease is also frequently seen in pSS patients [21], even in nonsmokers [22,23].

Histology and imaging studies

Epithelial cell tissue infiltration by lymphocytes is the primary histopathologic finding in SS. The composition of the monocytic infiltrate appears to differ depending on lesion severity [1], with T lymphocytes characterizing mild lesions

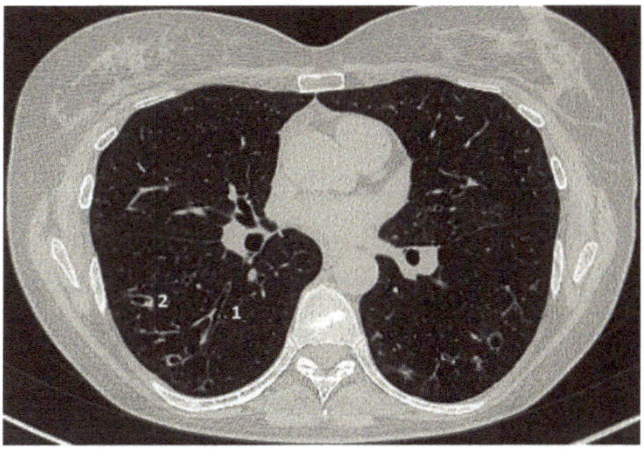

FIGURE 4.2 Bronchiectasis in a pSS patient presented with hemoptysis. See the tram track sign (number 1, cylindrical bronchiectasis) as well as the signet sign (number 2, dilated bronchus compared to the adjacent artery).

and B cells predominating in severe disease. In the setting of SS-related airway disease, several histopathologic patterns have been described such as peribronchial lymphoid infiltrates, mainly consisting of CD4+ T cells that can lead to small-airway obstruction [24,25], and bronchiolitis, either constrictive or follicular. Constrictive bronchiolitis is a result of submucosal fibrous tissue deposition, while follicular bronchiolitis is characterized by B cell hyperplasia of lymphoid follicles along with reactive germinal centers [26]. Pathology consistent with bronchiolitis is frequently seen in small airway disease [26].

Chest radiography is not very helpful in the detection of airway disease in SS patients, thus, upon clinical suspicion, high-resolution computed tomography (HRCT) should be obtained [12]. While reticular or reticulonodular abnormalities in chest X-rays generally indicate the presence of interstitial disease, Papiris et al. demonstrated that in the setting of SS, these abnormalities could suggest thickened bronchioles, as a result of bronchial inflammation [25]. Airway disease in HRCTs can be depicted as bronchial wall thickening (8%–68%), bronchiectasis (5%–54%), mosaic attenuation (22%), as well as centrilobular nodules and nodular opacities (6%–29%) [4,6,11,27–29]. Radiologically, bronchiectasis is an irreversible abnormal bronchial dilation, wider than the bronchial artery or visible within 1 cm of the pleural surface (Fig. 4.2), while mosaic attenuation is a term implemented to describe pulmonary regions of diverge attenuation [30]. Air cysts and interstitial thickening are often seen in follicular bronchiolitis, a finding that further confirms the close relationship of this entity with lymphocytic interstitial pneumonia (LIP) [31], a disease primarily of the interstitium. Hence, bronchiolitis is often described in both airway and interstitial disease (Fig. 4.1).

Pulmonary function tests in airway disease

Pulmonary function tests (PFTs) in airway disease may reveal an obstructive pattern of ventilation with reduced forced expiratory volume in one second

(FEV1) to forced vital capacity (FVC) ratio and increased total lung capacity (TLC) [32]. Typically, most SS patients display a pattern of small airway involvement characterized by reduced maximal mid-expiratory flows [15,33]. In general, clinically significant distal airway disease as evaluated by PFTs is seen in 22%–46% of SS patients [4,15,25,34,35].

BHR, mainly expressed as episodic dry cough/dyspnea following exposure to certain irritants, is quite common in SS, reported in about 42%–60% of patients [18,36,37], and especially among those with small airway disease [18]. Patients with BHR are particularly sensitive to the methacholine challenge but do not respond as well to inhaled glucocorticoids or sodium cromoglycate, compared to those with asthma, with eosinophilia being uncommon in SS-BHR [18,38]. In about a third of SS patients with BHR, a significant reduction in PFTs at eight-year follow-up was observed [39].

Treatment

Treatment of SS-related airway disease is rather empirical, mostly based on therapeutic regimens implemented in other airway disorders. In 2020, a consensus expert panel of rheumatologists and pulmonologists developed guidelines for the evaluation and management of lung disease in SS patients [12]. In the presence of persistent dry cough due to xerotrachea, humidification, secretagogues, and guaifenesin are suggested. Moreover, short course steroids and macrolides are recommended for the management of previously untreated small airway disease, as are inhaled bronchodilators/corticosteroids. Management of bronchiectasis includes any of the treatments used in primary or secondary bronchiectasis, such as mucolytic agents, nebulized or hypertonic saline, postural drainages, positive expiratory pressure, mechanical high frequency chest wall oscillation, and macrolides on a chronic basis (having excluded active or latent mycobacterium tuberculosis infection) [12].

Interstitial lung disease

Overview

ILD is rather common type of pulmonary involvement in pSS, ranging between 6% and 70% in several studies [40]. Although LIP portrays a classic association with pSS [41], it does not appear to be the most frequent pathological subtype. Nonspecific interstitial pneumonia (NSIP) is recognized as the most typical pSS-ILD disorder [9,32] followed by organizing pneumonia (OP), usual interstitial pneumonia (UIP), and pleuroparenchymal fibroelastosis [42–44]. Other pulmonary abnormalities in pSS patients that manifest as cystic lesions of the lung include amyloidosis [41], lymphoma [27], and LIP [45].

Most pSS-ILD patients exhibit pulmonary symptoms such as dyspnea, cough, expectoration, or chest pain [9]. The severity of the symptoms varies.

Some patients are asymptomatic whereas others appear with minimal to severe dyspnea on exertion. Time of ILD onset appears to increase over time, with a reported prevalence of 10% within the primary year of diagnosis and 20% after five years [10]. Physical examination may reveal fine bibasilar, end-inspiratory, "velcro-like" crackles at auscultation or may even more commonly be unremarkable.

Acute exacerbation of ILD is often reported in patients with CTD-ILD, including pSS [46,47]. The definition of acute exacerbation is that of an acute, clinically significant respiratory deterioration characterized by evidence of widespread alveolar abnormalities [48]. Histologically, the predominant pattern is diffuse alveolar damage superimposed on a chronic ILD. Some studies compared the prevalence of acute exacerbation across the spectrum of CTD-ILD [49] showing that a UIP pattern seems to be a greater risk for this complication, regardless of the underlying disease [50]. The incidence and therefore the clinical characteristics of acute exacerbation in CTD-ILD appear to be almost like those of idiopathic pulmonary fibrosis (IPF) patients, with a high fatality rate (about 80%) [47,49]. Ito et al. [27] reported that mortality is related to decreased baseline PaO_2 and presence of microscopic honeycombing. An outsized retrospective cohort from Taiwan [51] of 4954 SS patients reported that this group displayed increased incidence of respiratory failure compared to non-SS patients, irrespective of sex, age, and comorbidities. Respiratory failure in pSS was most typically attributed to ILD (25%), followed by small airway disease (22%), desiccation of upper tract (17%), and airway obstruction (8%).

Histology and imaging studies

pSS-ILD appears to be complex, and areas of patterns of interstitial pneumonia or airway abnormalities often coexist. Among SS patients with ILD, specific subtypes that are reported include: NSIP (45%), respiratory bronchiolitis (i.e., chronic bronchiolitis, obliterative bronchiolitis, and panbronchiolitis, 25%) [52], UIP (16%), LIP (15%), OP (7%), amyloid deposition (6%), and lymphoma (4%) [9]. Fig. 4.3 shows characteristic imaging findings of chest computed tomography (CT) in symptomatic patients with primary Sjögren's syndrome (pSS) [20].

Nonspecific interstitial pneumonia

NSIP is characterized histopathologically by interstitial involvement of varying degrees with chronic inflammation or fibrosis [53,54]. Furthermore, bilateral areas of ground-glass attenuation and reticulation, traction bronchiectasis and loss of volume, with both basal and peribronchovascular predominance are observed at the HRCT scan [53]. Findings in patients with pSS are similar to those with idiopathic NSIP [53].

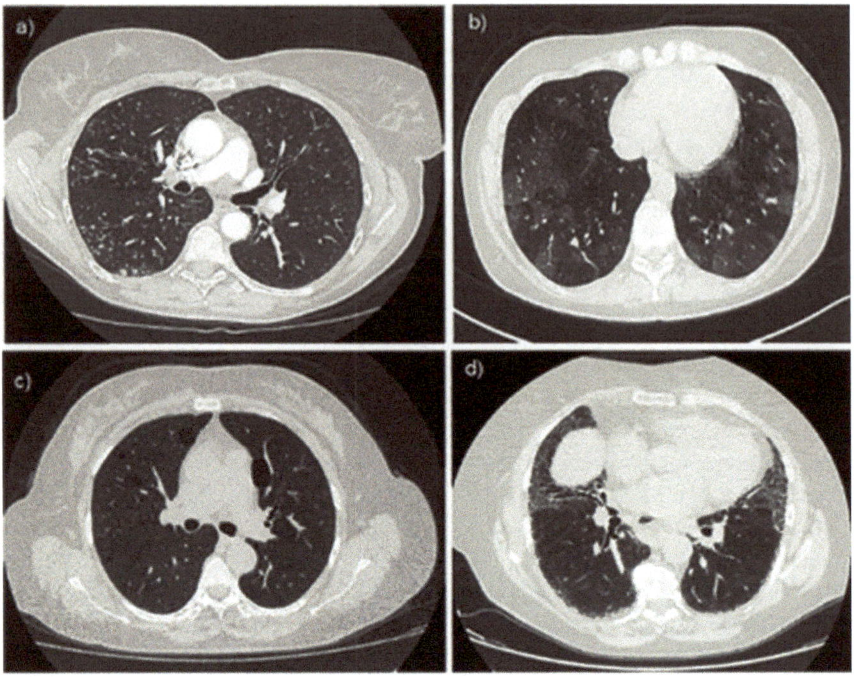

FIGURE 4.3 Chest computed tomography (CT) findings in symptomatic primary SS patients. a) small centrilobular nodules and bronchiectasis, b) expiratory air trapping, c) Multiple lung cysts, d) honeycombing, septal thickening, traction bronchiectases, compatible with interstitial lung disease. *Image from Kampolis CF, et al. Prevalence and spectrum of symptomatic pulmonary involvement in primary Sjögren's syndrome, courtesy of "Clinical and Experimental Rheumatology".*

Usual interstitial pneumonia

UIP is characterized by a variable distribution of patchy interstitial fibrosis, inflammation, honeycombing, and normal lung. Histologically, the diagnosis is established when small aggregates of fibroblasts and myofibroblasts, termed fibroblast foci, are observed [54]. Bilateral areas of intralobular reticular attenuation in the course of traction bronchiectasis and little cystic change, with both basal and peripheral predominance and temporal heterogeneity are seen with HRCT [54]. UIP cases have also been reported in the studies of Deheinzelin and Yamadori by surgical biopsies [55,56].

Organizing pneumonia

OP is a pathological subtype of ILD characterized by intra-alveolar buds of connective tissue. At high-resolution CT, OP is depicted as multiple patchy areas of consolidation with a subpleural and/or peribronchovascular distribution [57,58], as areas of ground-glass attenuation or fine centrilobular nodules. In addition, reversed-halo sign can be seen in patients with pSS [59,60]. While

OP has been described previously within the setting of several autoimmune disorders—mainly rheumatoid arthritis—it occurs quite rarely in pSS [61]. Since the clinical and radiological features of OP are similar to those of community-acquired pneumonia, diagnosis is often delayed, usually after one or more failed courses of antibiotics [62,63].

Lymphocytic interstitial pneumonia

Lymphocytic interstitial pneumonia, which may be considered both a lymphoproliferative disorder and an interstitial pneumonia [54,64] is characterized by a diffuse, polyclonal lymphoid cell infiltrate surrounding airways and expanding into the lung interstitium [41]. LIP usually presents as areas of ground-glass attenuation, air cysts, interlobular septal thickening, thickening of the peribronchovascular interstitium, and poorly defined centrilobular or subpleural nodules [64]. The natural history of LIP is variable, starting from a benign course (stabilization or improvement) to the evolution of lymphoma [65,66].

Cystic lung disease

pSS patients are often diagnosed with parenchymal bullae and cysts. They are presumably associated with a check-valve mechanism because of peribronchiolar mononuclear cell infiltration or amyloid deposition [45,67]. In pSS patients with abnormal CT findings, the presence of bullae or cysts ranged from 20% to 30% [4,29]. In some early reports, lung cysts coexisted with amyloidosis [67,68]. In a recent study, lung cysts were related to anti-SSB/La seropositivity and occurrence of lymphoproliferative disease (LPD) [69]. Lechtman et al. [70] also reported the high frequency of anti-SSB/La antibody in these patients. However, patients with cystic lung disease displayed neither PFT deterioration nor significant radiographic progression after a median follow-up of four years. On the other hand, Martinez-Balzano et al. [71] reported that cystic lung disease was related to older age, a diagnosis of secondary SS, and elevated anti-SSA/Ro antibody.

Pulmonary function tests in interstitial lung disease

PFTs are a significant tool for diagnosing and monitoring pulmonary involvement in pSS patients. Typically, PFTs will detect a restrictive pattern of ventilatory failure, characterized by reduced TLC and FVC, with a normal FEV_1/FVC ratio [2,27] and an often reduced D_{LCO}. If ILDs and airway disease coexist, spirometry can be normal [72], but a disproportionate reduction in D_{LCO} may occur [73]. In some patients the course of the illness may be benign. Furthermore, it has to be noted that early lung involvement can be detected by HRCT and PFTs in asymptomatic patients with pSS, but HRCT abnormalities do not necessarily connote significant functional impairment [4].

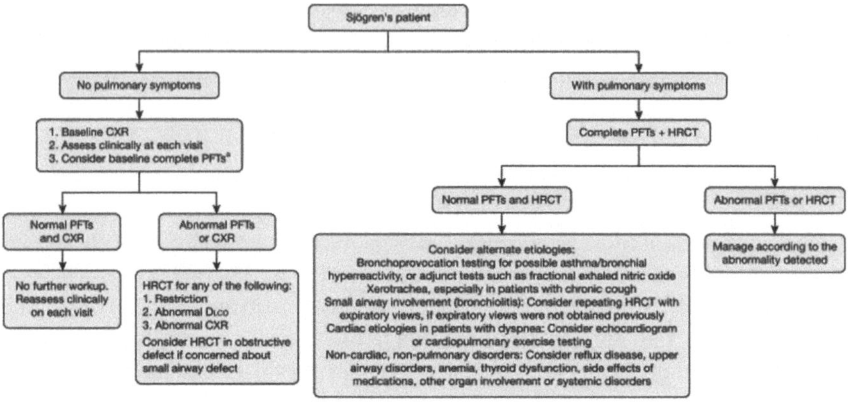

FIGURE 4.4 Complete PFTs include spirometry, DLCO, and lung volumes, ideally measured by body plethysmography. *CXR*, chest radiograph; *DLCO*, diffusing capacity of the lung for carbon monoxide; *HRCT*, high-resolution CT; *PFTs*, pulmonary function tests.

The most accurate tool for evaluating CTD-ILD progression is serial PFT measurements. As FVC is extremely reproducible, with the exception of major extrapulmonary restriction due to pleural disease or muscle weakness, changes in FVC are specific to ILD [74]. Relying on data regarding ILD evaluation in systemic sclerosis, disease progression in pSS patients is also detected by PFT changes that include a decline in FVC of $\geq$10% or a decrease within the DLCO of $\geq$15% over 6–12 months. Several studies have shown that 6-min walk distance (6MWD) and/or decline in 6MWD are strong independent predictors of mortality in patients with IPF [75,76] and CTD-ILD [77]. It is an easy test that could also be applied in pSS-ILD patient evaluation.

Clinical practice guidelines for pulmonary manifestations of SS were developed by the SS Foundation in October of 2020 [12]. Fig. 4.4 shows respiratory evaluation for both symptomatic and asymptomatic SS patients (Image taken from "Consensus Guidelines for Evaluation and Management of Pulmonary Disease in Sjögren's" by AS Lee et al., courtesy of Elsevier Publisher).

Bronchoalveolar lavage

Bronchoalveolar lavage (BAL) cell count patterns in SS are nonspecific, thus the main role of BAL in a patient who is suspected of SS-ILD is to exclude other causes of diffuse parenchymal lung disease, such as eosinophilic pneumonia, infection, lymphangitic tumor, and hemorrhage. Therefore, BAL is sometimes performed in patients with SS-ILD when respiratory symptoms have an acute onset or display fever, hemoptysis, or peripheral eosinophilia. Increased numbers of BAL lymphocytes or neutrophils are common among pSS patients [55,78]. However, data are conflicting about whether the degree of lymphocytosis or neutrophilia predicts the presence or severity of ILD. In a study of 23 patients with pSS, patients with over 15% BAL lymphocytosis were more likely to present with pulmonary symptoms (cough and dyspnea), radiographic evidence of ILD, and decreased pulmonary function than those with less than 15% lymphocytes [78]. BAL cell counts do not appear to have prognostic value in SS-ILD and it is unknown whether patients with subclinical disease supported by the BAL results will develop symptomatic pulmonary disease.

Lung biopsy

Lung biopsy is deemed unnecessary when evaluating patients with SS and radiographic and/or physiologic evidence of ILD. The standard indications for lung biopsy are suspicion of malignancy, atypical HRCT pattern, and worsening clinical and radiographic abnormalities. Circumscribed or nodular areas of consolidation that are persistent and not because of infection generally require histopathologic evaluation. Based on the location of the abnormality and local expertise, transbronchial or cryobiopsy, video-assisted thoracoscopic, or surgical lung biopsy is also performed. Transbronchial lung biopsy is useful in the diagnosis of sarcoidosis or lymphangitic carcinomatosis, whereas a larger biopsy obtained via video-assisted thoracoscopic or even open thoracotomy is required to differentiate the subtypes of ILD [58].

Treatment

Many of the pharmacological interventions are guided by the severity of the ILD. EULAR SS Disease Activity Index, which uses symptoms defined by the New York Heart Association (NYHA) Functional Classification, imaging, and PFT results, stages the disease as either low, moderate, or severe/high. Low is used to describe the presence of persistent cough with no radiographic abnormalities and normal lung function test, moderate disease includes shortness of breath on exercise (NYHA II) or PFTs with FVC between 60% and 80% predicted or DLCO between 40% and 70% predicted, and finally severe disease is manifested as shortness of breath at rest (NYHA III, IV) or PFTs with FVC <60% predicted or DLCO <40% predicted [9].

As previously stated, the severity of symptoms and lung function capacity determine the treatment of pSS-ILD. For patients with asymptomatic mild or nonprogressive ILD without significant abnormalities on PFTs, a "see and wait" approach may be acceptable, while in patients with progressive or severe disease, first-line therapy typically consists of glucocorticoids, at the initial dose of 0.5−1 mg/kg of prednisone daily [79,80] alone or together with immunosuppressive drugs like cyclophosphamide (CYC), mycophenolate mofetil (MMF), or azathioprine (AZA), in order to reduce the cumulative dose of steroids and improve the effectiveness of the treatment [46]. The dose and duration of corticosteroids in SS-ILD is not standardized. The panel of the SS Foundation proposes a dose that does not exceed 60 mg of daily prednisone with a slow taper over weeks or months. In rapidly progressive ILD, or acute respiratory failure, pulse dose IV corticosteroids or high-dose oral corticosteroids up to 60 mg daily of prednisone should be considered [12].

Saraux et al. [81] reported that AZA in some case series improved FVC values after a six-month follow-up in seven out of 11 pSS-ILD patients while FVC values remained unchanged in three patients and worsened in one. Roca et al. [79] reported an improvement of pulmonary disease in three out of four patients treated with AZA with steroid-refractory ILD and also reported an improvement of pulmonary status in one patient treated with CYC (0.7 g/m^2 every four weeks for six cycles). Shi et al. [58] found that there was improvement or stability during the follow-up period (median 38 months) in 14 patients with pSS and biopsy-proven pulmonary involvement treated with prednisone and CYC. Treatment with MMF has still not been related to either stable or improved pulmonary findings in pSS patients.

Regarding rituximab (RTX), data are limited. However, a registry-based study from France showed improvement in lung function in six out of eight patients with pSS-ILD treated with RTX, already evident after the primary cycle of the therapy [82].

Nintedanib, an antifibrotic agent, was recently approved for "progressive" fibrotic ILD phenotypes, which can also include those related to SS and other CTDs [12]. The efficacy and safety of nintedanib in subjects with ILD in the context of systemic sclerosis (SSc-ILD) was explored in the SENSCIS trial, where the rate of FVC decline was reduced in patients treated with nintedanib compared to patients enrolled in the placebo group. The effect of nintedanib was lower in patients with SSc-ILD than in patients with IPF (INPULSIS trials), but the relative reduction in the rate of FVC decline observed with nintedanib versus placebo was similar (44% and 49%, respectively) [83]. The other antifibrotic drug, pirfenidone, was tested in the open-label LOTUSS study where pirfenidone related to MMF also had an appropriate safety and tolerability profile in subjects with SSc-ILD. There was not a comparator group, however, so it needs to be further investigated in clinical trials [84]. The SS Foundation in October of 2020 proposes an evaluation and management of patients with SS who exhibit symptoms and/or physical examination signs of ILD as shown in Fig. 4.5 [12] .

Finally, data regarding survival after lung transplantation in CTD and specifically in patients with pSS are poor and conflicting. However, recent studies seem to suggest that post-transplant outcomes in patients with CTD-ILD, including pSS, do not differ significantly from those in patients with non-CTD-ILD [85].

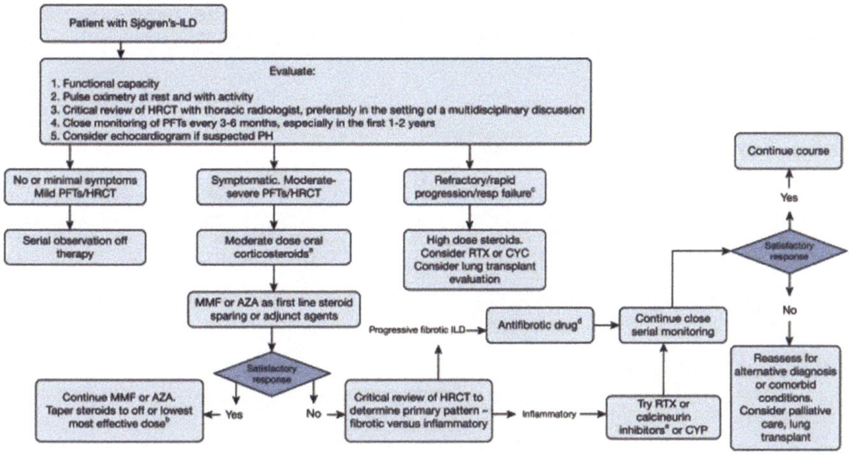

FIGURE 4.5 Consensus guidelines for evaluation and management of ILD in the setting of Sjögren's Syndrome. *AZA*, azathioprine; *CYP*, cyclophosphamide; *HRCT*, high-resolution CT; *ILD*, interstitial lung disease; *MMF*, mycophenolate mofetil; *PFTs*, pulmonary function tests; *PH*, pulmonary hypertension; *RTX*, rituximab. *Image taken from Lee AS, et al. Consensus guidelines for evaluation and management of pulmonary disease in Sjögren's, courtesy of Elsevier Publisher.*

Other pulmonary manifestations

Lymphoma

LPD is a well-known complication of pSS, reported in approximately 5%–10% of pSS patients. Non-Hodgkin's lymphoma is the most common LPD in pSS, with diffuse large B cell lymphoma and mucosa-associated lymphoid tissue (MALT) being the most frequent subtypes [86]. MALT that affects the bronchial lymphoid tissue is commonly referred to as BALT. As previously mentioned, LIP may progress to pulmonary lymphoma [65,66]. Imaging CT findings consistent with MALT lymphoma include solitary or multiple nodules, masses, with areas of airspace consolidation or ground-glass attenuation [87–89]. Typically, MALT lymphomas are found along a bronchovascular bundle accompanied with traction bronchiectasis and interlobular septal thickening [90]. It is also important to emphasize that multiple nodules and cystic lesions or septal thickening with small randomly distributed nodules, which can calcify can be due to amyloidosis related to pSS [91].

Pleural disease

Pleural disease is relatively uncommon in pSS and only a few cases of isolated pleural effusions have been described [92–94]. Therefore, pleural disease in SS should lead to a careful evaluation for the presence of a probable underlying concomitant autoimmune disease, such as rheumatoid arthritis and systemic lupus erythematosus. In pSS, pleural effusion is most commonly exudative in nature, with lymphocytosis and normal lactate dehydrogenase and glucose levels [93,94].

Pulmonary arterial hypertension

Pulmonary arterial hypertension (PAH), i.e., grade I pulmonary hypertension, is a rare complication of pSS, with few cases described worldwide. PAH in pSS has been associated with the presence of Raynaud's phenomenon and cutaneous vasculitis indicating underlying substantial vasculopathy [95].

Pulmonary amyloidosis

Amyloid deposition in the lungs of pSS patients is a histopathologic diagnosis and thus a rather rarely recognized entity, affecting almost entirely women. Of the few described cases, radiological manifestations mainly included diffuse nodules and/or cysts, while definitive therapeutic approaches are not yet available [96].

References

[1] Mavragani CP, Moutsopoulos HM. Sjogren's syndrome. Annu Rev Pathol 2014;9:273–85.

[2] Flament T, Bigot A, Chaigne B, Henique H, Diot E, Marchand-Adam S. Pulmonary manifestations of Sjogren's syndrome. Eur Respir Rev 2016;25(140):110–23.

[3] Garcia-Carrasco M, Ramos-Casals M, Rosas J, Pallares L, Calvo-Alen J, Cervera R, et al. Primary Sjogren syndrome: clinical and immunologic disease patterns in a cohort of 400 patients. Medicine 2002;81(4):270–80.

[4] Uffmann M, Kiener HP, Bankier AA, Baldt MM, Zontsich T, Herold CJ. Lung manifestation in asymptomatic patients with primary Sjogren syndrome: assessment with high resolution CT and pulmonary function tests. J Thorac Imag 2001;16(4):282–9.

[5] Ramos-Casals M, Solans R, Rosas J, Camps MT, Gil A, Del Pino-Montes J, et al. Primary Sjogren syndrome in Spain: clinical and immunologic expression in 1010 patients. Medicine 2008;87(4):210–9.

[6] Palm O, Garen T, Berge Enger T, Jensen JL, Lund MB, Aalokken TM, et al. Clinical pulmonary involvement in primary Sjogren's syndrome: prevalence, quality of life and mortality–a retrospective study based on registry data. Rheumatology 2013;52(1):173–9.

[7] Fauchais AL, Martel C, Gondran G, Lambert M, Launay D, Jauberteau MO, et al. Immunological profile in primary Sjogren syndrome: clinical significance, prognosis and long-term evolution to other auto-immune disease. Autoimmun Rev 2010;9(9):595–9.

[8] Flores-Chavez A, Kostov B, Solans R, Fraile G, Maure B, Feijoo-Masso C, et al. Severe, life-threatening phenotype of primary Sjogren's syndrome: clinical characterisation and outcomes in 1580 patients (GEAS-SS Registry). Clin Exp Rheumatol 2018;36(Suppl. 112(3)):121–9.

[9] Ramos-Casals M, Brito-Zeron P, Seror R, Bootsma H, Bowman SJ, Dorner T, et al. Characterization of systemic disease in primary Sjogren's syndrome: EULAR-SS Task Force recommendations for articular, cutaneous, pulmonary and renal involvements. Rheumatology 2015;54(12):2230–8.

[10] Nannini C, Jebakumar AJ, Crowson CS, Ryu JH, Matteson EL. Primary Sjogren's syndrome 1976–2005 and associated interstitial lung disease: a population-based study of incidence and mortality. BMJ Open 2013;3(11):e003569.
[11] Lohrmann C, Uhl M, Warnatz K, Ghanem N, Kotter E, Schaefer O, et al. High-resolution CT imaging of the lung for patients with primary Sjogren's syndrome. Eur J Radiol 2004;52(2):137–43.
[12] Lee AS, Scofield RH, Hammitt KM, Gupta N, Thomas DE, Moua T, et al. Consensus guidelines for evaluation and management of pulmonary disease in Sjogren's. Chest 2021;159(2):683–98.
[13] Manfredi A, Sebastiani M, Cerri S, Cassone G, Bellini P, Casa GD, et al. Prevalence and characterization of non-sicca onset primary Sjogren syndrome with interstitial lung involvement. Clin Rheumatol 2017;36(6):1261–8.
[14] Moutsopoulos HM. Sjogren's syndrome: autoimmune epithelitis. Clin Immunol Immunopathol 1994;72(2):162–5.
[15] Constantopoulos SH, Papadimitriou CS, Moutsopoulos HM. Respiratory manifestations in primary Sjogren's syndrome. A clinical, functional, and histologic study. Chest 1985;88(2):226–9.
[16] Bloch KJ, Buchanan WW, Wohl MJ, Bunim JJ. Sjoegren's syndrome. A clinical, pathological, and serological study of sixty-two cases. Medicine 1965;44:187–231.
[17] Mathieu A, Cauli A, Pala R, Satta L, Nurchis P, Loi GL, et al. Tracheo-bronchial mucociliary clearance in patients with primary and secondary Sjogren's syndrome. Scand J Rheumatol 1995;24(5):300–4.
[18] Gudbjornsson B, Hedenstrom H, Stalenheim G, Hallgren R. Bronchial hyperresponsiveness to methacholine in patients with primary Sjogren's syndrome. Ann Rheum Dis 1991;50(1):36–40.
[19] Gupta S, Ferrada MA, Hasni SA. Pulmonary manifestations of primary Sjogren's syndrome: underlying immunological mechanisms, clinical presentation, and management. Front Immunol 2019;10:1327.
[20] Kampolis CF, Fragkioudaki S, Mavragani CP, Zormpala A, Samakovli A, Moutsopoulos HM. Prevalence and spectrum of symptomatic pulmonary involvement in primary Sjogren's syndrome. Clin Exp Rheumatol 2018;36(Suppl. 112(3)):94–101.
[21] Mandl T, Diaz S, Ekberg O, Hesselstrand R, Piitulainen E, Wollmer P, et al. Frequent development of chronic obstructive pulmonary disease in primary SS–results of a longitudinal follow-up. Rheumatology 2012;51(5):941–6.
[22] Linstow M, Kriegbaum NJ, Backer V, Ulrik C, Oxholm P. A follow-up study of pulmonary function in patients with primary Sjogren's syndrome. Rheumatol Int 1990;10(2):47–9.
[23] Nilsson AM, Diaz S, Theander E, Hesselstrand R, Piitulainen E, Ekberg O, et al. Chronic obstructive pulmonary disease is common in never-smoking patients with primary Sjogren syndrome. J Rheumatol 2015;42(3):464–71.
[24] Papiris SA, Saetta M, Turato G, La Corte R, Trevisani L, Mapp CE, et al. CD4-positive T-lymphocytes infiltrate the bronchial mucosa of patients with Sjogren's syndrome. Am J Respir Crit Care Med 1997;156(2 Pt 1):637–41.
[25] Papiris SA, Maniati M, Constantopoulos SH, Roussos C, Moutsopoulos HM, Skopouli FN. Lung involvement in primary Sjogren's syndrome is mainly related to the small airway disease. Ann Rheum Dis 1999;58(1):61–4.

[26] Nakanishi M, Fukuoka J, Tanaka T, Demura Y, Umeda Y, Ameshima S, et al. Small airway disease associated with Sjogren's syndrome: clinico-pathological correlations. Respir Med 2011;105(12):1931–8.

[27] Ito I, Nagai S, Kitaichi M, Nicholson AG, Johkoh T, Noma S, et al. Pulmonary manifestations of primary Sjogren's syndrome: a clinical, radiologic, and pathologic study. Am J Respir Crit Care Med 2005;171(6):632–8.

[28] Franquet T, Gimenez A, Monill JM, Diaz C, Geli C. Primary Sjogren's syndrome and associated lung disease: CT findings in 50 patients. Am J Roentgenol 1997;169(3):655–8.

[29] Koyama M, Johkoh T, Honda O, Mihara N, Kozuka T, Tomiyama N, et al. Pulmonary involvement in primary Sjogren's syndrome: spectrum of pulmonary abnormalities and computed tomography findings in 60 patients. J Thorac Imag 2001;16(4):290–6.

[30] Hansell DM, Bankier AA, MacMahon H, McLoud TC, Muller NL, Remy J. Fleischner Society: glossary of terms for thoracic imaging. Radiology 2008;246(3):697–722.

[31] Howling SJ, Hansell DM, Wells AU, Nicholson AG, Flint JD, Muller NL. Follicular bronchiolitis: thin-section CT and histologic findings. Radiology 1999;212(3):637–42.

[32] Luppi F, Sebastiani M, Sverzellati N, Cavazza A, Salvarani C, Manfredi A. Lung complications of Sjogren syndrome. Eur Respir Rev 2020;29(157).

[33] Vitali C, Tavoni A, Viegi G, Begliomini E, Agnesi A, Bombardieri S. Lung involvement in Sjogren's syndrome: a comparison between patients with primary and with secondary syndrome. Ann Rheum Dis 1985;44(7):455–61.

[34] Gardiner P, Ward C, Allison A, Ashcroft T, Simpson W, Walters H, et al. Pleuropulmonary abnormalities in primary Sjogren's syndrome. J Rheumatol 1993;20(5):831–7.

[35] Segal I, Fink G, Machtey I, Gura V, Spitzer SA. Pulmonary function abnormalities in Sjogren's syndrome and the sicca complex. Thorax 1981;36(4):286–9.

[36] La Corte R, Potena A, Bajocchi G, Fabbri L, Trotta F. Increased bronchial responsiveness in primary Sjogren's syndrome. A sign of tracheobronchial involvement. Clin Exp Rheumatol 1991;9(2):125–30.

[37] Potena A, La Corte R, Fabbri LM, Papi A, Trotta F, Ciaccia A. Increased bronchial responsiveness in primary and secondary Sjogren's syndrome. Eur Respir J 1990;3(5):548–53.

[38] Stalenheim G, Gudbjornsson B. Anti-inflammatory drugs do not alleviate bronchial hyperreactivity in Sjogren's syndrome. Allergy 1997;52(4):423–7.

[39] Ludviksdottir D, Valtysdottir ST, Hedenstrom H, Hallgren R, Gudbjornsson B. Eight-year follow-up of airway hyperresponsiveness in patients with primary Sjogren's syndrome. Ups J Med Sci 2017;122(1):51–5.

[40] Kreider M, Highland K. Pulmonary involvement in Sjogren syndrome. Semin Respir Crit Care Med 2014;35(2):255–64.

[41] Liebow AA, Carrington CB. Diffuse pulmonary lymphoreticular infiltrations associated with dysproteinemia. Med Clin N Am 1973;57(3):809–43.

[42] Enomoto Y, Nakamura Y, Colby TV, Johkoh T, Sumikawa H, Nishimoto K, et al. Radiologic pleuroparenchymal fibroelastosis-like lesion in connective tissue disease-related interstitial lung disease. PLoS One 2017;12(6):e0180283.

[43] Wang Y, Zhao S, Du G, Ma S, Lin Q, Lin J, et al. Acute fibrinous and organizing pneumonia as initial presentation of primary Sjogren's syndrome: a case report and literature review. Clin Rheumatol 2018;37(7):2001–5.

[44] Ryerson CJ, Collard HR. Update on the diagnosis and classification of ILD. Curr Opin Pulm Med 2013;19(5):453–9.

[45] Hubscher O, Re R, Iotti R. Cystic lung disease in Sjogren's syndrome. J Rheumatol 2002;29(10):2235–6.

[46] Parambil JG, Myers JL, Lindell RM, Matteson EL, Ryu JH. Interstitial lung disease in primary Sjogren syndrome. Chest 2006;130(5):1489–95.

[47] Suda T, Kaida Y, Nakamura Y, Enomoto N, Fujisawa T, Imokawa S, et al. Acute exacerbation of interstitial pneumonia associated with collagen vascular diseases. Respir Med 2009;103(6):846–53.

[48] Collard HR, Ryerson CJ, Corte TJ, Jenkins G, Kondoh Y, Lederer DJ, et al. Acute exacerbation of idiopathic pulmonary fibrosis. An international working group report. Am J Respir Crit Care Med 2016;194(3):265–75.

[49] Manfredi A, Sebastiani M, Cerri S, Vacchi C, Tonelli R, Della Casa G, et al. Acute exacerbation of interstitial lung diseases secondary to systemic rheumatic diseases: a prospective study and review of the literature. J Thorac Dis 2019;11(4):1621–8.

[50] Luppi F, Cerri S, Taddei S, Ferrara G, Cottin V. Acute exacerbation of idiopathic pulmonary fibrosis: a clinical review. Intern Emerg Med 2015;10(4):401–11.

[51] Yeh JJ, Chen HJ, Li TC, Wong YS, Tang HC, Yeh TC, et al. Association between Sjogren's syndrome and respiratory failure: put airway, interstitia, and vessels close together: a national cohort study. PLoS One 2014;9(10):e110783.

[52] American Thoracic S, European Respiratory S. American Thoracic Society/European Respiratory Society international multidisciplinary consensus classification of the idiopathic interstitial pneumonias. This joint statement of the American Thoracic Society (ATS), and the European Respiratory Society (ERS) was adopted by the ATS board of directors, June 2001 and by the ERS Executive Committee, June 2001. Am J Respir Crit Care Med 2002;165(2):277–304.

[53] Travis WD, Hunninghake G, King Jr TE, Lynch DA, Colby TV, Galvin JR, et al. Idiopathic nonspecific interstitial pneumonia: report of an American Thoracic Society project. Am J Respir Crit Care Med 2008;177(12):1338–47.

[54] Demedts M, Costabel U. ATS/ERS international multidisciplinary consensus classification of the idiopathic interstitial pneumonias. Eur Respir J 2002;19(5):794–6.

[55] Deheinzelin D, Capelozzi VL, Kairalla RA, Barbas Filho JV, Saldiva PH, de Carvalho CR. Interstitial lung disease in primary Sjogren's syndrome. Clinical-pathological evaluation and response to treatment. Am J Respir Crit Care Med 1996;154(3 Pt 1):794–9.

[56] Yamadori I, Fujita J, Bandoh S, Tokuda M, Tanimoto Y, Kataoka M, et al. Nonspecific interstitial pneumonia as pulmonary involvement of primary Sjogren's syndrome. Rheumatol Int 2002;22(3):89–92.

[57] Ujita M, Renzoni EA, Veeraraghavan S, Wells AU, Hansell DM. Organizing pneumonia: perilobular pattern at thin-section CT. Radiology 2004;232(3):757–61.

[58] Shi JH, Liu HR, Xu WB, Feng RE, Zhang ZH, Tian XL, et al. Pulmonary manifestations of Sjogren's syndrome. Respiration 2009;78(4):377–86.

[59] Lee JW, Lee KS, Lee HY, Chung MP, Yi CA, Kim TS, et al. Cryptogenic organizing pneumonia: serial high-resolution CT findings in 22 patients. Am J Roentgenol 2010;195(4):916–22.

[60] Marchiori E, Zanetti G, Escuissato DL, Souza Jr AS, de Souza Portes Meirelles G, Fagundes J, et al. Reversed halo sign: high-resolution CT scan findings in 79 patients. Chest 2012;141(5):1260–6.

[61] Ioannou S, Toya SP, Tomos P, Tzelepis GE. Cryptogenic organizing pneumonia associated with primary Sjogren's syndrome. Rheumatol Int 2008;28(10):1053–5.

[62] Cordier JF. Update on cryptogenic organising pneumonia (idiopathic bronchiolitis obliterans organising pneumonia). Swiss Med Wkly 2002;132(41–42):588–91.

[63] Myers JL, Colby TV. Pathologic manifestations of bronchiolitis, constrictive bronchiolitis, cryptogenic organizing pneumonia, and diffuse panbronchiolitis. Clin Chest Med 1993;14(4):611–22.

[64] Johkoh T, Muller NL, Cartier Y, Kavanagh PV, Hartman TE, Akira M, et al. Idiopathic interstitial pneumonias: diagnostic accuracy of thin-section CT in 129 patients. Radiology 1999;211(2):555–60.

[65] Papiris SA, Tsonis IA, Moutsopoulos HM. Sjogren's syndrome. Semin Respir Crit Care Med 2007;28(4):459–71.

[66] Parke AL. Pulmonary manifestations of primary Sjogren's syndrome. Rheum Dis Clin N Am 2008;34(4):907–20 [viii].

[67] Sakamoto O, Saita N, Ando M, Kohrogi H, Suga M, Ando M. Two cases of Sjogren's syndrome with multiple bullae. Intern Med 2002;41(2):124–8.

[68] Bonner Jr H, Ennis RS, Geelhoed GW, Tarpley Jr TM. Lymphoid infiltration and amyloidosis of lung in Sjogren's syndrome. Arch Pathol 1973;95(1):42–4.

[69] Watanabe M, Naniwa T, Hara M, Arakawa T, Maeda T. Pulmonary manifestations in Sjogren's syndrome: correlation analysis between chest computed tomographic findings and clinical subsets with poor prognosis in 80 patients. J Rheumatol 2010;37(2):365–73.

[70] Lechtman S, Debray MP, Crestani B, Bancal C, Hourseau M, Dossier A, et al. Cystic lung disease in Sjogren's syndrome: an observational study. Jt Bone Spine 2017;84(3):317–21.

[71] Martinez-Balzano CD, Touray S, Kopec S. Cystic lung disease among patients with Sjogren syndrome: frequency, natural history, and associated risk factors. Chest 2016;150(3):631–9.

[72] Cottin V, Nunes H, Mouthon L, Gamondes D, Lazor R, Hachulla E, et al. Combined pulmonary fibrosis and emphysema syndrome in connective tissue disease. Arthritis Rheum 2011;63(1):295–304.

[73] Mejia M, Carrillo G, Rojas-Serrano J, Estrada A, Suarez T, Alonso D, et al. Idiopathic pulmonary fibrosis and emphysema: decreased survival associated with severe pulmonary arterial hypertension. Chest 2009;136(1):10–5.

[74] Davidson BK, Kelly CA, Griffiths ID. Ten year follow up of pulmonary function in patients with primary Sjogren's syndrome. Ann Rheum Dis 2000;59(9):709–12.

[75] du Bois RM, Albera C, Bradford WZ, Costabel U, Leff JA, Noble PW, et al. 6-Minute walk distance is an independent predictor of mortality in patients with idiopathic pulmonary fibrosis. Eur Respir J 2014;43(5):1421–9.

[76] Caminati A, Bianchi A, Cassandro R, Mirenda MR, Harari S. Walking distance on 6-MWT is a prognostic factor in idiopathic pulmonary fibrosis. Respir Med 2009;103(1):117–23.

[77] Vandecasteele E, De Pauw M, De Keyser F, Decuman S, Deschepper E, Piette Y, et al. Six-minute walk test in systemic sclerosis: a systematic review and meta-analysis. Int J Cardiol 2016;212:265–73.

[78] Dalavanga YA, Constantopoulos SH, Galanopoulou V, Zerva L, Moutsopoulos HM. Alveolitis correlates with clinical pulmonary involvement in primary Sjogren's syndrome. Chest 1991;99(6):1394–7.

[79] Roca F, Dominique S, Schmidt J, Smail A, Duhaut P, Levesque H, et al. Interstitial lung disease in primary Sjogren's syndrome. Autoimmun Rev 2017;16(1):48–54.

[80] Ramos-Casals M, Brito-Zeron P, Siso-Almirall A, Bosch X, Tzioufas AG. Topical and systemic medications for the treatment of primary Sjogren's syndrome. Nat Rev Rheumatol 2012;8(7):399–411.

[81] Saraux A, Pers JO, Devauchelle-Pensec V. Treatment of primary Sjogren syndrome. Nat Rev Rheumatol 2016;12(8):456–71.

[82] Gottenberg JE, Cinquetti G, Larroche C, Combe B, Hachulla E, Meyer O, et al. Efficacy of rituximab in systemic manifestations of primary Sjogren's syndrome: results in 78 patients of the AutoImmune and Rituximab registry. Ann Rheum Dis 2013;72(6):1026–31.

[83] Distler O, Highland KB, Gahlemann M, Azuma A, Fischer A, Mayes MD, et al. Nintedanib for systemic sclerosis-associated interstitial lung disease. N Engl J Med 2019;380(26):2518–28.

[84] Khanna D, Albera C, Fischer A, Khalidi N, Raghu G, Chung L, et al. An open-label, phase II study of the safety and tolerability of pirfenidone in patients with scleroderma-associated interstitial lung disease: the LOTUSS trial. J Rheumatol 2016;43(9):1672–9.

[85] Mathai SC, Danoff SK. Management of interstitial lung disease associated with connective tissue disease. BMJ 2016;352:h6819.

[86] Fragkioudaki S, Mavragani CP, Moutsopoulos HM. Predicting the risk for lymphoma development in Sjogren syndrome: an easy tool for clinical use. Medicine 2016;95(25):e3766.

[87] Rodallec M, Guermazi A, Brice P, Attal P, Zagdanski AM, Frija J, et al. Imaging of MALT lymphomas. Eur Radiol 2002;12(2):348–56.

[88] Lee DK, Im JG, Lee KS, Lee JS, Seo JB, Goo JM, et al. B-cell lymphoma of bronchus-associated lymphoid tissue (BALT): CT features in 10 patients. J Comput Assist Tomogr 2000;24(1):30–4.

[89] Bae YA, Lee KS, Han J, Ko YH, Kim BT, Chung MJ, et al. Marginal zone B-cell lymphoma of bronchus-associated lymphoid tissue: imaging findings in 21 patients. Chest 2008;133(2):433–40.

[90] Shah RM, Friedman AC. CT angiogram sign: incidence and significance in lobar consolidations evaluated by contrast-enhanced CT. Am J Roentgenol 1998;170(3):719–21.

[91] Jeong YJ, Lee KS, Chung MP, Han J, Chung MJ, Kim KI, et al. Amyloidosis and lymphoproliferative disease in Sjogren syndrome: thin-section computed tomography findings and histopathologic comparisons. J Comput Assist Tomogr 2004;28(6):776–81.

[92] Kawamata K, Haraoka H, Hirohata S, Hashimoto T, Jenkins RN, Lipsky PE. Pleurisy in primary Sjogren's syndrome: T cell receptor beta-chain variable region gene bias and local autoantibody production in the pleural effusion. Clin Exp Rheumatol 1997;15(2):193–6.

[93] Hosoda C, Hosaka Y, Ryu K, Kinoshita A, Saito K, Kuwano K. Pleuritis associated with primary Sjogren syndrome. Respirol Case Rep 2018;6(2):e00285.

[94] Ma D, Lu H, Qu Y, Wang S, Ying Y, Xiao W. Primary Sjogren's syndrome accompanied by pleural effusion: a case report and literature review. Int J Clin Exp Pathol 2015;8(11):15322–7.

[95] Launay D, Hachulla E, Hatron PY, Jais X, Simonneau G, Humbert M. Pulmonary arterial hypertension: a rare complication of primary Sjogren syndrome: report of 9 new cases and review of the literature. Medicine 2007;86(5):299–315.

[96] Rajagopala S, Singh N, Gupta K, Gupta D. Pulmonary amyloidosis in Sjogren's syndrome: a case report and systematic review of the literature. Respirology 2010;15(5):860–6.

Chapter 5

Lung involvement in systemic sclerosis

Corrado Campochiaro,[1,2] Cosimo Bruni,[3] Sara Tomassetti,[4] Lorenzo Dagna[1,2] and Marco Matucci-Cerinic[1,3,*]

[1]*Unit of Immunology, Rheumatology, Allergy and Rare diseases (UnIRAR), IRCCS San Raffaele Hospital, Milan, Italy;* [2]*Vita-Salute San Raffaele University, Milan, Italy;* [3]*Department of Experimental and Clinical Medicine, University of Florence, Florence, and Division of Rheumatology, AOUC, Florence, Italy;* [4]*Department of Experimental and Clinical Medicine, University of Florence, and Division of Interventional Pneumology, AOUC, Florence, Italy*

**Corresponding author at: marco.matuccicerinic@unifi.it.*

Epidemiology

Interstitial lung disease

The exact prevalence of interstitial lung disease (ILD) in systemic sclerosis (SSc) patients is highly variable and depends on the diagnostic tool used to confirm ILD [8]. Other factors may help to understand the heterogeneity found in the literature such as the cohorts of patients selected (nationwide studies usually include small centers with a low prevalence of SSc-ILD patients compared to referral centers where an enrichment in SSc-ILD patients is common) and the disease duration of included patients [9,10]. The Scleroderma Patient-Centered Intervention Network has estimated an overall prevalence of physician-reported SSc-ILD of 36.2% [11]. Though, the prevalence of SSc-ILD is significantly different according to disease subset as it is more prevalent in dcSSc (ranging from 30% to 71% of patients) compared to lcSSc (ranging from 21% to 53%) [12]. Moreover, specific autoantibodies (antitopoisomerase I and anticentromere) increase or reduce the risk of ILD in SSc. Definitively, antitopoisomerase I antibody is a risk factor for ILD while anticentromere antibody seems protective for ILD [12]. Nonetheless antitopoisomerase I positivity is not always associated with ILD as up to 50% of antitopoisomerase I positive patients do not have ILD, nor it is associated with a more rapid ILD progression [13]. Some other rarer SSc-specific antibodies have also been associated with the risk of ILD development: anti-Th/To

The Lung in Autoimmune Diseases. https://doi.org/10.1016/B978-0-323-91083-5.00009-8

antibody is associated to ILD in lcSSc [14] and the anti-PM/Scl, usually found in myositis overlap syndromes, is also associated with an increased prevalence of ILD but with a better functional outcome [15]. The data about the anti-U3-RNP antibody are still controversial and it is not clear whether the antibody may confer an increased risk of pulmonary arterial hypertension (PAH) and ILD prevalence [16,17].

It is commonly accepted that the first 3–4 years from the disease onset are most critical as in this time interval, the greatest lung function loss is observed [18]. More recently, studies, such as the Scleroderma Lung Study I (SLS I) [19], have questioned this paradigm in SSc-ILD progression because in the placebo arm, a similar rate of lung function decline was observed independently from their disease duration [20]. The impact of gender and other features on ILD development and progression is not entirely clear yet [21]. Indeed, while male gender, impaired lung function at the time of SSc diagnosis, presence of respiratory symptoms (cough and dyspnea), honeycombing, and extent of disease on high-resolution computed tomography (HRCT) scan, elevated KL-6 values, and increased alveolar epithelial permeability have been identified as predictors of mortality and ILD progression, none of these variables has been clearly associated with ILD [21]. The SSc-ILD has been associated with non-Caucasian and African American race which also confers an increased risk of PH [22,23].

Pulmonary arterial hypertension

In SSc-PH, the reported prevalence is highly dependent on the disease duration and the used diagnostic technique, especially when right heart catheterization is compared to echocardiography. For SSc-PAH diagnosis, only right heart catheter is acceptable. Recent studies suggest a prevalence of SSc-PAH of at least 10% when the disease duration is longer than 10 years [24]. Moreover, retrospective studies in monocentric cohorts have highlighted an annual incidence of 1% to 2%, with a higher incidence of PAH in lcSSc patients and a slightly higher incidence of SSc-PH (postcapillary or ILD-associated) in dcSSc patients [25].

Pathogenesis

Over the last 30 years, an enormous amount of data has been produced over the possible pathogenetic mechanisms of lung involvement in SSc. Nonetheless, the exact pathogenesis of lung disease in SSc is far from being completely understood as it is hard to distinguish between epiphenoma and central pathogenetic pathways. In addition, it should be first noticed that although the underlying pathogenetic mechanism can be shared among different lung complications, beside lung fibrosis and PAH, other rarer manifestations can occur in SSc patients such as organizing pneumonia (OP), thromboembolic and veno-occlusive disease (PVOD).

Lung fibrosis

Lung fibrosis in SSc has been historically considered the terminal phase of a previous inflammatory process which then has left a scar in the lungs [26]. Gradually, this disease paradigm has evolved and now it is commonly accepted in SSc-ILD fibrosis and different degrees of inflammation coexist [27]. Fibrosis, which is one the hallmark of SSc pathogenesis, derives from the excessive accumulation of extracellular matrix produced by activated fibroblasts in response to tissue injury, inflammation, or as a part of a more complex and orchestrated process called fibrogenesis [28,29]. This latter refers to a peculiar ability of fibroblasts to transform into myofibroblasts that are the cells producing extracellular matrix. Likely, SSc lung fibrosis shares common pathogenic momenta with other ILD such as idiopathic lung fibrosis (IPF) or rheumatoid arthritis (AR)-associated ILD. Moreover, similar processes can take place in different systems and organs such skin, kidney, and heart in SSc patients. Different cell types and cellular mediators have been implicated in the development of lung fibrosis including lung epithelial cells (pneumocytes), innate immunity cells (neutrophils, macrophages, and eosinophils), adaptive immunity cells (B cells, T cells, and NK), and mesenchymal cells (fibroblasts and myofibroblasts) [5,30].

Genetic susceptibility toward SSc-ILD is mainly driven by two key elements: genetic predisposition and epigenetic factors. Association studies and direct sequencing studies have shown that candidate immunological and inflammatory genes are associated with SSc-ILD in large independent cohorts. These include the connective tissue growth factor (CTGF) [31] linked to a functional polymorphism and interleukin-6 (IL-6) whose polymorphism and serum levels are strongly linked to SSc-ILD development and progression [32,33]. Nonetheless, given the heterogeneity of the disease, and the complex gene-environment interactions, single-cohort studies are sometimes not replicable across different cohorts. This is the example of CTGF polymorphism which, while it was positively associated with SSc-ILD development in two independent single-center studies, it was confirmed in a large multinational study. This suggests a role for this polymorphism in specific populations (UK and Japanese patients) but not in the entire SSc-ILD population [31,34,35]. Moreover, epigenetic factors can also influence the fibrogenesis in SSc-ILD. This is the case of microRNAs that can modulate the activation of lung fibroblasts, especially miR-155 [36].

As previously stated, myofibroblasts are active profibrotic contractile cells characterized by the expression of α-smooth muscle actin, are crucial for the development of fibrosis [37]. In SSc, lung myo fibroblasts have a profibrotic phenotype [37] and three major pathways and regulators which are the transforming growth factor-β (TGFβ), the CC-chemokine ligand 2 (CCL2), and interleukin (IL)-13, regulate their fibrotic ability as their enhanced extracellular matrix production, and also increase fibroblasts contractility and induce myofibroblasts differentiation [37–40]. *In vitro* studies on SSc-ILDc epithelial and endothelial cells deriving have shown a fundamental role for endothelial-mesenchymal and epithelial-mesenchymal transition in the pathogenesis of SSc-ILD. This suggests that the culprit cell (myofibroblast) can derive for the differentiation of cell from other lineages of origin [41–43]. Specific inflammatory cytokines and chemokines, in particular, IL-6, CCL2, and CXCL4 have also been associated with the presence of ILD and with the progression of the disease [32,44,45]. Gastro-oesophageal reflux disease (GORD) with chronic aspiration and microaspiration of stomach gastric content has also been hypothesized as a major contributor in ILD progression [46]. Indeed, in mice genetically predisposed to lung injury, the aspiration of an acidic saline solution can induce lung fibrosis [47]. Moreover, some studies have also observed how the severity of ILD could be linked to GORD severity [46,48].

All local and systemic triggers that can cause lung epithelial injury can then induce a profibrotic environment with the induction and perpetuation of the TGFβ signaling pathways [49]. This pathway is crucial for the abnormal repair of injured connective tissue—the "defective lung fibrogenesis" typical of SSc-ILD—and can be induced either by local activation of TGFβ via integrin pathways or via postnatal activation of canonical receptor-mediated signaling [49,50]. The essential role of TGFβ signaling in SSc-ILD pathogenesis has also been confirmed in experimental studies in genetically modified mice with an attenuation of TGFβ signaling. In the studies by Hoyles et al., it was also found that a population of the resident lung fibroblasts with lineage-specific deletion of high-affinity type II TGFβ receptor are responsible for the orchestration of lung fibrosis contributing to the exaggerated lung tissue repair and being able to recruit and regulate other fibrogenic cells from the bloodstream such as fibrocytes [51,52]. Epithelial injury as fundamental momentum associated with SSc-ILD has also been shown by the association of rapid diethylene triamine pentaacetate clearance and the elevated serum levels of serum Krebs con den Lungen 6 (KL-6) with SSc-ILD progression [47,53].

More recently, the circulating and local resident monocyte-macrophage lineage has attracted the attention of the medical community in the pathogenesis of SSc-ILD. Indeed, analysis of genes expressed in the skin were found to correlate with the severity of lung fibrosis and a gene and protein analysis has highlighted an altered monocyte and macrophage function in SSc-ILD pathogenesis, possibly due to an antigen-driven process [54].

Pulmonary arterial hypertension

Pulmonary endothelial cell injury and dysfunction are key elements in the pathogenesis of SSc-PAH. This process progressively leads to excessive fibroproliferative repair and eventually to the typical obliterative pulmonary vasculopathy found in SSc-PAH patients [55]. Evidence from pathology shows that SSc-PAH features are muscularization of intrapulmonary arterioles and medial wall thickening with perivascular inflammatory changes, similar to those observed in other PAH conditions. It is not surprising that bone morphogenetic protein receptor type 2 (BMPR2), which is implicated in the heritable forms of PAH, has also been associated with SSc-PAH [56,57]. Mouse models have shown that together with endothelial injury, defect in BMPR2 expression and function are associated with SSc-PAH thus suggesting that SSc itself might be a susceptibility phenotype for PAH [56]. Similarly to SSc-ILD, in SSc-PAH multiple mechanisms and cellular compartments interplay one with another. Among immune cells, dysfunctional monocyte and macrophage with M2 polarization have been associated with SSc-PAH development. Moreover, endothelial-mesenchymal transition has been accounted for the fibroproliferative alterations observed in the pulmonary vessels of SSc-PAH patients [58]. Other mediators that are considered relevant for SSc-PAH include IL-6, platelet-derived growth factor (PDGF), and CTGF [59]. Mitochondrial dysfunction with high oxidative stress levels have also been linked to the inflammation-induced damage in SSc-PAH.

Clincal presentation

Interstitial lung disease

The clinical presentation of patients with a clinically significant SSc-ILD is similar to those affected by IPF and idiopathic nonspecific interstitial pneumonia (NSIP). Usually exertional dyspnea is the first symptom which can be progressive and it is often found in association with cough [60]. Unfortunately, the presence of ILD can be completely clinically silent, either in patients with ILD of limited extension or in patients that cannot exert themselves enough to induce dyspnea such as those with limited daily activities due to concomitant musculoskeletal problems. In SSc patients, the presence of exertional dyspnea is not merely associated with ILD, but can be the manifestation of other conditions that can complicate SSc patients such as musculoskeletal abnormalities, loss of fitness, anemia, cardiac involvement, and PAH [61].

Physical examination may disclose basal inspiratory velcro-like crackles [62]. Crackles can be present early in SSc-ILD, with an initial appearance in the basal areas of the lung where the disease process starts, but can then become evident also in the upper zones according to the extension of the disease. Given the limited diagnostic power of standard chest X-ray, it is important to remember that the presence of crackles, together with dyspnea or gas exchange abnormalities, may indicate ILD even if the chest radiograph is normal. Finger clubbing is usually a manifestation of advanced lung fibrosis as it suggests the presence of long-standing hypoxia. In patients with normal findings at physical examination, further screening is recommended.

Pulmonary arterial hypertension

Clinical presentation of PAH can be similar to that of patients with SSc-ILD as the presence of exertional dyspnea is a shared presenting symptom. The presence of PAH can also be associated with a number of symptoms that reflect the reduced cardiac output, especially on exertion. These include lethargy, fatigue, exertional chest pain due to subendocardial hypoperfusion, exertional syncope, peripheral oedema, signs of hepatic congestion such as ascites, cough, and hemoptysis. At physical examination, the most typical signs include an increased intensity of the pulmonary component of the second heart sound, a right-sided third or fourth heart sound (gallop rhythm), wide splitting of the second heart sound, and hepatomegaly with signs or right-heart failure in advanced cases (peripheral oedema, ascites, pleural effusion) [63].

Diagnosis of ILD

Abnormalities in clinical examination and chest X-ray findings have a low sensibility for detecting SSc-IL, while a restrictive ventilatory defect in pulmonary function tests (PFTs) is more specific for ILD involvement [61]. Nonetheless, the presence of extrapulmonary causes of restrictions such as pleural disease, respiratory muscle weakness, or severe cutaneous involvement might cause a similar restrictive pattern [64,65]. Moreover, the presence of an isolated reduction in diffuse lung CO (DLCO) is highly nonspecific as it may reflect the presence of interstitial lung involvement or the presence of SSc-PAH [5]. It is also important to remember that lung volumes are highly different among individuals with normal lung capacity as the range of % predicted values can go from 80% to 120% of the average value for a person of the same gender, weight, and height. This is why a value considered normal such as FVC of 90% could represent in an SSc patient either the absence of any ILD involvement or a dramatic reduction from a premorbid condition of 120%. Thus, the delta changes over time are more informative and a mild reduction of FVC over time might be the result of a more significant ILD extension.

In SSc, the sensitivity of pulmonary function as a screening tool for ILD can be increased with the inclusion of other parameters beside % predicted FVC such as DLCO, total lung capacity, and/or functional residual capacity. The positivity for specific antibodies (especially anti-Scl70) or the SSc subset (dcSSc) should warrant further investigations with a lower threshold. As LFTs parameters are not specific for ILD involvement in SSc patients, it is important to learn how the relative changes of single parameters can be informative. As an example, a patient with a disproportionate reduction in DLCO as compared to FVC, in absence of emphysema, may be more in keeping with the development of SSc-PAH rather than ILD.

Typically, ILD results in a restrictive ventilatory defect with reduced lung volumes (including both FVC and TLC) and normal or increased forced expiratory volume in 1 s FEV1 with a FEV1/FVC ratio >0.80. In patients with SSc-ILD but with no other overlapping conditions such PAH or emphysema, the DLCO/alveolar volume (VA) ratio is usually normal or only slightly decreased [61].

Other tests to assess SSc-ILD include routine chest x.ray, exercise tolerance tests, and dyspnea scores, but they have all significant limitations for detecting early lung fibrosis because of poor sensibility and specificity for ILD.

For this reason, it is now widely accepted that the diagnosis of SSc-ILD should rely on CT to identify the presence of even minimal lung abnormalities, and furthermore define the ILD pattern such as NSIP versus usual interstitial pneumonia (UIP) and to better quantify the degree of ILD extension. Moreover, the use of CT is fundamental for a differential diagnosis to rule out other diseases, especially in immunosuppressed individuals such as infections, malignancies, and drug-induced lung diseases.

Bronchoalveolar lavage (BAL) and lung biopsy (Lbx) can also provide useful insights for the diagnosis and for the management of SSc-ILD patients. Both BAL and LBx are helpful to exclude infections, drug-related ILD, and in the differential diagnosis with other ILDs (environmental, hypersensitivity pneumonitis, idiopathic ILD, etc.). Usually, BAL and transbronchial biopsy are combined and performed during the same bronchoscopy, but BAL can be performed alone depending on the clinical suspicion (e.g., likelihood of infectious etiology) or the patient's underlying conditions (increased risks for LBx). Currently, the value of BAL and LBx in the characterization of SSc-ILD is low, mainly because they do not provide yet a significant diagnostic or prognostic information. However, recent trials showing that antifibrotic drugs can be useful in slowing SSc-ILD progression open a new scenario in which physicians needs to choose between multiple drugs (biologics, immunosuppressive, and antifibrotic) either as single agents or in combinations [66]. The need to refine the capacity to choose the best tailored therapy fuels a renewed interest in what informations BAL and Lbx might add onto the underlying prevalence of inflammation or fibrosis. Therefore, BAL and LBx utility today in SSc-ILD can be summarized in: (1) to help physicians to make more timely and appropriate treatment decisions; (2) to allow a better understanding of SSc-ILD pathogenetic mechanisms.

High-resolution computed tomography

For the diagnosis of SSc-ILD, HRCT represents the current gold standard as it has a high correspondence with pathological patterns and has a higher sensitivity vesus chest X-ray and PFTs [67,68]. The HRCT detection of SSc-ILD is also part of the American College of Rheumatology/European League Against Rheumatism 2013 classification criteria for SSc. In this context, ILD is defined as the presence of pulmonary fibrosis at HRCT or X-ray or non-otherwise determined Velcro sign on auscultation [69]. A recent European consensus has recommended the performance of chest HRCT at the time of diagnosis in all SSc patients, as a form of baseline screening for SSc-ILD [70]. Despite this recommendation, there is no strong agreement among SSc-treating physicians when to perform HRCT in SSc patient. In this context, chest HRCT is still considered more a diagnostic tool, to confirm clinical and functional suspicion of SSc-ILD, compared to a screening assessment to be performed also in asymptomatic or at-risk patients [71].

NSIP (Fig. 5.2, left section) represents the most frequently detected SSc-ILD pattern, characterized by the presence of bilateral peripheral ground glass opacities, with basal prevalence and frequent subpleural sparing, seldom associated to reticulation and traction bronchiectasis [72]. Conversely, the lack of ground glass opacities and the simultaneous presence of reticular and honeycombing changes is the hellmark of the UIP (Fig. 5.2, left section) pattern [72]. Despite the NSIP is usually 6–8 times more frequent than the UIP pattern, the prevalent ILD pattern has shown no impact on the patient prognosis [21]. Conversely, the presence of specific HRCT features, such as honeycombing and reticulation, are associated with a worse prognosis, while the proportion of ground glass opacities with lower mortality [73].

Recent literature supports the usefulness of chest HRCT in the follow-up of patients with SSc-ILD. A recently published post-hoc analysis of the SLS II, comparing the effect of cyclophosphamide (CYC) and mycophenolate mofetil (MMF) for the treatment of SSc-ILD, compared the evolution of SSc-ILD patterns under treatment. When computerized texture analysis was applied to these images, it was possible to study the transition between of different ILD patterns, including normal to ground glass opacities or to reticulation or the evolution between ground glass and reticulation, and vice versa [74].

In addition to the diagnosis and the characterization of the parenchymal involvement, HRCT allows the quantification of the ILD extent. This can be achieved through visual semi-quantitative and computer-based qualitative methods. Different studies showed a weak correlation between pulmonary functional parameters (such as FVC% and DLCO%) and the extent of ground glass and fibrotic ILD assessment through the visual scoring [75] and similar results were obtained also with computerized whole-lung assessments, such as histogram-based densitometry analysis [76] and texture analysis [77]. These results stress the importance of chest HRCT performance in the stratification of anatomical involvement related to SSc-ILD, despite there is currently no radiation-free substitute of PFTs to monitor the longitudinal evolution of SSc-ILD.

Among the visual scores for ILD extent, the system proposed by Wells et al. is the most frequently used [64]: it quantifies the extent of ground glass opacities and reticulation, as well as coarseness of reticulation and total disease extent at five predefined levels (origin of the great vessels, main carina, pulmonary venous confluence, halfway between the third and the fifth section, immediately above the right hemi-diaphragm). The score is assigned to the closest 5% of each alteration, after the mean between the five levels is calculated. This evaluation of ILD patterns and total extent has been adopted in many research studies [73]. In their studies, the total disease extent is dichotomized according to a 20% value, with limited disease for extent <20% and extensive disease when >20%. In case of indeterminate ILD extent, an FVC<70% is considered as a surrogate of extensive disease, otherwise as limited if above this cut-off. This staging system has shown significant prognostic implication in SSc-ILD patient, with significantly impaired prognosis for the patients with increased ILD extent [73]. The superiority of SSc-ILD extent and patterns evaluation on HRCT to the functional impairment in terms of mortality prediction has been shown for both the visual evaluation [75], the histogram-based quantitative parameters [78] and the texture analysis [79].

In addition to the computerized quantitative evaluation of SSc-ILD extent and patterns, lung texture analysis has also allowed the identification and quantification of pulmonary vascular volumes. Recent studies have shown a strong direct correlation between lung vascular volumes and parenchymal patterns in SSc-ILD [79], both significantly impacting on patient prognosis in other fibrosing conditions [80]. The link between the two components, in terms of timing and pathogenetic connection, still remains to be elucidated.

HRCT still carries a significant radiation exposure burden, which limits its repeatability in time and also its application as a screening tool [81]. In this context, reduced slice number and radiation protocols have been proposed as SSc-ILD screening algorithm: in the study from Frauenfelder et al., a direct comparison between standard and 9-slice reduced HRCT protocol showed similar performance in terms of image quality, diagnostic accuracy, and diagnostic confidence, with good performance also for the detection of limited/minimal ILD [82].

Different techniques have emerged thanks to their radiation-free nature. Lung ultrasound (LUS) identifies the presence of hyperechoic reverberation artefacts starting from the pleural lines, called B-lines. Different counting systems applied to different numbers of intercostal spaces have been proposed so far [83]. Despite differences in terms of feasibility, the different LUS protocols have shown the potential of B-Lines' quantification in SSc-ILD, may be a tool for screening, quantification, and prognostication. Gargani et al. first showed that a total of >10 B-lines can be considered as a reliable cut-off to predict for ILD presence of HRCT, with very high sensitivity and negative predictive value even for subclinical early disease [84]. Following this, B-lines numbers was correlated with the severity and the extent of ILD, as well as with its functional impairment in terms of FVC% and DLCO% decline [85–87]. Finally, LUS may also carry as a significant predictive prognostic value, as Gargani et al. have shown in a large cohort of patients that an increased value of B-Lines was associated with pulmonary progression [88].

Lung magnetic resonance imaging (LMRI) has been more recently proposed as a possible tool combining morphological and functional assessments [89]. Similar to LUS, no standardized protocol is applied to SSc-ILD and LMRI is currently performed mostly for research purposes, with similar performance on morphological ILD detection when compared to chest HRCT. In fact, ultra-short time (UTE) LMRI sequences have shown very good performance in the anatomical definition of SSc-ILD, when compared to HRCT (See Figs. 5.1 and 5.2, comparing HRCT and LMRI in two cases of NSIP and UIP SSc-ILD patient) [90]. Similarly, LMRI allowed to identify significantly different short tau inversion recovery (STIR) and T1 mapping values between areas of affected and unaffected lung in SSc, possibly reflecting different amount of fibrotic and inflammatory changes, respectively [91]. Moreover, the altered STIR signal may predict the development or the progression of ILD, therefore identifying LMRI also as a possible prognostic assessment.

With a similar target of identifying active inflammatory disease in the lung tissue, positron emission tomography (PET), combined with CT acquisitions (PET/CT) was applied as a research tool in SSc and SSc-ILD, using different tracers, i.e., radioactive fluor-deoxy-glucose [92]. As seen for LMRI, a different signal intensity in terms of standardized uptake value was seen when comparing SSc patients and healthy controls and SSc-ILD positive and negative cases [92]. In addition, the standardized uptake values were also shown to be significantly different in unaffected lung areas of SSc patients with and without ILD, as a possible marker of preradiologic activity [93], and

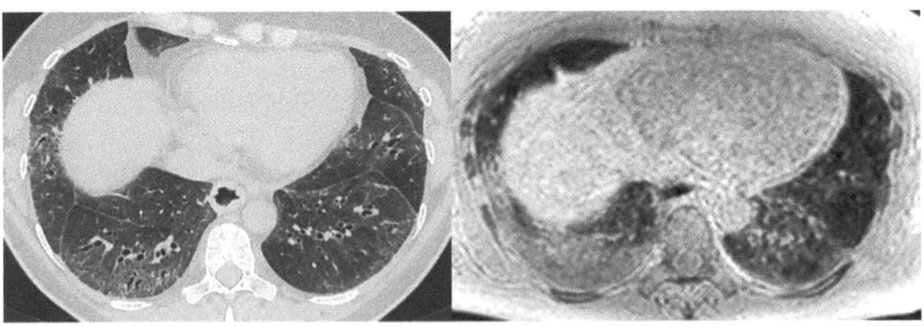

FIGURE 5.1 - HRCT (left) and Ultra-Short Echo Time (UTE) MRI (right) images, lower lung field: both CT and MRI show ground glass opacities, consistent with NSIP pattern.

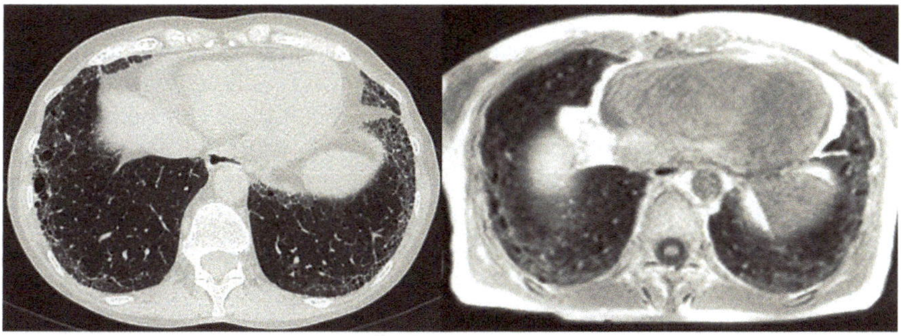

FIGURE 5.2 – HRCT (left) and Ultra-Short Echo Time (UTE) MRI (right) images, lower lung field: both CT and MRI show subpleural interstitial lung diease. MRI may also recognize fibrotic cists, resembling honeycombing.

to parallel the presence of HRCT detected reticulation and ground glass opacities on HRCT [94]. As for all the other above-mentioned assessment, PET/CT detected signal was also identified as a predictor of ILD worsening progression [95].

Acknowledgments: We thank Dr. Nicholas Landini for providing us the HRCT and lung MR images.

Bronchoalveolar lavage

BAL is useful in SSc to document infections, noninfective complications (drug-related ILD or malignant disease [96]), but its utility in the assessment of disease activity has not been established and serial BAL to monitor disease course are currently discouraged [96]. The BAL procedure is performed during standard flexible bronchoscopy, good sampling retrieves at least 30% of instilled volume. Safety of BAL is its major advantage compared to other more invasive techniques such as LBx. BAL is easily performed, well tolerated, and can be done in acutely ill patients (e.g., patients with ARDS or intubated). The safety of BAL has been confirmed in a recent prospective cohort of 223 IPF patients who underwent bronchoscopy in the PROFILE study. All subjects tolerated the procedure well, a cell differential could be obtained in all, and there were no immediate (<72 h) complications [97].

BAL is a safe technique for the diagnosis of pulmonary infections in SSc-ILD providing the clinician with accurate guidance for antibiotic or antiviral treatment. In the complex scenario of SSc-ILD (esophageal dysmotility predisposing to aspiration and bronchopneumonia, immunosuppressive drug treatment predisposing to opportunistic infections), the exclusion of infections is one of the most common clinical indications for BAL. In CTD-ILD, Sun et al. [98] documented on BAL opportunistic infections (*Aspergillus* sp., *Pneumocystis Jirovecii*), mycobacterial infections, and both gram-negative bacilli and gram-positive cocci (*Klebsiella pneumoniae*, *Sternotrophomonas maltophilia*, Corynebacterium, one MRSA). Both the presence of clinically relevant symptoms and the presence of ground glass or consolidation on HRCT increased significantly the BAL diagnostic yield (symptomatic vs. asymptomatic: 25.6% vs. 3.7%, $P = .042$ and ground glass/consolidations vs. reticular pattern: 20.3% vs. 0, $P < .001$).

In the diagnosis of ILD, BAL cellular analysis narrows the differential diagnosis with the identification or exclusion of a predominant inflammatory cellular pattern [99,100]. The normal values of differential cytology in non-smokers are: macrophages >80%, lymphocytes <15%, neutrophils <3%, eosinophils <0.5%, mast cells <0.5%. Neoplastic diseases can occasionally present with radiological ILD appearance and, most notably, in some cases of SSc-ILD, areas of dense fibrosis on CT raise the problem of differential diagnosis with malignancy which can be ruled out by BAL in combination with biopsy. Both SSc-ILD and drug-induced lung disorders may present with any type of patterns (lymphocytic, neutrophilic, eosinophilic, and mixed). Therefore, the differentiation between the two processes based on BAL alone is not possible though a pronounced eosinophilia and is rather suggestive of a drug reaction, in particular, when lymphocytosis with foamy macrophages and plasma cells of hypersensitivity pneumonitis are present [96]. No convincing results have shown a superiority of BAL on HRCT and pulmonary function in the evaluation of disease severity, prognosis, and treatment response of SSc-ILD. The role of BAL in SSc has been investigated in several studies and fibrotic-related ILD neutrophilia resulted the most prevalent abnormality linked to greater pulmonary function impairment [101]. In earlier studies, BAL neutrophilia seemed related to SSc-ILD worse outcome, but after adjustment for disease severity, BAL neutrophilia had no independent prognostic significance. Bouros et al. [102] reported an increased mortality in SSc-NSIP with lower DLco and higher BAL eosinophils levels at baseline. Indeed, other trials showed no additional value of BAL compared to HRCT and PFTs in predicting disease progression or treatment response to CYC [103–105]. When comparing IPF to SSc-ILD, after adjustment for disease severity, BAL neutrophilia did not differ between these two diseases, making difficult to find a link between BAL neutrophilia and diseases progression [106]. Thus, it appears that in SSc-ILD, BAL neutrophilia is a marker of disease severity [107]. The study results are limited and at present there is insufficient evidence to support the routine use of BAL for SSc prognosis prediction or disease activity evaluation. However, further larger collaborative trials should address BAL usefulness in assessing SSc-ILD.

Many attempts have been made to find in BAL fluid valuable biomarkers for CTD-ILD. The discovery of a biomarker or a combination of biomarkers for the diagnosis, prognosis, treatment response, and ILD endotyping would be of great clinical relevance. To date large prospective studies are lacking and the current evidence comes from retrospective, single center studies. Autoantibodies play a crucial role in CTD-ILD as their presence is related to the pathogenesis of the lung tissue damage, nevertheless their presence in BAL has been poorly investigated, particularly in SSc-ILD. Other biomarkers that are increased in BAL of SSc-ILD include: KL-6 [108], CCL18 [109], CCL2 [110], MMP-9 [111], IL-6, endothelin-1 [112]. The available studies are mainly of serum and a clear correlation with BAL and histopathology is lacking. Many questions about the true pathogenic role of those markers remain unanswered and open a path for future clinical and basic research.

Lung biopsy

The most frequently observed SSc-ILD pathologic patterns are: NSIP 80% (two-thirds are fibrotic), UIP, OP, DAD. Lung biopsy in SSc-ILD shows histological features that are often indistinguishable from those of idiopathic counterparts, except for the presence of pleural fibrosis. NSIP, OP, and DAD differentials include drug toxicity or infections. Coexistent findings may include the presence of microaspiration which is related to esophageal dysmotility. Pulmonary hypertension in 40% of patients: pulmonary arteriopathy, with medial hypertrophy and concentric laminar intimal thickening. Plexiform lesions can be seen and occasionally occlusive venopathy (pulmonary veno-occlusive disease). Preliminary studies suggested that the better prognosis of SSc-ILD could be primarily linked to the high prevalence of NSIP compared to UIP [113,114]. However, subsequent observations showed appreciable differences between idiopathic and SSc-ILD within the same histologic patterns (i.e., different appearance of myofibroblast, lower profusion of fibroblastic foci) and demonstrated also that the better prognosis of SSc-ILD compared to the idiopathic group was not linked solely to the presence of an NSIP pattern. In fact CTD-UIP overall had a better prognosis compared to IPF [113,115,116]. Among those studies, the one with the largest UIP population was that published by Park et al. [115] in 2007 (203 IPF patients, 36 UIP-CTD, 66 idiopathic fibrotic NSIP and 57 CTD-NSIP). Patients with UIP-CTD survived longer than IPF (mean 125.5 months compared to 66.9 months, $P = .001$), with connective tissue disease being an independent factor of better survival in UIP patients by multivariate Cox analysis, along with age and more preserved pulmonary function. Studies focused on histopathologic subsets of SSc patients, and the results of those studies SSc patients (approximately 70% had limited cutaneous SSc in all subgroups) into NSIP (N = 62, of whom 47 were fibrotic) and UIP/ESL (total N = 12: UIP, N = 6/End Stage Lung, N = 6) and found that the outcome was linked more strongly to disease severity at presentation and serial DLco trends rather than to histopathologic findings (five year survival for NSIP was 90% and for UIP/ESL was 82%, $P = .33$). Even, the survival between cellular and fibrotic NSIP did not differ. The authors caution against over-interpretation of their results that were limited by the small number of UIP, mixed with ESL patients, and by the mortality from lung cancer and severe systemic disease that considering overall mortality may have obscured the prognostic distinction between UIP and NSIP. The prognostic distinction between SSc-UIP and SSc-NSIP was found relevant in a study conducted by Fischer at al [117]. that on 22 scleroderma patients (all Scl-70 negative), 14 NSIP (13 fibrotic), and 8 UIP, found a trend toward a significant survival difference, 15.3 years compared to 3 years, respectively, $P = .07$, but on multivariate Cox analysis, histopathological subtypes failed to demonstrate any significant prognostic differences. The small populations and the retrospective design of those studies, along with the heterogeneity of SSc patients and the variable immunosuppressive drug regimens used, make very difficult to extrapolate solid conclusions on the prognostic utility of lung biopsy in SSc-ILD. However, taking into account those negative results and the risks of surgery, LBx in CTD-ILD has been abandoned and recent trials on drug treatment for CTD-ILD, including the recent SENSCIS trial on antifibrotic drugs, relied on the sole clinical-radiological evaluation of cases.

Steps forward should guide the path through a more accurate definition and characterization of CTD-ILD with the intention to explore whether there are subgroups of patients for whom antifibrotics can be more beneficial. In conclusion, the distinction between NSIP and UIP does not seem to carry significant prognostic information. However, those findings have been extrapolated mainly from small studies conducted in the preantifibrotic era, and with a very small prevalence of UIP cases therefore should be interpreted with great caution. Nowadays less invasive biopsy techniques are available, most notably cryobiopsy is overcoming the needs for surgery, allowing to take lung samples with a simple bronchoscopy in an outpatient setting [118]. These less invasive biopsy methods, along with the increased therapeutic armamentarium for SSc-ILD, are motivating physicians and researcher to dive deeper into the submerged ocean of information that LBx can provide. Whether histologic patterns impact SSc-ILD prognosis remains to be proven by larger prospective trials and we hope that the availability of cryobiopsy in many referral centers will allow in the future the design of innovative trials evaluating also histology. To note that, even if the available evidence revolves mainly around the distinction between UIP and not-UIP, histopathology is a precious font of information and the use of more sophisticated technologies rather than traditional hematoxylin-eosin staining could lead in the future to the development of much more accurate theragnostic biomarkers and to a deeper understanding of SSc-ILD pathogenesis.

Screening for ILD

Given the high prevalence and its impact of patients' mortality, it is now widely accepted that all SSc patients should be screened for ILD at time of SSc diagnosis and on a regular basis over time [119]. The frequency of screening should be guided by likelihood of developing ILD combined with new symptoms. Nonetheless an ideal screening protocol for SSc-ILD is yet to be validated. This is why there is still a degree of disagreement on whether CT should be routinely performed in all SSc patients at diagnosis or their use should be reserved for SSc patients with clinical or pulmonary function abnormalities suggestive of SSc-ILD or even if it should be performed in all high-risk individuals (i.e., anti-Scl70 positive patients).

As already stated above, typical respiratory symptoms of ILD include dyspnea, nonproductive cough, and fatigue. However, not all patients experience symptoms related to SSc-ILD regardless of the severity ILD, especially in the early phases of the disease. As a consequence, even in absence of specific respiratory symptoms, further screening for ILD is recommended. The current local and national screening algorithms differ between expert centers and countries; and several different algorithms have been suggested. Here we report the recently published expert consensus recommendations where it was agreed that all SSc patients should be screened with the following tools [70]:

1) LFTs including FVC and DLCO: They should be performed in all new SSc patients to provide baseline parameters and should be repeated regularly as screening in all patients with SSc.
2) HRCT: All patients with SSc should be screened at baseline with HRCT. This is particularly true for patients who belong to the group with an increased risk of SSc-ILD such as patients with anti-Scl70 autoantibody positivity, rapidly progressive dcSSc subset, and with overt respiratory symptoms at baseline. HRCT has been shown to be superior to PFTs in detecting SSc-ILD due to existing mismatches of findings on HRCT and reduced FVC (40). Indeed, among all patients with SSc-ILD, it was found that only 37.5% also had an FVC <80% predicted. Interestingly, even in SSc-ILD patients with >10% fibrosis on HRCT, up to 17% had FVC >100% predicted. This is why in the recently published expert consensus recommendations, a baseline HRCT of the lungs was justified in all SSc patients. It should also be remembered that new techniques have minimized radiation exposure. However, the drawback of HRCT is represented by its high sensitivity that can complicate management. This is the case of patients presenting with very limited abnormalities that will not necessarily evolve to clinical significant ILD.
3) Physical examination: All SSc patients should receive an auscultation as part of their usual evaluation. The presence of inspiratory velcro-like crackles should immediately warrant further tests.
4) Respiratory symptoms: Dyspnea assessed by the New York Heart Association (NYHA) functional class and the presence of cough are fundamental for the early detection of SSc-ILD. However, as already discussed,

these symptoms are not universally present and are not specific for the presence of ILD.

5) Chest X-ray has low sensitivity for ILD and a normal chest X-ray does not exclude the presence of SSc-ILD. The value of chest X-ray at baseline might allow repetition to identify major changes of the development of some comorbidities.

ILD monitoring and progression

LFTs represent the cornerstone of monitoring in patients with SSc-ILD. Similarly to other ILDs, a serial change in FVC is considered the cardinal functional parameter to evaluate the progression of SSc-ILD, thanks to its reproducibility. Conversely, DLCO, which might correlate even better to the extent of SSc-ILD at HRCT at a single time point, is less reliable as it might also be influenced by the development of SSc-PAH and are more variable over time. As already stated above, it is important to evaluate the serial decline over time of both parameters as a decline of FVC paralleled by even a lesser degree of decline of DLCO might be more in keeping with SSc-ILD progression compared to a significant decline in DLCO, paralleled by a lesser or no degree of decline of FVC which might reflect a SSc-PAH development or progression [64].

Follow-up LFT testing is often conducted for follow-up every 3–6 months for the first 3–5 years and thereafter at least once a year [120]. However, monitoring needs to be tailored to the single patient after assessment of all predictive factors (i.e., newly diagnosed, anti-Scl70 positive SSc-ILD patients with signs of inflammation should be monitored every 3–6 months over the first years, while a long-standing ACA positive patient with mild ILD can be monitored on an annual basis). The comparison of LFTs parameters over time (especially with premorbid values) can provide useful information to evaluate the severity of ILD. While no valid definition of SSc-ILD disease progression exists, a decline in FVC relative of $\geq$10%, or an FVC decline of 5%–9% in association with a DLCO decline of $\geq$15% (in a patient with normal proBNP and without SSc-PAH) are the most indicative for suggesting SSc-ILD progression. Nonetheless, there is no validated definition of the threshold for a relevant decline and it should be remembered that an accurate monitoring requires a multimodal assessment and multidisciplinary discussion. For instance, a reduction of FVC between 5% and 10% with a worsening of respiratory symptoms might indicate a true SSc-ILD progression and in this case the monitoring should always be integrated with HRCT, echocardiography, or other evaluations to rule out secondary causes of worsening such as cardiac involvement, SSc-PAH development or progression, infections, and so on.

Based on this, HRCT should be repeated to resolve uncertainties when there is a clinically meaningful decline in LFTs or when patients develop new symptoms that could be attributed to SSc-ILD. No consensus exists on whether HRCT should be repeated for screening purpose [121].

It should also be remembered that the SSc subset is a prognostic factor for patients with SSc-ILD as dcSSc patients are at higher risk for SSc-ILD development and progression compared to lcSSc patients. Moreover, the progression of skin fibrosis within 12 months is associated with decline in FVC and reduced survival in dcSSc patients. Lastly, also laboratory parameters are crucial for the monitoring of SSc-ILD patients. Anti-Scl70 antibody is a prognostic marker for SSc-ILD progression and, especially in the first 3 to 5 years poses the patients at risk of developing severe SSc-ILD. Anti-RNA-polymerase III has also been associated with ILD progression. The only other clinically available laboratory marker of SSc-ILD is represented by C-reactive protein which has been shown to correlate with SSc-ILD prognosis. The two most promising biomarkers of SSc-ILD progression (KL-6 and CCl-18) are currently still investigated [5].

Prognosis

The natural history of ILD in SSc is highly variable as it can span from mild disease with no significant impact on patients' survival or quality of life to rapidly progressing disease leading to respiratory failure and death in few years. It was previously believed that the greatest decline in lung function in SSc-ILD patients occurred early in the course of the disease, and this is still true for the majority of individuals. Nonetheless, it has also become clearer that SSc-ILD patients may also show ILD progression later on in the disease course. Moreover, it has now become evident that the rate of decline can be extremely different as some patients can have a slow decline and other a very rapid disease course [12]. These rapid progressors are a small subgroup of SSc-ILD patients but are critical to be identified and in order to receive early an aggressive treatment and should be monitored very closely for response to therapy and for further ILD progression. Extensive ILD is defined by extension on HRCT >20% of the total lung volume or an HRCT extension >10% but <20% and an FVC threshold of 70% [73]. Patients with extensive disease have an increased likelihood of progression over time. While this definition has been proposed for the introduction of immunosuppressive treatment in patients with SSc-ILD, even in patients with lSSc (<10% on HRCT) there will be progressors who deserve treatment as early as possible. Two other characteristics should then be taken into account to evaluate the need for treatment introduction: (1) disease duration (first 3–4 years); (2) clinical significant pulmonary disease evident within the first 6–12 months; and (3) a decline in FVC and DLCO levels over the first 1–2 years.

Treatment

Cyclophosphamide and mycophenolate mofetil

Immunosuppression represents the cornerstone of treatment in patients with SSc-ILD [122]. Since the first retrospective studies on CYC and/or azathioprine, it emerged that the strategy of targeting the immune system could be effective in SSc-ILD patients. The first studies had though no stringent inclusion criteria and showed that only a minority of patients had a clear benefit from the immunosuppression and this benefit was lost once the treatment was withheld [123]. The first study who clearly paved the way for the use of immunosuppressive drugs in SSc-ILD was the SLS I [19] in which SSc-ILD patients were treated with oral CYC compared to placebo for 12 months. This study demonstrated that oral CYC was effective in terms of FVC, symptoms scores, and radiological quantification of fibrosis in patients with active symptomatic SSc-ILD. Unfortunately, though, CYC treatment was associated with significant adverse events including leukopenia and hematuria. Moreover, it was observed that the benefit of the 12 month of treatment continued to 18 months but dissipated at 24 months suggesting that prolonged immunosuppression was needed in these patients. The toxicity profile of CYC prevented though for a more prolonged use and alternative immunosuppressive drugs were therefore pursued. In the subsequent Fibrosing Alveolitis in Scleroderma Trial (FAST) [124], the design of the SLS I trial was surpassed with the introduction of intravenous monthly CYC for six months followed by oral azathioprine as maintenance therapy. The study failed to demonstrate any statistically significant benefit and only a marginal trend toward FVC improvement was observed in the treatment group with placebo. The intravenous route of administration of CYC was found to be better tolerated compared to the oral one. In 2016 the SLS II [125] showed that MMF was as efficacious as oral CYC for SSc-ILD patients. In this study patients were treated with either two years of MMF at a target dose of 1.500 mg twice daily or with one year of oral CYC. In both arms an improvement in LFTs was observed. The most important finding of the study was that MMF was extremely better tolerated compared to CYC with fewer haematological adverse events. The results of post-hoc analyses performed comparing the MMF-treated group of the SLS II study and the placebo group of the SLS I study further confirmed the efficacy of MMF for the treatment of SSc-ILD and confirmed the role of immunosuppression in these patients [126]. As stated above, the MMF which was found to be effective was 3 gr daily but for patients who struggle to tolerate 3 gr daily, 2 gr daily might be considered. Thanks to the result of this study MMF was identified as the preferred initial treatment for the majority of SSc-ILD patients with CYC (especially the intravenous route) being a reasonable option.

Targeted therapies

The use of the anti-CD20 rituximab (RTX) in SSc-ILD is supported by several retrospective case series and preclinical studies where the role of B cell depletion was shown to be beneficial not only for skin involvement but also for lung involvement in SSc patients [127–129]. Unfortunately, to date, the evidence base for RTX of SSc-ILD is limited due to the absence of significant randomized-controlled trials (RCTs). However, controlled clinical trials are ongoing. In 2018 a cohort study including SSc patients from the European Scleroderma Trials and Research (EUSTAR) network treated with RTX and who were compared to 9575 matched untreated SSc patients and selected using a propensity score matching strategy was published [130]. The study assessed the real-life safety and efficacy profile of RTX in 254 patients because of lung (58%) and skin (32%) involvement. After a median time of two years of follow-up, 70% of RTX-treated patients showed no side effects and no significant rate of decline was observed for % predicted FVC or DLCO. Moreover, a significant higher steroid withdrawal or tapering was found in RTX-treated patients (odds ratio 2.34, $P < .0001$) and a significant better lung outcome was found for ILD patients concomitantly treated with MMF (delta % pFVC 5.22, $P = .019$). More recently, a 24-week, open-label, randomized, controlled trial was performed to compare the efficacy and safety of RTX compared to intravenous CYC in early (<3 years) anti-Scl70 positive dcSSc patients with SSc-ILD. In this study no background immunosuppressive treatment was allowed [131]. The primary endpoint of the study was the change in % predicted FVC, but it also included other secondary endpoints were such as absolute FVC change, 6-minute walking test, and Medsger's score. Sixty patients were randomized to either monthly pulses of CYC 500 mg/m^2 or two infusions of RTX of 1000 mg two weeks apart. At 24 weeks, a significant improvement of the % predicted FVC was observed in the RTX group compared to the CYC (61% to 67% vs. 59% to 58%, respectively, $P = .003$). No significant differences were observed for the other secondary endpoints. Serious adverse events such as pneumonia, premature ovarian failure, and malignancy were more commonly observed in the CYC-treated group. Goswami et al. [132] in a systematic literature review showed that RTX was associated with a significant improvement compared to baseline in FVC of 4.49% at 6 months and of 7.03% at 12 months, whereas DLCO improvement was of 3.47% at 6 months and of 4.08% at 12 months: the safety of RTX in SSc-ILD patients was confirmed as patients were less likely to develop infections compared with controls (odds ratio = 0.256, 95% CI: 0.104, 0.626). The optimal timing for treatment with RTX in SSc-ILD is yet to be defined and in the recent consensus statements for the identification and treatment of SSc-ILD RTX escalation was recommended when treatment with CYC and MMF is not appropriate. Lastly, the use of RTX-biosimilar as a more economic option has been supported by a recent Italian study [133].

Tocilizumab (TCZ) is an interleukin-6 (IL-6) receptor-inhibitor. As already discussed in the pathogenesis section, IL-6 has been deeply implicated in SSc-ILD. In 2016, the first phase two RCT investigating the safety and efficacy of subcutaneous (sc) TCZ in SSc patients was published [134]. Patients with disease duration ≤5 years and with raised inflammatory serum markers were assigned to TCZ 162 mg sc weekly or placebo, without concomitant immunosuppression. The primary endpoint of the study was the change of mRSS and even if the primary endpoint was not met at 24 weeks, a significantly smaller decrease in FVC in the TCZ group compared to placebo was observed (TCZ −34 mL vs. placebo −171 mL; $P = .0368$). The incidence of serious adverse events was similar between the two groups (33% vs. 34%), but the incidence of serious infections was higher in the TCZ group (16% vs. 5%). The results of this trial paved the way to the phase 3 trial focuSSced trial [135]. The trial has similar characteristics (early dcSSC with no concomitant immunosuppression) and even in this case the primary endpoint of the study was the change in the mRSS at week 48. Secondary endpoint of the study was the change in % predicted FVC at week 48 and time to treatment failure, defined as the time from first study drug treatment to the occurrence of the following SSc-related complications: death, decline in FVC>10%, increase in mRSS >20% and mRSS>5, and other predefined SSc-related complications. A total of 212 SSc patients were enrolled. And although the primary endpoint was not met, the cumulative distribution of change in %predicted FVC favored TCZ compared to placebo (−3.9 vs. −0.6, $P = .0015$) and the mean difference in FVC change from baseline was 167 mL in favor of TCZ. Adverse events and serious adverse events were similar between the two groups. A post-hoc analysis was then performed, stratifying treatments arms according to the degree of lung involvement evaluated as quantitative ILD and fibrosis scores assessed by computer software [136]. Patients participating to the focuSSced trial were then classified into the following categories: mild (>5%−10%), moderate (>10%−20%), and severe (>20%). The results of the analysis showed that TCZ-treated patients had a preservation of % predicted FVC over the 48 weeks of the study compared to placebo (−0.1% vs. −6.3%). More specifically for mild QILD at 48 weeks, the mean change in % predicted FVC was −4.1 ± 2.5% versus 10.0 ± 2.6%, for moderate QILD it was 0.7 ± 1.9% versus −5.7 ± 1.6%, and for severe QILD it was 2.1 ± 1.6% versus −6.7 ± 2.0%. TCZ was therefore shown to preserve lung function especially in severe SSc-ILD patients. The placing of TCZ and its use in combination with other immunosuppressive drugs is yet to be identified.

Abatacept (ABT) is recombinant fusion protein that binds to CD80 and CD86 thus preventing T cell co-stimulation by CD28. The use of ABT in SSc-ILD patients is quite recent and only partially supported by retrospective and prospective data. In a recent EUSTAR retrospective study on 15 SSc-ILD patients, no change in lung function was observed [137]. The results of a 12-month, phase two RCT on ABT in dcSSc patients was published in 2020

[138] and the subsequent open-label 6-month extension phase was recently published [139]. As the primary endpoint of the study was the change in the mRSS, the cohort of patients was not selected for SSc-ILD. Patients were randomized to ABT 125 mg weekly sc or placebo and even in this study no background immunosuppression was allowed. At 12 months % predicted FVC declined compared to baseline value in both groups during the double-blind trial ($-2.7 \pm 5.5\%$ in the ABT group vs. $1.6 \pm 8.0\%$ in the placebo group). However, during the open-label extension, both treatment groups had improvements in % predicted FVC so that the mean change from baseline to month 18 was small ($-0.3 \pm 6.3\%$ in the placebo–ABT group vs. $0.9 \pm 9.9\%$ in the ABT–ABT group). Moreover, a minimal clinically important difference for % predicted FVC (>3%) was observed at 12 months in 19% of ABT patients and 16% of placebo patients. These percentages increased to 30% in the placebo–ABT group and 28% in the ABT-ABT group at 18 months.

Antifibrotic therapies

Pirfenidone (PRF) is a synthetic antifibrotic agent already approved by the FDA for the treatment of patients with IPF. In vitro studies have shown that PRF could be of benefit in patients with SSc-ILD as it can inhibit myofibroblast differentiation blocking TGF-β and STAT-3 activation [140]. A phase II open-label, 16-week trial investigated the safety and efficacy of PFR in SSc-ILD patients randomized to either a two- or four-week PRF titration starting at 801 mg daily and titrating up to 2403 mg daily maintenance dose (LOTUSS trial) or placebo [141]. In this study the use of concomitant immunosuppressive therapy was allowed. Patients included in the study needed to have a disease duration <7 years, a % predicted FVC >50%, and a DLCO >40%. In this study no change in disease outcomes was observed but the drug was globally well tolerated in SSc-ILD patients especially in patients treated with four-week titration scheme. This study paved the way to the ongoing SLS III where PRF is used in combination with MMF (clinicaltrials.gov NCT03221257).

Nintedanib (NTB) is a multi-tyrosine kinase inhibitor which blocks FGF receptor-1, VEGF receptor-2, and PDGF receptor-α and β52 [142]. Preclinical models of SSc-ILD had already shown a significant potential as an antifibrotic and antiinflammatory agent [143]. NTB was approved for the treatment of idiopathic pulmonary fibrosis in 2014 and has become the only treatment approved for the treatment of SSc-ILD after the publication of an RCT in SSc-ILD [144]. In the SENSCIS trial, patients with a disease duration <7 years, regardless of their disease subset, but with a SSc-ILD >10% as assessed by HRCT were enrolled to oral NTB 150 mg twice a day or placebo. In this case, concomitant immunosuppression was allowed. The primary endpoint of the study was the annual rate of decline in FVC. SENSCIS trial has been so far the one with highest number of SSc patients enrolled (576 patients). Of these, 52%

of patients were dcSSc and 48% were on stable MMF therapy at baseline. Over the study period, the adjusted annual rate of change in FVC was significantly lower in the NTB group compared to the placebo group (−52 mL/year vs. −93 mL/year, $P = .04$). Of note, as the primary endpoint of the study was the annual rate of decline in FVC, both lcSSc (with low mRSS) and dcSSc patients were included in the study. No subgroup was identified as better responders although the combination of MMF plus NTB was observed as the best scenario for the prevention of decline. The most common adverse event reported, experienced by 76% of patients was diarrhea which was usually mild with transient reduction of NTB dose and/or the use of anti-diarrheic drugs. This study led to the approval of NTB for the treatment of SSc-ILD by the FDA in 2019 and EMA in April 2020.

Haematopoietic Stem cell transplantation

Haematopoietic stem cell transplantation (HSCT) has also been attempted in patients with SSc and post-hoc analysis have tried to evaluate a role for SCT in SSc-ILD patients. The American Scleroderma Stem Cell versus Immunosuppression Trial (ASSIST) [145], the Autologous Stem Cell Transplantation International Scleroderma (ASTIS) [146] trial, and the Scleroderma Cyclophosphamide or Transplantation (SCOT) [147] trial have all compared HSCT to intravenous CYC in SSc patients. In all three studies, it was observed that HSCT was superior to CYC alone in FVC and mRSS improvement. In ASSIST it was observed that improvement in FVC with HSCT was also evident in SSc-ILD patients who progressed despite initial CYC treatment. Whereas in the SCOT trial, which was designed with a focus on ILD, a significant decrease in lung fibrosis evaluated at computer-assisted quantitative CT analysis was observed, suggesting that HSCT could actually reserve lung fibrosis in some patients. Nonetheless, given the toxicity associated with HSCT, this option remains a major undertaking. Patient selection, conditioning regimens, and timing are critical determinants of prognosis and mortality post-HSCT [148].

COVID-19 and systemic sclerosis

There is still a paucity of data about the prognosis of COVID-19 in SSc patients and how COVID-19-related interstitial lung involvement can be differentiated from SSc-related ILD involvement [149]. The biggest cohort of SSc patients with COVID-19 patients published so far derives from a cohort of Italian patients [150]. In this retrospective study, a total of 14 patients with definite SARS-CoV-2 infection and 47 patients with highly suspected infection were described. Clinically mild-to-moderate COVID-19 manifestations were observed in the majority of cases and only 15% of patients required hospital admission for respiratory symptoms. Four of these patients died and all were older than 80 years. More recently, an EUSTAR study performed among

European SSc patients who got COVID-19 [151] shown that among clinical features older age, SSc-related renal disease, and ILD are risk factors for severe outcome. Interestingly a case of rapid SSc progression was also reported in a young woman after SARS-CoV-2 infection [152]. Longer follow-up is needed to clearly identify the risk of future relapses in SSc patients and the residual lung damage in those affected by ILD.

Summary

ILD involvement is a major SSc challenge and it still represents the leading cause of death in SSc patients. Nonetheless, thanks to both retrospective and prospective studies, over the last years our knowledge about SSc-ILD has significantly improved and nowadays we have a clearer idea on which SSc-specific features can be associated with ILD involvement, ILD severity, and progression. HRCT represents the imaging modality of choice for assessing ILD involvement while LFTs are deemed crucial for follow-up evaluations. International collaborative studies have also paved the way for a standardized approach toward SSc-ILD patients for both early diagnosis and follow-up. The last years have represented a turning point for what concerns the treatment of SSc-ILD patients as two placebo-controlled RCTs specifically assessing the use of targeted therapies (tocilizumab and NTB) in SSc-ILD patients have been published. As a result, NTB, a multi-tyrosine kinase inhibitor has been the first drug approved by the FDA and the EMA for the treatment of SSc-ILD patients. It is a rapidly evolving and exciting time for SSc-ILD and physicians who look after SSc patients should more than ever be updated to be able to correctly manage their patients.

Take-home messages

- SSc-ILD is the leading cause of death in SSc patients
- A number of SSc-specific features are associated with ILD involvement
- HRCT is the imaging modality of choice for assessing ILD involvement in SSc
- LFTs are fundamental for SSc-ILS patients' follow-up
- Targeted therapies including tocilizumab and NTB have been shown to positively impact on SSc-ILD progression.

References

[1] Denton CP, Khanna D. Systemic sclerosis. Lancet 2017. https://doi.org/10.1016/S0140-6736(17)30933-9.

[2] Hao Y, et al. Early mortality in a multinational systemic sclerosis inception cohort. Arthritis Rheum 2017;69:1067–77.

[3] Steen VD, Medsger TA. Changes in causes of death in systemic sclerosis, 1972–2002. Ann Rheum Dis 2007;66:940–4.

[4] Allanore Y, et al. Systemic sclerosis. Nat Rev Dis Prim 2015. https://doi.org/10.1038/nrdp.2015.2.

[5] Denton CP, Wells AU, Coghlan JG. Major lung complications of systemic sclerosis. Nat Rev Rheumatol 2018;14:511–27.

[6] van den Hoogen F, et al. 2013 classification criteria for systemic sclerosis: an American college of rheumatology/European league against rheumatism collaborative initiative. Ann Rheum Dis 2013;72:1747–55.

[7] Denton CP. Advances in pathogenesis and treatment of systemic sclerosis. Clin Med 2015;15:s58–63.

[8] Distler O, Volkmann ER, Hoffmann-Vold AM, Maher TM. Current and future perspectives on management of systemic sclerosis-associated interstitial lung disease. Expet Rev Clin Immunol 2019;15:1009–17.

[9] Nihtyanova SI, Denton CP. Scleroderma lung involvement, autoantibodies, and outcome prediction: the confounding effect of time. J Rheumatol 2017;44:404–6.

[10] Mackintosh JA, Stainer A, Barnett JL, Renzoni EA. Systemic sclerosis associated interstitial lung disease: a comprehensive overview. Semin Respir Crit Care Med 2019;40:208–26.

[11] Dougherty DH, et al. The scleroderma patient-centered intervention network cohort: baseline clinical features and comparison with other large scleroderma cohorts. Rheumatology 2018;57:1623–31.

[12] Nihtyanova SI, et al. Prediction of pulmonary complications and long-term survival in systemic sclerosis. Arthritis Rheum 2014;66:1625–35.

[13] Nihtyanova SI, et al. Using autoantibodies and cutaneous subset to develop outcome-based disease classification in systemic sclerosis. Arthritis Rheum 2020;72:465–76.

[14] Mitri GM, Lucas M, Fertig N, Steen VD, Medsger TA. A comparison between anti-TH/To- and anticentromere antibody-positive systemic sclerosis patients with limited cutaneous involvement. Arthritis Rheum 2003;48:203–9.

[15] Lazzaroni M-G, et al. The clinical phenotype of systemic sclerosis patients with anti-PM/Scl antibodies: results from the EUSTAR cohort. Rheumatology 2021. https://doi.org/10.1093/rheumatology/keab152.

[16] Tall F, et al. The clinical relevance of antifibrillarin (anti-U3-RNP) autoantibodies in systemic sclerosis. Scand J Immunol 2017;85:73–9.

[17] Aggarwal R, Lucas M, Fertig N, Oddis CV, Medsger TA. Anti-U3 RNP autoantibodies in systemic sclerosis. Arthritis Rheum 2009;60:1112–8.

[18] Cottin V, Brown KK. Interstitial lung disease associated with systemic sclerosis (SSc-ILD). Respir Res 2019;20.

[19] Tashkin DP, et al. Cyclophosphamide versus placebo in scleroderma lung disease. N Engl J Med 2006;354:2655–66.

[20] Furst DE, et al. Adverse events during the scleroderma lung study. Am J Med 2011;124:459–67.

[21] Winstone TA, et al. Predictors of mortality and progression in scleroderma-associated interstitial lung disease: a systematic review. Chest 2014;146:422–36.

[22] Moore DF, Kramer E, Eltaraboulsi R, Steen VD. Increased morbidity and mortality of scleroderma in African Americans compared to non–African Americans. Arthritis Care Res 2019;71:1154–63.

[23] Gelber AC, et al. Race and association with disease manifestations and mortality in scleroderma: a 20-year experience at the johns hopkins scleroderma center and review of the literature. Medicine 2013;92:191–205.

[24] Morrisroe K, et al. Validity of the workers productivity and activity impairment questionnaire: specific health problem (WPAI:SHP) in patients with systemic sclerosis. Clin Exp Rheumatol 2017;35:S130–7.

[25] Hachulla E, et al. Early detection of pulmonary arterial hypertension in systemic sclerosis: a French nationwide prospective multicenter study. Arthritis Rheum 2005;52:3792–800.

[26] Hinz B, et al. Recent developments in myofibroblast biology: paradigms for connective tissue remodeling. Am J Pathol 2012;180:1340–55.

[27] Nihtyanova SI, Denton CP. Pathogenesis of systemic sclerosis associated interstitial lung disease. J Scleroderma and Relat Disord 2020;5:6–16. https://doi.org/10.1177/2397198320903867.

[28] Silver RM, Feghali-Bostwick CA. Molecular insights into systemic sclerosis-associated interstitial lung disease. Arthritis Rheum 2014;66:485–7.

[29] Denton CP. Systemic sclerosis: from pathogenesis to targeted therapy. Clin Exp Rheumatol 2015;33:3–7.

[30] Hsu E, et al. Lung tissues in patients with systemic sclerosis have gene expression patterns unique to pulmonary fibrosis and pulmonary hypertension. Arthritis Rheum 2011;63:783–94.

[31] Fonseca C, et al. A polymorphism in the CTGF promoter region associated with systemic sclerosis. N Engl J Med 2007;357:1210–20.

[32] De Lauretis A, et al. Serum interleukin 6 is predictive of early functional decline and mortality in interstitial lung disease associated with systemic sclerosis. J Rheumatol 2013;40:435–46.

[33] Cénit MC, et al. Influence of the IL6 gene in susceptibility to systemic sclerosis. J Rheumatol 2012;39:2294–302.

[34] Rueda B, et al. A large multicentre analysis of CTGF -945 promoter polymorphism does not confirm association with systemic sclerosis susceptibility or phenotype. Ann Rheum Dis 2009;68:1618–20.

[35] Kawaguchi Y, et al. Association study of a polymorphism of the CTGF gene and susceptibility to systemic sclerosis in the Japanese population. Ann Rheum Dis 2009;68:1921–4.

[36] Christmann RB, et al. miR-155 in the progression of lung fibrosis in systemic sclerosis. Arthritis Res Ther 2016;18.

[37] Scleroderma lung fibroblasts exhibit elevated and dysregulated type I collagen biosynthesis. Arthritis Rheum 1997;40. https://pubmed.ncbi.nlm.nih.gov/9214423/.

[38] Shi-wen X, et al. Endothelin is a downstream mediator of profibrotic responses to transforming growth factor β in human lung fibroblasts. Arthritis Rheum 2007;56:4189–94.

[39] Liu F, et al. Mechanosignaling through YAP and TAZ drives fibroblast activation and fibrosis. Am J Physiol Lung Cell Mol Physiol 2015;308:L344–57.

[40] Shi-Wen X, et al. Endogenous endothelin-1 signaling contributes to type I collagen and CCN2 overexpression in fibrotic fibroblasts. Matrix Biol 2007;26:625–32.

[41] Gilbane AJ, Denton CP, Holmes AM. Scleroderma pathogenesis: a pivotal role for fibroblasts as effector cells. Arthritis Res Ther 2013;15.

[42] Manetti M, et al. Endothelial-to-mesenchymal transition contributes to endothelial dysfunction and dermal fibrosis in systemic sclerosis. Ann Rheum Dis 2017;76:924–34.

[43] Mendoza FA, Piera-Velazquez S, Farber JL, Feghali-Bostwick C, Jiménez SA. Endothelial cells expressing endothelial and mesenchymal cell gene products in lung tissue from patients with systemic sclerosis-associated interstitial lung disease. Arthritis Rheum 2016;68:210–7.

[44] Wu M, et al. CCL2 in the circulation predicts long-term progression of interstitial lung disease in patients with early systemic sclerosis: data from two independent cohorts. Arthritis Rheum 2017;69:1871–8.

[45] van Bon L, et al. Proteome-wide analysis and CXCL4 as a biomarker in systemic sclerosis. N Engl J Med 2014;370:433–43.

[46] Richardson C, et al. Esophageal dilatation and interstitial lung disease in systemic sclerosis: a cross-sectional study. Semin Arthritis Rheum 2016;46:109–14.

[47] Denton CP, et al. Fibroblast-specific expression of a kinase-deficient type II transforming growth factor β (TGFβ) receptor leads to paradoxical activation of TGFβ signaling pathways with fibrosis in transgenic mice. J Biol Chem 2003;278:25109–19.

[48] Goh NSL, et al. Increased epithelial permeability in pulmonary fibrosis in relation to disease progression. Eur Respir J 2011;38:184–90.

[49] Henderson NC, et al. Targeting of αv integrin identifies a core molecular pathway that regulates fibrosis in several organs. Nat Med 2013;19:1617–24.

[50] Sonnylal S, et al. Postnatal induction of transforming growth factor β signaling in fibroblasts of mice recapitulates clinical, histologic, and biochemical features of scleroderma. Arthritis Rheum 2007;56:334–44.

[51] Hoyles RK, et al. An essential role for resident fibroblasts in experimental lung fibrosis is defined by lineage-specific deletion of high-affinity type II transforming growth factor β receptor. Am J Respir Crit Care Med 2011;183:249–61.

[52] Hoyles RK, et al. Fibroblast-specific perturbation of transforming growth factor β signaling provides insight into potential pathogenic mechanisms of scleroderma-associated lung fibrosis: exaggerated response to alveolar epithelial injury in a novel mouse model. Arthritis Rheum 2008;58:1175–88.

[53] Denton CP, et al. Activation of key profibrotic mechanisms in transgenic fibroblasts expressing kinase-deficient type II transforming growth factor-β receptor (TβRIIΔk). J Biol Chem 2005;280:16053–65.

[54] Taroni JN, et al. A novel multi-network approach reveals tissue-specific cellular modulators of fibrosis in systemic sclerosis. Genome Med 2017;9.

[55] Hemnes AR, Humbert M. Pathobiology of pulmonary arterial hypertension: understanding the roads less travelled. Eur Respir Rev 2017;26.

[56] Gilbane AJ, et al. Impaired bone morphogenetic protein receptor II signaling in a transforming growth factor-β-dependent mouse model of pulmonary hypertension and in systemic sclerosis. Am J Respir Crit Care Med 2015;191:665–77.

[57] Davies RJ, et al. BMP type II receptor deficiency confers resistance to growth inhibition by TGF-β in pulmonary artery smooth muscle cells: role of proinflammatory cytokines. Am J Physiol - Lung Cell Mol Physiol 2012;302.

[58] Good RB, et al. Endothelial to mesenchymal transition contributes to endothelial dysfunction in pulmonary arterial hypertension. Am J Pathol 2015;185:1850–8.

[59] Garcia-Rivas G, Jerjes-Sánchez C, Rodriguez D, Garcia-Pelaez J, Trevino V. A systematic review of genetic mutations in pulmonary arterial hypertension. BMC Med Genet 2017;18.

[60] Wells AU, Denton CP. Interstitial lung disease in connective tissue disease - mechanisms and management. Nat Rev Rheumatol 2014;10:728–39.

[61] Wells A, Devaraj A, Renzoni EA, Denton CP. Multidisciplinary evaluation in patients with lung disease associated with connective tissue disease. Semin Respir Crit Care Med 2019;40:184–93.
[62] Cottin V, Cordier JF. Velcro crackles: the key for early diagnosis of idiopathic pulmonary fibrosis? Eur Respir J 2012;40:519–21.
[63] Fayed H, Coghlan JG. Pulmonary hypertension associated with connective tissue disease. Semin Respir Crit Care Med 2019;40:173–83.
[64] Wells AU, et al. Fibrosing alveolitis in systemic sclerosis: indices of lung function in relation to extent of disease on computed tomography. Arthritis Rheum 1997;40:1229–36.
[65] Antoniou KM, Wells AU. Scleroderma lung disease: evolving understanding in light of newer studies. Curr Opin Rheumatol 2008;20:686–91.
[66] Seibold JR, et al. Safety and tolerability of nintedanib in patients with systemic sclerosis-associated interstitial lung disease: data from the SENSCIS trial. Ann Rheum Dis 2020;79:1478–84.
[67] Ya S, et al. Brief report: pulmonary function tests: high rate of false-negative results in the early detection and screening of scleroderma-related interstitial lung disease. Arthritis Rheum 2015;67:3256–61.
[68] A P, et al. High resolution computed tomography in systemic sclerosis. Real diagnostic utilities in the assessment of pulmonary involvement and comparison with other modalities of lung investigation. Clin Rheumatol 1992;11:465–72.
[69] van den H. F, et al. 2013 classification criteria for systemic sclerosis: an American College of Rheumatology/European League against rheumatism collaborative initiative. Arthritis Rheum 2013;65:2737–47.
[70] Hoffmann-Vold AM, et al. The identification and management of interstitial lung disease in systemic sclerosis: evidence-based European consensus statements. Lancet Rheum 2020;2:e71–83.
[71] Bernstein EJ, et al. Screening high-resolution computed tomography of the chest to detect interstitial lung disease in systemic sclerosis: a global survey of rheumatologists. Arthritis Rheum 2018;70:971–2.
[72] Desai SR, et al. CT features of lung disease in patients with systemic sclerosis: comparison with idiopathic pulmonary fibrosis and nonspecific interstitial pneumonia. Radiology 2004;232:560–7.
[73] Goh NSL, et al. Interstitial lung disease in systemic sclerosis: a simple staging system. Am J Respir Crit Care Med 2008;177:57–9.
[74] Kim GHJ, et al. Using transitional changes on high-resolution computed tomography to monitor the impact of cyclophosphamide or mycophenolate mofetil on systemic sclerosis-related interstitial lung disease. Arthritis Rheum 2020;72:316–25.
[75] Jhajj A, et al. Pulmonary physiology is poorly associated with radiological extent of disease in systemic sclerosis-associated interstitial lung disease. Eur Respir J 2019;53.
[76] Saldana DC, et al. Association of computed tomography densitometry with disease severity, functional decline, and survival in systemic sclerosis-associated interstitial lung disease. Ann Am Thorac Soc 2020;17:813–20.
[77] Goldin JG, et al. Longitudinal changes in quantitative interstitial lung disease on computed tomography after immunosuppression in the scleroderma lung study II. Ann Am Thorac Soc 2018;15:1286–95.
[78] Ariani A, et al. Quantitative chest computed tomography is associated with two prediction models of mortality in interstitial lung disease related to systemic sclerosis. Rheumatology 2017;56:922–7.

[79] Occhipinti M, et al. Quantitative analysis of pulmonary vasculature in systemic sclerosis at spirometry-gated chest CT. Ann Rheum Dis 2020;79:1210–7.
[80] Jacob J, et al. Predicting outcomes in rheumatoid arthritis related interstitial lung disease. Eur Respir J 2019;53.
[81] Picano E, et al. Rheumatological diseases and cancer: the hidden variable of radiation exposure. Ann Rheum Dis 2014;73:2065–8.
[82] Frauenfelder T, et al. Screening for interstitial lung disease in systemic sclerosis: performance of high-resolution CT with limited number of slices: a prospective study. Ann Rheum Dis 2014;73:2069–73.
[83] Hughes M, et al. The role of ultrasound in systemic sclerosis: on the cutting edge to foster clinical and research advancement. J Scleroderma Relat Disord 2020. https://doi.org/10.1177/2397198320970394.
[84] Barskova T, et al. Lung ultrasound for the screening of interstitial lung disease in very early systemic sclerosis. Ann Rheum Dis 2013;72:390–5.
[85] Hassan RI, et al. Lung ultrasound as a screening method for interstitial lung disease in patients with systemic sclerosis. J Clin Rheumatol 2019;25:304–7.
[86] Gargani G, et al. Ultrasound lung comets in systemic sclerosis: a chest sonography hallmark of pulmonary interstitial fibrosis. Rheumatology 2009;48:1382–7.
[87] Gutierrez M, et al. Utility of a simplified ultrasound assessment to assess interstitial pulmonary fibrosis in connective tissue disorders—preliminary results. Arthritis Res Ther 2011;13.
[88] Gargani L, et al. Prognostic value of lung ultrasound B-lines in systemic sclerosis. Chest 2020;158:1515–25.
[89] Romei C, et al. The use of chest magnetic resonance imaging in interstitial lung disease: a systematic review. Eur Respir Rev 2018;27.
[90] de Souza Müller C, et al. Pulmonary magnetic resonance imaging is similar to chest tomography in detecting inflammation in patients with systemic sclerosis. Rev Bras Reumatol 2017;57:419–24.
[91] Gargani L, et al. Lung magnetic resonance imaging in systemic sclerosis: a new promising approach to evaluate pulmonary involvement and progression. Clin Rheumatol 2021;40:1903–12.
[92] Ledoult E, et al. 18 F-FDG positron emission tomography scanning in systemic sclerosis-associated interstitial lung disease: a pilot study. Arthritis Res Ther 2021;23.
[93] Bellando-Randone S, et al. 18F-fluorodeoxyglucose positron-emission tomography/CT and lung involvement in systemic sclerosis. Ann Rheum Dis 2019;78:577–8.
[94] Peelen DM, et al. The quantitative assessment of interstitial lung disease with positron emission tomography scanning in systemic sclerosis patients. Rheumatology 2020;59:1407–15.
[95] Broens B, Zwezerijnen BGJC, van der Laken CJ, Voskuyl AE. Quantification of 68Ga-FAPI-04 in systemic sclerosis-associated interstitial lung disease. Lancet Rheum 2021;3:e475.
[96] Costabel U, Uzaslan E, Guzman J. Bronchoalveolar lavage in drug-induced lung disease. Clin Chest Med 2004;25:25–35.
[97] Molyneaux PL, et al. BAL is safe and well tolerated in individuals with idiopathic pulmonary fibrosis: an analysis of the PROFILE study. Am J Respir Crit Care Med 2021;203:136–9.

[98] Sun XF, Liu YJ, Xiao Y, Xu WB. Role of bronchoalveolar lavage for diagnosing pulmonary infection in patients with rheumatic autoimmune diseases and lung infiltrates. J Clin Rheumatol 2014;20:369–72.
[99] Hetzel J, et al. Transbronchial cryobiopsy increases diagnostic confidence in interstitial lung disease: a prospective multicentre trial. Eur Respir J 2020;56.
[100] Tomassetti S, et al. Bronchoscopic lung cryobiopsy increases diagnostic confidence in the multidisciplinary diagnosis of idiopathic pulmonary fibrosis. Am J Respir Crit Care Med 2016;193:745–52.
[101] Goh NSL, et al. Bronchoalveolar lavage cellular profiles in patients with systemic sclerosis-associated interstitial lung disease are not predictive of disease progression. Arthritis Rheum 2007;56:2005–12.
[102] Bouros D, et al. Histopathologic subsets of fibrosing alveolitis in patients with systemic sclerosis and their relationship to outcome. Am J Respir Crit Care Med 2002;165:1581–6.
[103] Strange C, et al. Bronchoalveolar lavage and response to cyclophosphamide in scleroderma interstitial lung disease. Am J Respir Crit Care Med 2008;177:91–8.
[104] Tashkin DP, et al. Effects of 1-year treatment with cyclophosphamide on outcomes at 2 years in scleroderma lung disease. Am J Respir Crit Care Med 2007;176:1026–34.
[105] Antoniu SA. Cyclophosphamide for scleroderma interstitial lung disease. Expet Opin Invest Drugs 2007;16:393–5.
[106] Wells AU, et al. Bronchoalveolar lavage cellularity: lone cryptogenic fibrosing alveolitis compared with the fibrosing alveolitis of systemic sclerosis. Am J Respir Crit Care Med 1998;157:1474–82.
[107] Wells AU. The clinical utility of bronchoalveolar lavage in diffuse parenchymal lung disease. Eur Respir Rev 2010;19:237–41.
[108] Zhu C, Zhao YB, Kong LF, Li ZH, Kang J. The expression and clinical role of KL-6 in serum and BALF of patients with different diffuse interstitial lung diseases. Zhonghua Jiehe He Huxi Zazhi 2016;39:93–7.
[109] Prasse A, et al. CCL18 as an indicator of pulmonary fibrotic activity in idiopathic interstitial pneumonias and systemic sclerosis. Arthritis Rheum 2007;56:1685–93.
[110] Schmidt K, et al. Bronchoalveoloar lavage fluid cytokines and chemokines as markers and predictors for the outcome of interstitial lung disease in systemic sclerosis patients. Arthritis Res Ther 2009;11.
[111] Andersen GN, et al. Bronchoalveolar matrix metalloproteinase 9 relates to restrictive lung function impairment in systemic sclerosis. Respir Med 2007;101:2199–206.
[112] Nielepkowicz-Goździńska A, et al. Exhaled cytokines in systemic lupus erythematosus with lung involvement. Pol Arch Med Wewn 2013;123:141–8.
[113] Flaherty KR, et al. Fibroblastic foci in usual interstitial pneumonia: idiopathic versus collagen vascular disease. Am J Respir Crit Care Med 2003;167:1410–5.
[114] Wells AU, et al. Fibrosing alveolitis associated with systemic sclerosis has a better prognosis than lone cryptogenic fibrosing alveolitis. Am J Respir Crit Care Med 1994;149:1583–90.
[115] Joo HP, et al. Prognosis of fibrotic interstitial pneumonia: idiopathic versus collagen vascular disease-related subtypes. Am J Respir Crit Care Med 2007;175:705–11.
[116] Yoshinouchi T, Ohtsuki Y, Ueda R, Sato S, Ueda N. Myofibroblasts and S-100 protein positive cells in idiopathic pulmonary fibrosis and rheumatoid arthritis-associated interstitial pneumonia. Eur Respir J 1999;14:579–84.
[117] Fischer A, et al. Clinically significant interstitial lung disease in limited scleroderma: histopathology, clinical features, and survival. Chest 2008;134:601–5.

[118] Hunninghake GM, et al. Detection and early referral of patients with interstitial lung abnormalities: an expert survey initiative. Chest 2021. https://doi.org/10.1016/j.chest.2021.06.035.

[119] Paschalaki KE, et al. Monitoring of lung involvement in rheumatologic disease. Respiration 2016;91:89–98.

[120] Volkmann ER. Natural history of systemic sclerosis-related interstitial lung disease: how to identify a progressive fibrosing phenotype. J Scleroderma Relat Disord 2020;5.

[121] Hoffmann-Vold AM, et al. Setting the international standard for longitudinal follow-up of patients with systemic sclerosis: a Delphi-based expert consensus on core clinical features. RMD Open 2019;5.

[122] Roofeh D, Distler O, Allanore Y, Denton CP, Khanna D. Treatment of systemic sclerosis–associated interstitial lung disease: lessons from clinical trials. J Scleroderma Relat Disord 2020;5:61–71. https://doi.org/10.1177/2397198320903208.

[123] Barnes H, Holland AE, Westall GP, Goh NS, Glaspole IN. Cyclophosphamide for connective tissue disease–associated interstitial lung disease. Cochrane Database Syst Rev 2018;2018.

[124] Hoyles RK, et al. A multicenter, prospective, randomized, double-blind, placebo-controlled trial of corticosteroids and intravenous cyclophosphamide followed by oral azathioprine for the treatment of pulmonary fibrosis in scleroderma. Arthritis Rheum 2006;54:3962–70.

[125] Tashkin DP, et al. Mycophenolate mofetil versus oral cyclophosphamide in scleroderma-related interstitial lung disease (SLS II): a randomised controlled, double-blind, parallel group trial. Lancet Respir Med 2016;4:708–19.

[126] Volkmann ER, et al. Mycophenolate mofetil versus placebo for systemic sclerosis-related interstitial lung disease: an analysis of scleroderma lung studies I and II. Arthritis Rheum 2017;69:1451–60.

[127] Daoussis D, et al. Experience with rituximab in scleroderma: results from a 1-year, proof-of-principle study. Rheumatology 2010;49:271–80.

[128] Keir GJ, et al. Rituximab in severe, treatment-refractory interstitial lung disease. Respirology 2014;19:353–9.

[129] Campochiaro C, Allanore Y. An update on targeted therapies in systemic sclerosis based on a systematic review from the last 3 years. Arthritis Res Ther 2021;23:155.

[130] Elhai M, et al. Outcomes of patients with systemic sclerosis treated with rituximab in contemporary practice: a prospective cohort study. Ann Rheum Dis 2019;78:979–87.

[131] Geetabali S, Rudra Prosad G, Dipankar S, Alakendu G, Parasar G. Intravenous cyclophosphamide vs rituximab for the treatment of early diffuse scleroderma lung disease: open label, randomized, controlled trial. Rheumatology 2018;57:2106–13.

[132] Goswami RP, et al. Rituximab in the treatment of systemic sclerosis-related interstitial lung disease: a systematic review and meta-analysis. Rheumatology 2021;60:557–67.

[133] Campochiaro C, et al. Safety and efficacy of rituximab biosimilar (CT-P10) in systemic sclerosis: an Italian multicentre study. Rheumatology 2020;59:3731–6.

[134] Khanna D, et al. Safety and efficacy of subcutaneous tocilizumab in adults with systemic sclerosis (faSScinate): a phase 2, randomised, controlled trial. Lancet 2016;387:2630–40.

[135] Khanna D, et al. Tocilizumab in systemic sclerosis: a randomised, double-blind, placebo-controlled, phase 3 trial. Lancet Respir Med 2020;8:963–74.

[136] Roofeh D, et al. Tocilizumab prevents progression of early systemic sclerosis-associated interstitial lung disease. Arthritis Rheum 2021;73.

[137] Castellví I, et al. Safety and effectiveness of abatacept in systemic sclerosis: the EUSTAR experience. Semin Arthritis Rheum 2020;50:1489–93.

[138] Khanna D, et al. Abatacept in early diffuse cutaneous systemic sclerosis: results of a phase II investigator-initiated, multicenter, double-blind, randomized, placebo-controlled trial. Arthritis Rheum 2020;72:125–36.

[139] Chung L, et al. Safety and efficacy of abatacept in early diffuse cutaneous systemic sclerosis (ASSET): open-label extension of a phase 2, double-blind randomised trial. Lancet Rheum 2020;2:e743–53.

[140] Xiao H, et al. Anti-fibrotic effects of pirfenidone by interference with the hedgehog signalling pathway in patients with systemic sclerosis-associated interstitial lung disease. Int J Rheum Dis 2018;21:477–86.

[141] Khanna D, et al. An open-label, phase II study of the safety and tolerability of pirfenidone in patients with scleroderma-associated interstitial lung disease: the LOTUSS trial. J Rheumatol 2016;43:1672–9.

[142] Huang J, et al. Nintedanib inhibits macrophage activation and ameliorates vascular and fibrotic manifestations in the Fra2 mouse model of systemic sclerosis. Ann Rheum Dis 2017;76:1941–8.

[143] Huang J, et al. Nintedanib inhibits fibroblast activation and ameliorates fibrosis in preclinical models of systemic sclerosis. Ann Rheum Dis 2016;75:883–90.

[144] Distler O, et al. Nintedanib for systemic sclerosis-associated interstitial lung disease. N Engl J Med 2019;380:2518–28.

[145] Burt RK, et al. Autologous non-myeloablative haemopoietic stem-cell transplantation compared with pulse cyclophosphamide once per month for systemic sclerosis (ASSIST): an open-label, randomised phase 2 trial. Lancet 2011;378:498–506.

[146] van Laar JM, et al. Autologous hematopoietic stem cell transplantation vs intravenous pulse cyclophosphamide in diffuse cutaneous systemic sclerosis: a randomized clinical trial. J Am Med Assoc 2014;311:2490–8.

[147] Sullivan KM, et al. Myeloablative autologous stem-cell transplantation for severe scleroderma. N Engl J Med 2018;378:35–47.

[148] Host L, et al. Autologous stem cell transplantation in systemic sclerosis: a systematic review. Clin Exp Rheumatol 2017;35(Suppl. 106):S198–207.

[149] Orlandi M, et al. The role of chest CT in deciphering interstitial lung involvement: systemic sclerosis versus COVID-19. SSRN Electron. J. 2021. https://doi.org/10.2139/SSRN.3790464.

[150] Ferri C, et al. COVID-19 and systemic sclerosis: clinicopathological implications from Italian nationwide survey study. Lancet Rheumatol 2021;3:e166–8.

[151] Hoffmann-Vold AM, et al. POS0054THEIMPACT and outcome of COVID -19ON systemic sclerosis patients from the European Scleroderma Trial and Research Group (EUSTAR). Ann Rheum Dis 2021;80:232–3.

[152] Severe acute respiratory syndrome coronavirus-2-induced flare of systemic sclerosis. Scand J Rheumatol 2021. https://doi.org/10.1080/03009742.2021.1932582.

Chapter 6

Inflammatory myopathy, mixed connective tissue disease, and antisynthetase syndrome

Albert Selva-O'Callaghan[1,*] and Ernesto Trallero-Araguás[2]
[1]*Internal Medicine Department, Vall d'Hebron General Hospital, Barcelona, Spain;*
[2]*Rheumatology Department, Vall d'Hebron General Hospital, Barcelona, Catalonia, Spain*
**Corresponding author at: aselva@vhebron.net.*

Introduction

Systemic autoimmune diseases, also known as connective tissue diseases or collagenopathies, are a group of entities that share certain characteristic features [1]. As their name clearly expresses, these disorders are systemic and can affect several organs. Well-defined manifestations are seen in musculoskeletal structures (arthritis and myositis), skin (characteristic rashes, as in dermatomyositis [DM] or lupus), kidney (mainly glomerulonephritis), gastrointestinal system (dysphagia or even chronic intestinal pseudo-obstruction), and heart (myocarditis or valvular heart disease in lupus or antiphospholipid syndrome). In particular, the lung seems to be commonly affected [2]. As these diseases are autoimmune in nature, several well-described autoantibodies are useful for diagnostic purposes and as biomarkers of specific features, as is the case of lung involvement [3].

In this chapter, the inflammatory myopathies (IM), which include DM, polymyositis, and antisynthetase syndrome, as well as mixed connective tissue diseases (MCTDs) are delineated and described with specific emphasis on lung involvement.

The lung in inflammatory myopathies

Overview of lung involvement in inflammatory myopathies

IM, often referred to as myositis, are a heterogeneous group of diseases of autoimmune origin and systemic nature [4]. An inflammatory infiltrate,

The Lung in Autoimmune Diseases. https://doi.org/10.1016/B978-0-323-91083-5.00005-0

usually detected by biopsy study, is characteristically observed in skeletal muscle of these patients, but other organs may be also affected, with lung involvement being particularly common [5].

Interstitial lung disease (ILD) is the main manifestation of lung disease in IM patients, but not the only one. Other disorders related with respiratory function are also acknowledged causes. These include pulmonary hypertension (PH) [6], venous thromboembolism [7,8], ventilatory insufficiency due to diaphragmatic dysfunction [9], and obstructive sleep apnea syndrome (OSAS) caused by involvement of nasopharyngeal muscles [10].

The various phenotypes included in the heterogeneous group of IM can develop different types of lung involvement. DM associated with melanoma differentiation-associated gene 5 antibodies (anti-MDA5), or myositis associated with some well-recognized antisynthetase antibodies (anti-ARS) can exhibit ILD in both its acute and chronic forms. In contrast, this manifestation is highly infrequent or undescribed in patients with immune-mediated necrotizing myopathy (IMNM) or sporadic inclusion body myositis (sIBM). On the other hand, OSAS or ventilatory insufficiency can appear in any type of muscle disease and is seen in all myositis phenotypes, excluding the amyopathic forms of DM.

These disease-related features and manifestations will be comprehensively reviewed in the following sections.

Obstructive sleep apnea syndrome

Sleep-disordered breathing events, among them OSAS, are common in neuromuscular disorders. Specifically in myopathies, these events are due to upper airway muscle involvement, mainly pharyngeal muscle dysfunction [11]. Muscle hypotonia seems to be mainly accountable in patients with acid maltase deficiency (Pompe disease) and dystrophies [12–14]. Upper airway collapse due to muscle weakness is an underlying mechanism to be considered in any type of myopathy. In the case of IM, upper airway muscle involvement has been well described and may contribute as a cause of OSAS in some patients [10,15].

To our knowledge, only two studies have explored the issue of OSAS in IM patients. Selva-O'Callaghan et al. [10] prospectively analyzed a cohort of 16 consecutive adult patients (12 DM and 4 polymyositis or sIBM) seeking the presence of OSAS and found that more than 80% had a hypopnea/apnea index >5 per hour, criteria establishing the diagnosis of OSAS. Treatment with continuous positive airway pressure (CPAP) was administered to seven patients. Four of them tolerated the procedure well and showed an improvement in the characteristic daytime sleepiness associated with OSAS. There was no improvement in the myositis activity, itself, however.

The second study focused only on sIBM patients. Rodriguez Cruz et al. [15] analyzed 15 consecutive patients with biopsy-proven sIBM, and reported hypopnea-apnea indexes ranging from 7 to 50.3 per hour, establishing the diagnosis of OSAS in all cases. Only four of these patients experienced excessive daytime sleepiness, whereas the remainder were asymptomatic.

Although OSAS is often misdiagnosed, it can be considered a lung function complication in IM patients. A proper diagnosis and CPAP therapy when indicated may improve the health and well-being of these patients.

Ventilatory failure

Respiratory muscles, mainly the diaphragm, but also auxiliary muscles, such as the intercostal and sternocleidomastoid muscles, can also be affected in myositis patients, as has been supported by necropsy findings [9,16]. It is reported that nearly 75% of patients with myositis develop some degree of respiratory muscle weakness [17], and this is also our experience [18]. Twenty-two per cent of individuals in our cohort of myositis patients have some degree of what we call *restrictive myopathic lung involvement*, in which the restriction results from muscle (mainly diaphragmatic) involvement rather than ILD. Clinicians should be aware that evidence of restriction on pulmonary function testing—that is, abnormally low forced vital capacity (FVC) values—may in part be due to diaphragmatic muscle weakness. Low muscle inspiratory pressure may account for these low values and should be determined when doubts arise: for example, an FVC of 45% with normal diffusion lung capacity for carbon monoxide (DLCO) and an absence of ILD on high-resolution computed tomography (HRCT) study. From the clinical viewpoint, lacking of respiratory crackles or worsening of dyspnea in the supine position (usually with a >10% FVC decrease when respiratory muscles are the culprit of restriction) are clues to detecting some degree of ventilatory failure. Bedside ultrasound of the diaphragm and electrophysiological testing, when possible, may be of assistance to reach the correct diagnosis.

Most patients with ventilatory failure respond to conventional immunosuppressive therapy; the lesser the proximal muscle weakness, the lesser is the myopathic restriction. There is a good correlation between these two features. Nevertheless, in less than 5% of patients, diaphragmatic involvement may be serious enough to require external ventilation with bilevel positive airway pressure as a bridge while waiting for a response to immunosuppressive therapy [10,19]. Occasionally ventilatory failure is the first manifestation of the disease [15,20].

Interstitial lung disease

ILD is related to increased morbidity and mortality, and is the most common form of pulmonary involvement in patients with IM. ILD is particularly linked to various myositis-specific autoantibodies and is the hallmark of certain specific IM phenotypes, such as the antisynthetase and anti-MDA5 syndromes.

Antisynthetase syndrome (ASS) is the paradigm of slowly progressive chronic IM-ILD, whereas anti-MDA5 syndrome is the archetype of rapidly progressive forms of IM-ILD (RP-ILD). The clinical assessment and treatment options for each of these situations serve as a reference for the management of similar ILD cases in other IM subtypes.

Diagnosis, severity assessment, and monitoring of ILD in IM

Diagnosis and main tools for diagnosing

Respiratory symptoms can vary in IM patients with ILD. Cough and dyspnea on exertion, often with an indolent and progressive course, are common at disease onset. In some patients, ILD has an aggressive presentation, with severe and rapidly progressive dyspnea, usually associated with nonproductive cough and fever, whereas other patients are completely asymptomatic. Pulmonary involvement is easily recognizable in symptomatic patients, but the ILD diagnosis in the latter group requires a high degree of suspicion and a thorough clinical assessment. Subtle fine crackles at the dorsal aspect of the lower lobes on auscultation or evidence of interstitial changes on chest X-ray may be the only abnormal findings in many asymptomatic patients. However, both auscultation and chest X-ray can be virtually normal in very early stages. In these cases, the presence of myositis-specific autoantibodies (MSAs) or myositis-associated autoantibodies (MAAs) can help clinicians identify patients at a high risk of developing ILD in whom further investigation is required.

Pulmonary functional testing (PFT) and HRCT are the main tools for determining the ILD diagnosis. IM-associated interstitial lung disease (IM-ILD) is characterized by a restrictive respiratory pattern, that is, reduced FVC, reduced DLCO, usually exceeding the FVC reduction, and increased forced expiratory volume in 1 s (FEV1)/FVC ratio. In ILD, the DLCO usually drops before the FVC or total lung capacity, and it may be the only abnormal parameter on PFT at very early stages [21]. However, it should be noted that mild ILD can be present even in the setting of normal PFT results. Up to now, HRCT has been the most sensitive and commonly used imaging test for diagnosing ILD [21]. HRCT scans provide detailed images of the lung architecture, enabling identification of characteristic ILD lesions, such as ground-glass opacities, a reticular pattern and pulmonary fibrosis, and yield information on their distribution, characteristics, and extent.

Disease severity assessment

Pulmonary function testing is superior to clinical assessment for evaluating ILD severity [22]. Functional status and exercise tolerance in IM patients can be highly conditioned by muscle weakness secondary to myositis, joint involvement, or general symptoms such as asthenia, and do not always reflect the severity of lung involvement. In addition, for the same reasons, these symptoms can also mask dyspnea on exertion, which may not be mentioned by the patient as a relevant symptom. PFT provides objective and reproducible information about lung functionality and HRCT yields information on the patterns and extent of lung involvement. Various HRCT scores have been proposed to determine the prognostic value of imaging at disease onset [23,24]. However, the usefulness of these scores in clinical practice is limited, as HRCT scoring is usually an arduous process that requires intense evaluation by skilled CT specialists and is related to significant interobserver variation [22].

Monitoring of ILD

Serial PFT is the cornerstone of routine monitoring in patients with ILD associated with IM. Spirometry and DLCO results have proved of value for determining the response to therapy and identifying disease progression in connective tissue diseases [22]. PFT should be repeated every 3–6 months, depending on the initial severity of pulmonary involvement, especially during the first years after the ILD diagnosis. A relative decline in the percent predicted FVC of $\geq 10\%$, or a $\geq 5\%$ to $<10\%$ relative decline in percent predicted FVC and a $\geq 15\%$ relative decline in percent predicted DLCO, have been proposed as markers of clinically meaningful progression [25]. Of note, PFT results should be carefully interpreted, as major confounding factors such as coexistence of pulmonary vascular complications (e.g., PH, pulmonary thromboembolism), extrapulmonary restriction (e.g., respiratory muscle weakness), intrinsic airway disease (e.g., bronchiectasis), lower respiratory tract infection, and even weight gain can cause PFT changes that are not secondary to ILD progression. Significant FVC or DLCO declines, or worsening of clinical symptoms should be thoroughly evaluated through HRCT to determine whether they are attributable to ILD progression. Serial HRCT for ILD monitoring is not recommended beyond these scenarios to avoid radiation burden.

Role and utility of myositis-related autoantibodies in ILD-IM

Several specific and associated autoantibodies have been described in patients with IM [26]. MSAs are solely found in patients with IM. Characteristically, MSAs are generally mutually exclusive and define distinct IM phenotypes and clinical associations. Paradoxically, the MSA concept may be questionable, as some of these autoantibodies are more biomarkers of specific manifestations, such as ILD, even in the absence of myositis itself. Myositis-associated autoantibodies (MAAs) can be found in other autoimmune conditions that can occur in overlap with myositis. Overall, two types of MAAs are described: the first, including anti-PM/Scl and anti-Ku, rarely occur together or in combination with MSAs and are also biomarkers of specific clinical features, such as the scleromyositis overlap syndrome; the second, including anti-Ro52/60, anti-La, and anti-RNP, are often seen in association with other MSAs or MAAs [26].

ILD in IM is especially linked to specific myositis autoantibodies [26]. Thus, among MSAs, the spectrum of antisynthetase antibodies and anti-MDA5 define two clinical syndromes that are characterized by ILD as a hallmark manifestation. The prevalence of ILD in patients with anti-ARS is around 80%, whereas up to 50% of patients with anti-MDA5 from Western countries and almost 75% from Asian countries develop this complication [27–29]. Anti-SAE has also been related to a high ILD rate in Asian patients (50%–70%) [30,31], while this association seems weaker in Western countries (0%–18%) [32,33]. Conversely, ILD is extremely rare in patients with other MSAs, such as anti-TIF1γ, anti-HMGCR, anti-Mi2, and anti-SRP [26]. Importantly, the type of MSA is also related with the specific ILD presentation and prognosis. Thus, RP-ILD is especially frequent in patients with anti-MDA5 antibodies, and is associated with high mortality despite intensive immunosuppressive therapy [34]. In contrast, ILD associated with ASS is typically characterized by a slowly progressive chronic course, with no severe complications in up to 70% of patients, although acute forms can also occur [35,36]. Finally, ILD associated with anti-SAE is generally mild and seems to be associated with a good prognosis [37,38].

ILD is also a common feature in patients with two MAAs, anti-PM/Scl and anti-Ku. Both autoantibodies are markers of overlap syndromes between myositis and scleroderma. Generally, ILD seems to be mild and have a better outcome in these patients, although severe cases are also reported [39]. The prevalence of ILD in patients with anti-PM/Scl and anti-Ku is high, around 35% to 87%, and 76%, respectively [40–42].

Anti-Ro52 has been described in association with other MSAs. It frequently co-occurs in patients with ASS, especially those with anti-Jo1 (58%–72%) [43,44] and anti-MDA5 antibodies [45]. Overall, this combination has been linked to more aggressive ILD, resistance to conventional treatment, and lower survival in both groups of patients, those with the anti-MDA5 and the anti-ARS antibodies [46,47]. In contrast, this deleterious effect is not observed in IM patients with ILD who have anti-Ro52 alone [48].

As IM syndromes are usually dynamic, with certain manifestations such as ILD presenting over time, the myositis autoantibody profile provides very useful information to identify patients at a higher risk of developing pulmonary complications. In these patients, baseline ILD screening, including PFT and HRCT, should be performed even in the absence of clinical evidence of pulmonary involvement [49].

Clinical spectrum of ILD in IM

Antisynthetase syndrome

Definition ASS was first described as a clinical condition characterized by a constellation of signs and symptoms associated with autoantibodies against different anti-ARS in patients with DM or PM [50]. ASS patients typically present with one or more of the following clinical features: IM, ILD, arthritis, Raynaud's phenomenon, fissured hyperkeratotic finger lesions known as *mechanic's hands* (Fig. 6.1), and fever [50].

The hallmark of this syndrome is the presence of circulating autoantibodies directed against any of the aminoacyl-tRNA synthetases, a family of cytoplasmic enzymes that play a crucial role in protein synthesis by binding amino acids to their cognate tRNA to form an aminoacyl tRNA. To date, eight different anti-ARS, almost always mutually exclusive [26], have been described, including antihistidyl-tRNA synthetase (anti-Jo1), antithreonyl-tRNA synthetase (anti-PL7), antialanyl-tRNA synthetase (anti-PL12), antiisoleucyl-tRNA synthetase (anti-OJ), antiglycyl-tRNA synthetase (anti-EJ), antiasparaginyl-tRNA synthetase (anti-KS), antityrosil-tRNA synthetase (anti-Ha), and antiphenylalanyl-tRNA synthetase (anti-Zo). Anti-Jo1 is the most frequent anti-ARS (60%–70%), and the most common autoantibody in most IM populations (20%–30% of adult patients with IM) [51]. Anti-PL7 and anti-PL12 are much less frequent (5% of IM), as are anti-OJ, anti-EJ, and anti-KS (<5%). Autoantibodies to anti-Ha and anti-Zo are very rare (<1%) [52].

For many years, ASS was considered a clinical syndrome affecting patients with different types of IM, such as DM or PM, and not a separate disease among the IM. In this regard, the features of patients with myopathic ASS are similar to those of DM, PM, and IMNM, including proximal muscle weakness, elevated muscle enzymes, and myopathic electromyography findings. Some patients may exhibit characteristic DM-like skin rashes. Muscle biopsies of

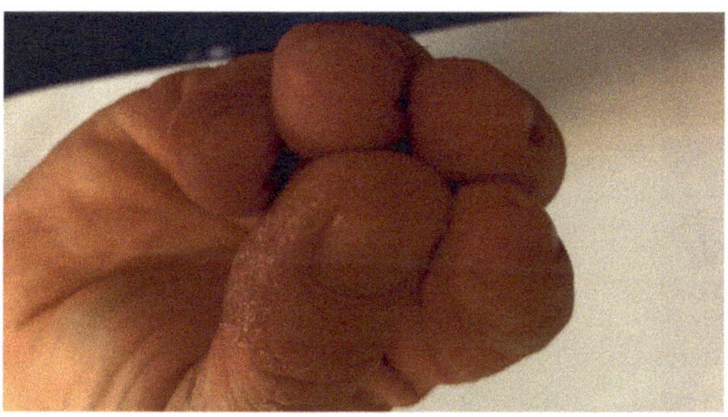

FIGURE 6.1 Hyperkeratotic finger lesions (mechanic's hands) in a patient with antisynthetase syndrome.

ASS patients have perimysial and perifascicular-predominant pathologic findings similar to those seen in DM, even in the absence of the DM cutaneous manifestations. However, thanks to recent advances in the pathological analysis of skeletal muscle biopsies, there is increasing evidence to consider ASS as a separate entity, different from other IM subtypes [53]. Perimysial fragmentation and perifascicular-predominant myofiber necrosis are especially prominent in ASS, whereas perifascicular-predominant atrophy is the most common finding in DM muscle biopsies [54]. Of note, ultrastructural analysis of ASS muscle biopsies with electron microscopy shows distinctive myonuclear actin filament inclusions, including rod formation, a feature that has not been described in other IM types [53]. In addition, muscle biopsies from ASS patients show strong myofiber MHC-II/HLA-DR expression with a unique perifascicular pattern that is not observed in DM. This feature is associated with C5b-9 deposition on sarcolemma of non-necrotic perifascicular fibers, whereas in DM, C5b-9 is mainly detected in endomysial capillaries. CD8+ cells are also more abundant in ASS than in DM and electively located in perimysium or in perifascicular endomysium, showing a good correlation with HLA-DR expression. Furthermore, muscle biopsies from DM patients exhibit several characteristics that are uncommon in ASS patients. For example, sarcoplasmic overexpression of myxovirus resistance A (MxA), one of the type-1 interferon-inducible proteins, now considered a highly specific feature of DM (98% specificity for the DM diagnosis), is not seen in ASS [55]. Overall, these features suggest distinct pathogenic mechanisms or antigenic targets leading to ASS, and have contributed to change the paradigm of the IM classification. Thus, recent classifications include ASS as a unique form of IM that can be distinguished from DM, PM, IMNM, and sIBM [4].

Clinical spectrum ASS is a heterogeneous and dynamic disease. Heterogeneity refers both to phenotype and severity and does not appear to be entirely attributable to the anti-ARS subset, as variability is also seen between each separate group [52]. The clinical presentation of ASS varies greatly, with most patients showing incomplete forms and developing subsequent manifestations along follow-up. The delay between appearance of the various manifestations can range from a few months to several years [27,36].

ILD, myositis, and arthritis are the most prevalent and relevant clinical features in ASS patients. Overall, the prevalence of ILD in ASS is around 71% to 82%, with slight differences between the available studies and groups [27]. According to data from the AENEAS cohort, ILD is the most common initial manifestation in patients with anti-PL7 (present in 54% of patients), anti-PL12 (69%), and anti-EJ (74%) [27]. Moreover, ILD alone is also the most frequent initial clinical feature in these groups (present in 36%, 43%, and 39% of patients, respectively) and the most common over time in anti-PL12 patients (36%). The frequency of myositis is quite homogeneous among anti-Jo1-, anti-PL7-, anti-OJ-, and anti-EJ-positive patients, occurring in approximately 80%.

In contrast, only 50% of patients with anti-PL12 develop myositis during follow-up. Of note, myositis alone seems to be the most frequent clinical feature both at disease onset (51%) and during follow-up (28%) in anti-OJ patients. Finally, the prevalence of arthritis is significantly higher in anti-Jo1 (75%) in comparison to non-Jo1 anti-ARS patients (40%–50%), with arthritis alone being the most common clinical feature at disease onset in the first group (22%). Focusing only on the three major features of ASS (ILD, myositis, and arthritis), complete forms are the most common pattern at the end of follow-up in anti-Jo1 (50%), anti-PL7 (29%), and anti-EJ (39%), whereas a complete triad is the main presentation form in only 18% of anti-Jo1 patients and in 3% to 9% of the remaining anti-ARS [27].

Other features such as mechanic's hands, Raynaud's phenomenon, fever, or DM-like rashes are less common, without significant differences between the anti-ARS subtypes. Although information on the frequency of these features is quite inconsistent, data from larger studies report rates of 36.6% to 38%, 38.2% to 51%, 35%, and 44%, respectively [27,36,56].

In addition, a broad spectrum of other manifestations, including sicca syndrome, gastrointestinal symptoms, and occasionally cardiovascular morbidity, has been described in ASS patients [56]. Sicca syndrome has been reported in up to 33%, occasionally accompanied by anti-Ro and anti-La antibodies, fulfilling the criteria of definite Sjogren's syndrome [57]. Gastrointestinal symptoms are also common, especially in anti-PL12- and anti-PL7-positive patients [58,59]. Dysphagia and regurgitation have been described in up to 25% and 19% of ASS patients in these groups [60]. As to cardiovascular disease, myocarditis and pericarditis have been described both at disease onset and during follow-up [61,62].

Several small series and case reports have reported conflicting results regarding the frequency of cancer and the need for cancer screening in ASS patients [63–65]. The information in these reports contrasts with the data reported in large cohorts, where both ILD and anti-ARS are considered protective factors for cancer within IM [66]. A recent systematic review and meta-analysis of 69 studies has concluded that the presence of any ASS-related autoantibody is significantly associated with a lower risk of cancer [67].

ASS recognition and diagnosis Recognition of ASS at disease onset is usually straightforward when myositis or typical DM-like rashes (Gottron's papules or heliotrope rash) are present. However, the ASS diagnosis can be challenging when only ILD, arthritis, or both these features are the first manifestations of disease. This is the case of almost 45% of anti-Jo1 patients and more than 50% to 60% of non-anti-Jo1 ARS patients [27]. A high diagnostic suspicion is needed to identify ASS in these situations, and diagnostic delays and misdiagnoses are frequent, especially in non-anti-Jo1 ARS patients. Of note, whereas anti-ENA screening tests, usually containing anti-Jo1 antibodies, are often performed in patients with arthritis or isolated ILD, non-anti-

Jo1 ARS are rarely tested. Some ASS patients may be first diagnosed with rheumatoid arthritis (RA), undifferentiated connective tissue disease, idiopathic ILD, or interstitial pneumonia with autoimmune features, among others. Fever, Raynaud's phenomenon, mechanic's hands, and other less typical DM-like rashes should be thoroughly investigated in patients receiving those diagnoses and, if present, should raise a red flag about possible ASS. Of interest, significant nailfold capillaroscopy abnormalities (i.e., a scleroderma-resembling pattern) can be found in up to one-third of ASS patients even in the absence of Raynaud's phenomenon [68], suggesting that this test could provide relevant diagnostic support in patients with equivocal clinical presentations. However, specific anti-ARS tests should be ordered even in the absence of these features. Thus, anti-ARS testing would be suitable especially in patients with RA (seronegative or not) and ILD, and in patients with idiopathic ILD harboring nonspecific interstitial pneumonitis (NSIP) patterns. To date, there are no validated criteria to diagnose patients with ASS. Two classification proposals were published in 2010 and 2011, both including the presence of anti-ARS as a mandatory criterion in addition to clinical symptoms (Table 6.1) [69,70]. Whereas the Solomon criteria are more restrictive, including myositis and/or ILD as necessary major criteria to classify ASS [70], Connors et al. proposed that the presence of one feature—myositis, ILD, arthritis, unexplained fever, Raynaud's phenomenon, or mechanic's hands—plus a positive anti-ARS result could suffice to classify a patient within ASS [69]. A project for classification of ASS sponsored by the ACR/EULAR is currently ongoing (the CLASS: Classification Criteria of Antisynthetase Syndrome).

Anti-ARS detection Determination of anti-ARS is essential for the AAS diagnosis. Anti-ARS can be detected by a variety of methods, some of them not universally available. One of the main problems of anti-ARS determination, beyond anti-Jo1, is that the current commercially available tests are not

TABLE 6.1 Proposed classification criteria for antisynthetase syndrome.

Connors et al. [69]	*Solomon et al.* [70]
Antisynthetase antibody plus one or more of: - Myositis - Interstitial lung disease not explained by other causes - Arthritis - Unexplained, persistent fever - Raynaud's phenomenon - Mechanic's hands	Antisynthetase antibody plus two major criteria or one major and two minor criteria. *Major criteria* - Myositis - Intersitial lung disease not explained by other causes *Minor criteria* - Arthritis - Raynaud's phenomenon - Mechanic's hands

well standardized and yield a variable percentage of false-positive and false-negative results.

Protein and RNA immunoprecipitation (IP) is currently recognized as the reference assay for identifying anti-ARS [51]. However, IP is costly, time-consuming, and not widely available. For those reasons, enzyme-linked immunosorbent assays (ELISA) or chemiluminescent immunoassays, and immunoblotting techniques (line blot and dot blot assays), including multiple testing of a panel of myositis antibodies (except for anti-Ha and anti-Zo), are the most widely used methods in many laboratories for anti-ARS detection in routine clinical practice. Multiplex immunoblotting techniques have varying sensitivity and specificity, and in some cases, poor agreement with IP results [51]. Thus, each positive anti-ARS result obtained with these assays should be carefully interpreted in the context of the overall clinical picture.

A cytoplasmic pattern detected by indirect immunofluorescence (IIF) using HEp-2 cells is often seen in patients with anti-ARS antibodies. Hence, this method can be used as an anti-ARS screening test that provides important data on the reliability of a positive anti-ARS result by immunoblotting. However, the absence of this cytoplasmic pattern does not exclude the presence of any anti-ARS. The lack of sensitivity of IIF techniques may be related to low relative antigen concentrations or variability between laboratory technical protocols. Of note, negative IIF staining of the nucleus is not uncommon, and this situation is reported as a negative antinuclear antibody (ANA) result by many laboratories, even when there is prominent cytoplasmic reactivity.

Detection of certain anti-ARS such as anti-OJ can be especially challenging using immunoblotting. Characteristically, multiplex assays show poor agreement with IP for anti-OJ [71,72]. Targoff et al. identified isoleucyl-tRNA synthetase as the major corresponding target of anti-OJ, although reactivity with other related synthetases was also described [73]. This situation is favored by the fact that isoleucyl-tRNA synthetase is a part of a multienzyme synthetase complex including eight other synthetases and three noncatalytic components. This potential reactivity of serum from patients with anti-OJ to these other components or to the three-dimensional structure of the complex could explain the lack of concordance between linear antigen assays such as immunoblotting and IP [74].

In clinical practice, when a positive or negative anti-ARS result is discordant with the clinical pattern, a separate assay or system for anti-ARS detection, preferably IP, is recommendable to confirm or rule out the laboratory result.

ILD in antisynthetase syndrome ILD is often the dominant clinical feature in ASS and the greatest contributor to AAS morbidity and mortality. Even so, in more than two-thirds of ASS patients, ILD is a nonprogressive disease that tends to improve or stabilize under immunosuppressive therapy [35,36]. Two main patterns of ILD onset have been described: acute and gradual. Although a precise definition of these terms has not been established, patients with acute onset are often diagnosed not more than 6–8 weeks after the initial respiratory symptoms, and are characterized by severe dyspnea, acute respiratory failure, and fever [35]. The frequency of acute ILD onset in ASS is less than 10%, whereas the great majority of patients present with slow, gradual, progressive dyspnea and cough, or even with asymptomatic ILD [36,75].

NSIP is the most frequent radiologic pattern in ASS patients (around 50%), followed by the organizing pneumonitis (OP) pattern [76–78]. Although less common, usual interstitial pneumonia (UIP) has also been described and associated with a poorer prognosis [76]. In a study including 32 ASS patients, Tille-Leblond et al. reported that an ILD pattern consisting of a combination of diffuse, patchy, ground-glass attenuation, basal predominance of irregular lines, and basal consolidations was significantly more frequent in patients with an acute onset than in those with a slow onset (80% vs. 35%, $P = .015$) [35]. Very few studies have evaluated the impact of ILD extent at disease onset on pulmonary outcomes and survival in ASS [79]. Strikingly, and contrary to scleroderma and idiopathic pulmonary fibrosis (IPF), these studies have failed to demonstrate any prognostic value of disease extent in patients with IM-ILD.

Invasive tests such as bronchoscopy and lung biopsy are not usually required in the ASS diagnostic process except when other, alternative etiologies are suspected, such as infection, cancer, or primary ILD. Bronchoalveolar lavage (BAL) findings are generally variable and nonspecific [80,81]. In the study by Tille-Leblond et al., a high percentage of neutrophils (>5%) was detected more often in BAL specimens of patients with a slow ILD onset than in those with an acute onset (86% vs. 27%, $P = .004$) [35]. Previous studies in IM have described a good correlation between HRCT findings and histological lung damage, an indication that lung biopsy is not useful in the context of known ASS [76]. According to the published data, NSIP is the most frequent histological pattern associated with ASS, although UIP has also been described in patients with a gradual onset. In patients with acute ILD, OP and diffuse alveolar damage are the most common patterns described [35]. Watanabe et al. reported that a higher frequency of lymphoid follicles were associated with NSIP and UIP patterns in ASS patients than in patients with similar patterns harboring idiopathic ILD, a feature that could be of interest in the differential diagnosis [80].

Prognostic factors The prognosis of ILD in ASS is variable. Whereas some patients with severe forms can significantly improve and stabilize, others with a milder and more progressive ILD onset may present rapid deterioration of lung function with progression to end-stage lung disease and a poor short-term outcome, even after long, stable follow-up periods [56]. Based on these observations, periodic lung function assessment should be maintained over time in ASS patients to promptly identify those at risk of ILD progression. The risk factors that most consistently correlate with poorer survival include acute ILD onset, severity of dyspnea at ILD onset, UIP pattern, older age, increased fibrosis score on HRCT, and the presence of anti-Ro52 antibodies and non-Jo1 anti-ARS [57].

Clinical vignette 1

A 47-year-old man, with no previous comorbidities and no past history of tobacco smoking was admitted to the emergency department with a 3-weeks history of progressive dyspnea, fever, stabbing chest pain, night sweats, and dry cough. He had been diagnosed of left basal pneumonia 12 days before and had received antibiotic therapy without any response. Physical examination revealed bilateral fine basal crepitation and oxygen saturation of 90% on room air, with no other remarkable findings. He presented an erythrocyte sedimentation rate of 100 (0–15 mm/h) and C-reactive protein of 8.20 (<5 mg/dL). A chest CT scan showed bilateral pulmonary interstitial involvement in the form of lung parenchymal reticulation and ground-glass density enhancements with some areas of condensation at bases. PFT showed FVC values of 50%. Complete microbiological study including virus, bacteria, and mycobacteria polymerase chain reaction and cultures of BAL were negative. A lung cryobiopsy showed a histological pattern of organized pneumonia. Rheumatology workup showed a positive result for ANAs 1/160 with cytoplasmic pattern, and positivity to anti-Ro52 and anti-EJ antibodies. The patient was diagnosed with ASS with anti-EJ with isolated pulmonary involvement. Corticosteroid treatment at a dose of 1 mg/kg/day and tacrolimus were started with a good clinical response. Three months later he had FVC of 60% and a DLCO of 40%. Six months later, while the patient was on 7.5 mg/d of prednisone and 2 mg of tacrolimus every 12h, he was admitted with muscle weakness, predominantly in the shoulder girdle and pelvis, and fever for 2 weeks. He reported no worsening of dyspnea. Laboratory tests showed an elevated CK level of 3554 UI/L (NV<195 IU/L). Muscle biopsy was compatible with a polymyositis pattern. The prednisone dose was increased and treatment with IVIG 0.4 mg/kg/day for 5 days on a monthly basis was started. The patient progressively improved with normalization of CK and muscle balance. In December 2020, the patient was readmitted for fever, arthromyalgia without arthritis, and worsening muscle weakness with elevated CK (2235 IU/L). With the guidance of a new disease flare, methylprednisolone bolus was administered and rituximab was added to the treatment. The patient again showed clinical improvement and normalization of CK. At the last follow-up, 6 months later, the patient was stable, with no reports of weakness and PFTs that had remained stable.

Comment

Several important messages can be drawn from this clinical vignette. Firstly, the dynamic nature of the ASS, with different manifestations occurring over time despite the patient receiving immunosuppressive treatment. Secondly, the presentation of the syndrome as an isolated ILD is noteworthy. In patients with idiopathic ILD, especially with NSIP or OP HRCT or histologic patterns, the possibility of an underlying connective tissue disease should be always considered. Hence, rheumatological evaluation, including detailed history and physical examination together with a complete rheumatological autoantibody panel

Continued

Clinical vignette 1—cont'd

testing, is strongly recommended. The assessment of anti-ARS in patients with isolated ILDs, even in the absence of other manifestations of the syndrome, is key to achieve an early diagnose of some ASS cases, particularly those associated to non-Jo1 anti-ARS. Positive ANA with cytoplasmic pattern may suggest this possibility. Finally, some patients may present with refractory disease, requiring a progressive escalation in the immunosuppressive therapy. Rituximab seems to be a good option to treat refractory major life-threatening manifestations such as ILD or myositis. The prognosis of these patients is uncertain and requires close monitoring and follow-up.

ILD associated with anti-MDA5 antibodies

Anti-MDA5 syndrome In a study in 2005, IP and immunoblotting identified anti-MDA5 antibodies as polypeptides of approximately 140 kD in size (termed CADM-140 in the study), associated with clinically amyopathic dermatomyositis (CADM) and RP-ILD in a cohort of Japanese patients [82]. Similar findings were subsequently described in other Asian populations and in Caucasian cohorts [29,83,84]. New data from these cohorts have contributed to amplify the clinical spectrum of anti-MDA5 patients. The target of anti-CADM-140 has been identified as a cytoplasmic RNA helicase encoded by MDA5 [85], which is a part of the family of retinoic acid-inducible gene I (RIG-I)-like receptors involved in the innate immune response against viruses [86]. RIG-I-like receptors recognize double-stranded RNA viruses and trigger production of type 1 interferon and proinflammatory cytokines. These findings highly suggest a role of viruses as triggers of this syndrome.

Anti-MDA5 is a specific autoantibody in DM/CADM. The prevalence of anti-MDA5 in DM/CADM varies and likely depends on ethnic or environmental features. Anti-MDA5 is reported in 10% to 48% of DM/CADM patients in Asian cohorts [29], but rates of less than 13% are reported in European/American cohorts [83,87,88]. Anti-MDA5 autoantibodies have also been reported in juvenile DM, with clinical associations similar to those of adult patients, including ILD [89]. However, whereas RP-ILD is frequent in Asian juvenile DM patients, this is not the case in Western countries [90].

Clinical spectrum and diagnosis of anti-MDA5 The main clinical features of patients with anti-MDA5 include DM rashes, ILD, RP-ILD, palmar papules, skin ulcers, calcinosis, mechanic's hands, and arthralgia/arthritis. Half the patients in Western countries show overt myositis, but this feature is less common in eastern Asian populations [91]. RP-ILD and severe cutaneous disease are the two main clinical hallmarks of the anti-MDA5 syndrome. Cutaneous disease includes unique manifestations, such as skin ulceration, palmar papules, and digital ischemia secondary to a characteristic cutaneous vasculitis, findings that are not usually seen in other DM subtypes [92]. The frequency and severity of these manifestations vary considerably in anti-MDA5 patients. Recently, Allenbach et al. described three main phenotypes within the anti-MDA5 spectrum: the first, patients with RP-ILD and very high mortality rates; the second, patients with pure dermato-rheumatologic symptoms (arthralgia/arthritis) and a good prognosis; and the third, mainly male patients (72.7%) with severe skin vasculopathy, frequent signs of myositis (68.2%), and an intermediate prognosis [93].

As anti-MDA5 syndrome is a heterogeneous disease, the diagnosis can be challenging, especially when patients are initially evaluated in nonspecialized centers. An absence of myositis and predominance of atypical DM cutaneous lessons (e.g., ulcers, palmar nodules, cutaneous vasculitis) can contribute to misdiagnoses. Some patients develop RP-ILD with no other clinical manifestations of the syndrome or with a mild and evanescent cutaneous disease that could be overlooked by doctors. Moreover, coexistence of ANCA autoantibodies has been occasionally reported, and when positive can also be a confounding finding. However, the full-blown syndrome is quite recognizable, and with a high clinical suspicion, the diagnosis is easily performed in most cases. Patients with anti-MDA5 syndrome usually fulfill the commonly used classification criteria for CADM or classical DM [94–96]. Furthermore, measurement of anti-MDA5 antibodies in clinical practice is broadly available in nonspecialized immunology laboratories and is currently performed with commercial assays that include ELISA-based assays and immunoblotting techniques. Overall, these methods show a good correlation with IP, which is considered the gold standard test.

ILD in anti-MDA5 Together with skin manifestations, ILD is the most characteristic feature related with anti-MDA5 antibodies. The clinical presentation varies, with RP-ILD being considered the most severe phenotype. RP-ILD in anti-MDA5 patients is associated with high mortality rates of up to 50%, especially within 6 months after the diagnosis [97,98]. The prevalence of RP-ILD in anti-MDA5 seems to be higher in Asian (83%) than in Western cohorts (40%–50%) [91], suggesting that ethnic or geographic differences likely contribute to the disease presentation and severity. Non-RP-ILD is also common, occurring in about one-third to one-half of anti-MDA5-ILD patients in most series [93,99]. Mild respiratory symptoms, slowly progressive ILD with a chronic course, and clinical features resembling those of ASS patients are usually seen in this ILD subset. In addition, some patients with anti-MDA5 have asymptomatic ILD or never develop ILD during follow-up.

Rapidly progressive ILD. Patients with RP-ILD usually present acutely, with worsening dyspnea or cough over days to weeks, associated with constitutional symptoms such as fever and malaise. These patients often experience rapid deterioration of lung function with escalating oxygen requirements leading to ICU admission and a need for ventilatory support. Spontaneous pneumomediastinum or pneumothorax is seen in 15% to 33% of these patients, and is reported to be a marker of a poor prognosis associated with higher mortality rates [97].

A few small studies have evaluated HRCT features in anti-MDA5 RP-ILD patients. Hozumi et al. reported that most cases have *unclassifiable* HRCT patterns at disease onset, consisting in consolidation/ground glass attenuation-based areas inconsistent with NSIP or OP. This unclassifiable pattern was significantly associated with short-term mortality, in contrast to other less frequent patterns also described in patients with anti-MDA5, such as NSIP or OP [100]. Tanizawa K et al. have suggested that lower lung zone consolidation on HRCT is an independent predictor of 90-day mortality, whereas it is not associated with overall mortality in anti-MDA5-positive DM [79]. Zou et al. described OP as the dominant radiological pattern in patients with anti-MDA5 and reported that lower lung zone consolidation on HRCT was associated with RP-ILD but not with the prognosis of these patients [101]. Finally, Chino et al. reported that perilobular opacities that thicken and progress to consolidation are the main radiological findings in RP-ILD with anti-MDA5 antibody [102]. Taken together, these various radiological patterns are not very helpful for the management of the patients. Furthermore, pathological evaluation of surgical lung biopsies and necropsies has shown diffuse alveolar damage [102], which has been reported as the main histological pattern in patients with anti-MDA5 RP-ILD [29,83].

It is not always possible to determine a patient's FVC due to fast, progressive respiratory failure, but when it is feasible, the FVC value at diagnosis as a subrogate marker of ILD severity seems to be helpful for risk stratification. In a validated categorical model including three categories—FVC $\geq$50%, FVC <50%, and FVC unable to perform—mortality associated with each of these categories was, respectively, 15.3%, 46.8%, and 97.4% in the discovery cohort, and 14.9%, 58.3%, and 86.4% in the validation cohort [103].

Prognostic biomarkers Several prognostic biomarkers have been described in patients with anti-MDA5 ILD. Longitudinal changes in anti-MDA5 titers have been associated with disease activity and relapse, suggesting a role of anti-MDA5 in the pathogenesis of ILD [82]. However, controversial data from other studies have limited the use of anti-MDA5 titers for evaluating treatment response [104]. Nonetheless, there is general agreement that anti-MDA5 monitoring seems useful for predicting disease flares in long-term follow-up [105]. Serum ferritin level is a widely recognized biomarker that correlates with disease activity, treatment response, and survival outcome. High ferritin values are associated with more severe disease and lower survival rates. Several cut-offs, from 450 to 1600 ng/mL, are described and provide similar results [24,106]. Krebs von de Lungen-6 (KL-6), a mucin-like glycoprotein expressed predominantly on type II alveolar pneumocytes and bronchiolar epithelial cells, is a sensitive marker of the activity of various types of ILD. High KL-6 levels positively correlate with ferritin, lactate dehydrogenase (LDH), and HRCT scores, and inversely correlate with FVC, total lung capacity, and DLCO percentages. High KL-6 levels (>792 UI/mL) predict a poor prognosis in patients in the early stage of anti-MDA5 ILD. Over follow-up, KL-6 levels increase with exacerbations and decrease in remission/stable phases. This pattern suggests that KL-6 could be a sensitive marker for predicting ILD and the response to treatment [107]. Other serum biomarkers such as LDH, lymphocytopenia, and high levels of IL-15 and IL-18 have also been associated with a poor prognosis in anti-MDA5 patients [106,108–110].

In a small cohort of Japanese patients, Yamaguchi et al. reported that coexistence of associated autoantibodies, such as ANAs, anticyclic citrullinated peptide (CCP), anti-SSA (Ro60), and anti-SSB, present in 37.5% of patients, was related to a favorable prognosis, lower incidence of RP-ILD, better treatment response, and lower mortality rate [111]. In a cohort of adult anti-MDA5 patients from China, Xu et al. reported that coexistence of anti-Ro52 was associated with a more aggressive disease phenotype, a higher RP-ILD rate, more frequent cutaneous ulcerations, a poorer prognosis, and lower survival rates [45]. A high prevalence of anti-Ro52 (around 70%–75%) has been described in both Asian and Western patients with anti-MDA5 [45,83,112].

Scleromyositis (anti-PM/Scl and anti-Ku)

Scleromyositis is currently considered a typical overlap syndrome with features of scleroderma and myositis [113]. The main biomarkers of the syndrome are anti-PM/Scl and to a lesser extent, anti-Ku antibodies. Both are MAAs that can be easily detected by ELISA or blot test, with high reliability in most cases, making the lengthy, complex IP techniques unnecessary. PM/Scl is an antigenic complex with 11 proteins identified as an exosome involved in RNA processing [114]. The two main antigens targeted by ELISA and blotting are 75 kD and 100 kD in size.

Patients with scleromyositis can show the triad of myositis, mechanic's hands and ILD, resembling patients with antisynthetase antibodies, but these features may be due more to a similar genetic background than to the antibody itself [115,116]. Raynaud phenomenon and arthritis may be present, and sclerodactyly or "puffy hands" as a manifestation of systemic sclerosis may also appear. Lung involvement is not uncommon in scleromyositis patients, with a prevalence of 35% to 87% in the reported series. In comparison with ILD in other systemic diseases, mainly systemic sclerosis with antibodies against topoisomerase I, the outcome seems to be better in scleromyositis, as has been reported by various research groups [117–121].

A recently published multicenter study has confirmed the association with ILD and better respiratory functional outcome in scleromyositis patients testing positive for anti-PM/Scl antibodies than in those with systemic sclerosis negative for anti-PM/Scl [121]. These data agree with the previous results reported by researchers in Barcelona [117].

Data on anti-Ku syndrome, another scleromyositis syndrome, is scarce. In the small number of available reports, ILD seems to be common, but has a good outcome [122]. Nonetheless the scanty related information precludes generalizations.

Clinical vignette 2

A 51-year-old woman came to our outpatient myositis clinic after being evaluated in another center. She mentioned breathlessness for the last 2 months. On clinical examination she showed "puffy" mechanic's hands, Gottron's papules, and bibasal lung crackles. No muscle weakness was identified at that time, but creatine kinase value was 1200 IU/L (normal <195 IU/L). HRCT disclosed an organizing pneumonia pattern, and PFT showed a restrictive pattern (FVC 69%, DLCO 39%). The patient was offered immunosuppressive therapy with glucocorticoids and cyclophosphamide, which she refused. She started homeopathic therapy, but after a 4-month period with no improvement of the symptoms, she reconsulted. At that time, she was referred to our unit, where mild proximal muscle weakness was detected, and muscle biopsy disclosed findings suggestive of autoimmune IM. Anti-PM/Scl antibodies were highly positive, and the patient was diagnosed with an overlap scleromyositis syndrome.

Considering the patient's interstitial lung involvement and reduced FVC and DLCO, we recommended starting glucocorticoids and tacrolimus, but again, she refused. Steroid therapy without immunosuppressive agents was finally accepted, and she received 1 mg/kg/day of prednisone for 1 month. Subsequently, the dose was progressively reduced over 4 months to 5 mg/d. With this steroid maintenance dose, she has remained asymptomatic for the last 4 years. At the latest visit, FVC was 96% and DLCO 44%, muscle strength was normal as were the creatine kinase values (240 IU/L). The remaining manifestations and HRCT findings also improved.

Comment

This case report is a good example of the better outcome in terms of respiratory involvement expected in scleromyositis patients testing positive for anti-PM/Scl antibodies. The case reported did well only with corticosteroid treatment and did not need long-term immunosuppressive therapy.

Thus, at least two lessons can be drawn from this clinical vignette. The first is that ILD-associated scleromyositis may not always need treatment with a high-intensity immunosuppressive schedule; and second, it is worth considering all available therapeutic options with the patient, as a conjoined decision between both parties can strengthen the physician–patient relationship. We should remember that there is no solid evidence-based knowledge about treating these specific manifestations, and that a wide spectrum of therapeutic options is available, from no intervention to intensive immunosuppressive treatment.

Pathogenesis of myositis-associated ILD

The etiopathogenic mechanisms causing ILD in IM are complex, probably heterogeneous, and involve the interactions between predisposing genetic and environmental factors, which lead to altered immune activation and tolerance breakdown.

In ASS, the lungs seem to be the environment in which autoimmunity against synthetases initiates and propagates. This idea emerged from the available evidence on the generation of autoimmunity against histidyl-RNA-synthetase (HisRS) antigen, the substrate against which anti-Jo1 antibodies are directed. Although HisRS is an ubiquitous antigen, the HisRS present in the microenvironment of the alveolar epithelium of the lung is more susceptible to cleavage by granzyme B than that present in other tissues such as muscle. This cleavage of the HisRS protein produces fragments that match the epitopes targeted by anti-Jo1 antibodies and are capable of generating autoimmunity. Respiratory infections, airborne contaminants, and various inhaled substances such as tobacco smoke may act as triggers of this process, causing initial nonspecific inflammatory changes in the lung microenvironment that lead to cellular stress and tissue damage, with a massive release of inflammatory mediators and cellular antigens, including HisRS. Concurrent activation of inflammatory cells (e.g., natural killer cells) can result in considerable production of granzyme B, leading to HisRS cleavage and generation of immunogenic neo-antigens. Tolerance breakdown is caused by the development of an efficient adaptive response against these self-antigens, including anti-ARS production, which requires a specific genetic background. The strongest genetic risk for disease susceptibility is the major histocompatibility complex, which is involved in antigen presentation. Various studies have identified HLA-DRB1*03:01 and HLA-B1*08:01 alleles as the major predisposing markers for ASS in Caucasian patients [116,123], whereas HLA-DRB*07:01 appears to have a protective effect for development of this syndrome [123]. In the Korean and Japanese populations, anti-ARS have been associated with HLA-DRB1*08:03 [124,125]. A similar association with HLA-DRB1*04:05 has been described in Japanese patients [125]. Once the immune system in the lung has been activated, T/B cells and autoantibodies enter the systemic circulation and the autoimmune response spreads to other organs. The mechanisms by which some organs and systems (e.g., muscles, skin, and joints) are affected but not others are not well understood [126]. However, the inflamed muscles of IM patients significantly overexpress HisRS both in immune cells and regenerating myofibers, which contrasts with the low HisRS expression seen in normal muscle [127].

Environmental factors may play a relevant role in the development of anti-MDA5 syndrome. In a recent multicenter study, Nishina et al. reported seasonal and geographic influences on disease onset. Thus, ILD associated with anti-MDA5 occurred predominantly from October to March, especially in individuals residing near freshwater. Viral infection has been proposed as a plausible trigger for these geographical and seasonal associations. Infectious agents could be transmitted by vectors inhabiting near freshwater. Moreover, MDA5 is a cytoplasmic RIG-like receptor involved in the innate immune defense against viruses. Specifically, MDA5 recognizes intracellular RNA of several viruses, including coxsackievirus, rhinovirus, polio, and dengue, among others. MDA5 activation triggers production of type-I IFN and other proinflammatory cytokines, such as IL-6, IL-8, IL-1, INF-α, INF-α, and TNFα, in an attempt to restrict viral replication. Of interest, most of these cytokines are upregulated in blood of RP-ILD patients and directly associated with disease activity. As occurs in ASS, anti-MDA5 syndrome is associated with HLA-DRB1*12:02 [124,128], HLA-DRB1*01:01, and HLA-DRB1*04:05 in Asian countries [129].

Management strategy and treatment approach

When and why to treat ILD in IM?

ILD is the most severe extramuscular involvement in IM and is associated with high morbidity and mortality [104]. As a life-threatening manifestation, ILD frequently guides the treatment strategy in IM-ILD patients. The low prevalence, wide phenotypic heterogeneity, and variable course of IM-ILD complicate assessment of the different treatment approaches. This is illustrated by the lack of controlled trials dealing with this topic. As a consequence, IM-ILD treatment is mainly based on historical clinical practice and case series, and guided by the opinion of experts. Hence, it is recommendable that treatment of IM-ILD patients be coordinated in specialized centers with broad experience in the management of these diseases. In addition, multidisciplinary collaboration is becoming increasingly necessary in the diagnosis and management of IM-ILD. Multidisciplinary committees facilitate interaction between the various professionals involved in ILD management (e.g., respiratory physicians, thoracic radiologists, pathologists, rheumatologists) and contribute to integrate clinical, functional, and imaging data not only in the diagnostic process but also in accurate staging of disease severity, evaluating the prognosis, identifying ILD progression, and formulating a treatment strategy [22].

Immunosuppressive agents are the first-line treatment of IM-ILD. However, the type, dose, and number of immunosuppressants must be tailored to different scenarios (Table 6.2). Risk factors can help to identify patients with more severe ILD and a poorer prognosis. The autoantibody profile, age at diagnosis, ILD pattern, and high levels of ferritin or KL-6, among others, have been associated with poor outcomes. In patients at higher risk, combination therapy is recommended. In addition, the use of antifibrotic agents and

TABLE 6.2 Management of interstitial lung disease in inflammatory myopathies.

Scenario 1	Scenario 2	Scenario 3	Scenario 4	
Complementary exams				
HRCT<10% FVC >70%	FVC <70% *or* decline >10% FVC	FVC <50%	RP-ILD	
Symptoms				
Asymptomatic (no dyspnea)	Exertional dyspnea Modest desaturation	Significant dyspnea Oxygen required	Significant dyspnea Oxygen required	
Management				
	1st option	**1st option**	**1st option**	
No treatment (control 3–6 m)	GC + CYC/TAC	GC + CYC/TAC	GC + CYC/TAC ± CYCLOP	
	Alternatives	*Alternatives*	*Alternatives*	
	MMF, AZA	MMF, AZA	MMF, AZA	
		Progressive	**Rapidly progressive**	
		+ RTX/CYCLOP	1	+ RTX/CYCLOP
			2	PMX-HP, PMF, ICU, OIT, ECMO
			3	LT

AZA: Azathioprine; CYC: Cyclosporine; CYCLOP: Cyclophosphamide; ECMO: Veno-venous extracorporeal membrane oxygenation; FVC: Forced vital capacity; GC: Glucocorticoids; HRCT: High resolution computer tomography; ICU: Intensive care unit; MMF: Mycophenolate mofetil; OIT: Oropharyngeal intubation; PMX-HP: Polymyxin B hemoperfusion; PMF: Plasmapheresis; RTX: Rituximab; RP-ILD: Rapidly progressive interstitial lung disease; TAC: Tacrolimus

nonpharmacologic therapies, such as plasmapheresis, intravenous immunoglobulin, and polymyxin B hemoperfusion, can be considered for progressive ILD and refractory patients with severe acute ILD.

In some selected settings, absence of treatment can even be an option. Patients with limited ILD (<10%), especially those with few clinical repercussions, small abnormalities on respiratory function tests, and no evidence of clinical progression, can benefit from expectant management. These patients should be tightly monitored with clinical assessment and PFT every 3–4 months to upgrade treatment requirements. PFT changes should be carefully evaluated to rule out confounding factors of false respiratory impairment, such as concomitant infections or respiratory muscle weakness, among others. CT study would be necessary to confirm true IM-ILD progression when integration of clinical and PFT data is suggestive, but inconclusive.

Immunosuppressive therapy in antisynthetase syndrome and other slowly progressive IM-associated ILD cases

Most patients with IM-ILD develop slowly progressive ILD. This is the main ILD presentation form in ASS, overlap syndromes with anti-PM/Scl or anti-Ku, and IM-ILD with no associated MSAs. Patients with anti-MDA5 autoantibodies can also show a slow ILD course.

Mildly symptomatic forms of ILD can be effectively treated with glucocorticoids (e.g., prednisone) alone [130]. These drugs are usually initiated at around 0.5 to 1 mg/kg to a maximum dose of 70 to 80 mg/day. The treatment is maintained for 4–6 weeks and is followed by a slow tapering of 20% to 25% of the existing dose monthly to achieve daily prednisone doses of around 5 to 10 mg/day within 6 months. Complete withdrawal of glucocorticoids is not a generalized practice. Most IM-ILD patients require a chronic low prednisone dose of 5 to 7.5 mg/day. Of note, the addition of steroid-sparing agents from the time of the diagnosis is highly recommended in patients with IM-ILD. This practice, in addition to its potential effect in reducing common glucocorticoid side effects such as osteoporosis, hypertension, hyperglycemia and weight gain, is associated with better survival in IM-ILD and fewer relapses when compared with prednisone monotherapy [131,132].

The immunosuppressive drugs generally used as first-line agents for treatment of IM-ILD include mycophenolate mofetil (MMF, 2–3 g/day divided into two doses), azathioprine (AZT, 2–3 mg/kg per day in patients with normal thiopurine methyltransferase activity), cyclosporine A (CYC, 3–4 mg/kg per day), and tacrolimus (TAC, 0.06 mg/kg per day). Although methotrexate (MTX) has also been used for this indication, the potential lung toxicity associated with this drug has limited its use in clinical practice. To date there is no evidence to support the superiority of any one of the aforementioned immunosuppressive agents in ASS-ILD [133–135]. Selection of glucocorticoid-sparing immunosuppressant agents is usually guided by the security profile of each drug in each patient's clinical setting. For example, calcineurin inhibitors should be used with caution in elderly patients because of their higher prevalence of hypertension and kidney disease, which may require dose adjustment according to serum concentrations of the drug. In these settings, MMF and AZT are commonly used in clinical practice because of their good tolerability and known efficacy in ILD associated with other connective tissue diseases. However, some observational studies and expert opinion suggest that calcineurin inhibitors could have an additional benefit on survival and functional outcomes in comparison to other treatments, especially in refractory and more severe cases [136]. For this reason, these drugs are also often used in combination with glucocorticoids as first-line treatment for ILD associated with anti-ASS or anti-MDA5, especially in young people and in Asian countries. Nevertheless, there are no randomized studies supporting this practice.

Cyclophosphamide and rituximab have been used as third-line therapies in progressive ILD and refractory cases, with good results in observational studies. Cyclophosphamide has proved useful for achieving stabilization or improvement of functional respiratory parameters in clinical trials and retrospective studies in IM-ILD patients [137]. The use of this drug is mainly restricted by common adverse events, including cytopenia, infertility, and increased infections. Rituximab use in severe or refractory IM-ILD is supported by several retrospective case reports and case series [138–140], particularly in patients with anti-Jo1 ASS and anti-Ro52 [46]. In a retrospective study comparing the effect of cyclophosphamide or rituximab in refractory anti-Jo1 ASS-ILD, the two drugs showed similar efficacy as induction therapy at 6 months. However, rituximab followed by AZT or MMF as maintenance therapy was associated with better two-year progression-free survival than cyclophosphamide [141].

Tofacitinib, a Janus kinase inhibitor, has been evaluated in combination with glucocorticoids in patients with early stage anti-MDA5 CADM-ILD [142]. All patients had a mild-moderate ILD disease with a mean predicted FVC (%) value of 73.4 ± 15.2. Survival 6 months after ILD onset was significantly higher in patients treated with tofacitinib than in those with similar characteristics from a historical cohort who were treated with intensive immunosuppression (100% vs. 78%, $P = .04$). Ferritin levels, FVC, DLCO, and HRCT findings in tofacitinib-treated patients were also considerably improved over time. These tentative results suggest a potentially relevant role of tofacitinib as first-line ILD treatment in anti-MDA5 patients [143].

Management of rapidly progressive ILD associated with anti-MDA5 antibodies

Rapidly progressive ILD is a hallmark of DM/CADM with anti-MDA5 antibodies and its most severe manifestation. Characteristically, RP-ILD in these patients is associated with high mortality and refractoriness to conventional treatments. Similar acute ILD presentations are sometimes seen in other types of IM, such as ASS, but these cases usually have a better prognosis and response treatment.

RP-ILD is a life-threatening complication that requires early identification and intensive therapeutic management. The initial therapy should include a combination of different immunosuppressive drugs. In a recent review focused on the evidence-based therapeutic recommendations [144], two different schedules were suggested: a combination of glucocorticoids plus a calcineurin antagonist (CYC or TAC, considered equally good options), or triple therapy adding intravenous cyclophosphamide to the previous schedule. The usefulness of triple therapy has been supported by several observational retrospective and prospective studies performed in Japanese patients [106,145,146]. Cytomegalovirus reactivation is common in these series and should be considered a drawback of combined immunosuppressive therapy [144]. When the use of calcineurin antagonists or cyclophosphamide is unfeasible, combination therapy with MMF or adding rituximab to any of the previous schedules should be considered. Other treatments such as basiliximab (an anti-CD25/sIL-2R monoclonal antibody) or tofacitinib have also been reported as possible options in these patients. According to the emerging results of recent studies [142,143], tofacitinib is a promising therapeutic option for patients with anti-MDA5 syndrome. The effect that JAK-STAT inhibition exerts over multiple cytokines involved in the physiopathology of anti-MDA5 RP-ILD, such as types I and II interferon and IL-6, supports the potential role of this treatment as a first-line agent in future schedules.

Management of anti-MDA5 RP-ILD patients who do not respond to the initial combination therapy can include stepwise addition of any of the other aforementioned immunosuppressive agents (MMF, basiliximab, tofacitinib, or rituximab) to the current therapy or switching one immunosuppressive drug to another. The choice of these drugs will depend on their safety profile and the patient's characteristics.

Alternative nonpharmacologic rescue therapies such as polymyxin B hemoperfusion [147–149], plasmapheresis [147,150], and intravenous immunoglobulins [144] might also be considered in refractory cases. The efficacy of these therapies is related to their capacity to adsorb and eliminate inflammatory cytokines, mediators, and activated leukocytes, and to remove anti-MDA5 antibodies from the blood [144]. Veno-venous extracorporeal membrane oxygenation (ECMO), a life-support technique aimed at maintaining lung function and blood oxygenation in patients with respiratory failure, may be useful in selected patients as a bridge to lung transplantation (LT) or to provide time for immunosuppressive therapy to act [144].

Clinical vignette 3

Before the onset of the COVID-19 pandemic, a 42-year-old man was admitted to our systemic autoimmune unit due to a clinical syndrome of dyspnea, fever, and cough that had started 2 weeks previously. Radiography showed a diffuse bilateral reticular pattern. Broad-spectrum antibiotic therapy was instituted, but there was no improvement. HRCT of the chest showed substantial diffuse pulmonary fibrosis, traction bronchiectasis, and septal thickening, with a significant pneumomediastinum (Fig. 6.2). Physical examination identified mechanic's hands and Gottron papules, as well as severe orthodeoxia, with an oxygen saturation drop to <80% in sitting position at rest. Thus, a diagnosis of a RP-ILD in a patient with amyopathic DM was suspected. Antibodies against MDA5 were highly positive by ELISA and confirmed by blot.

Clinical vignette 3—cont'd

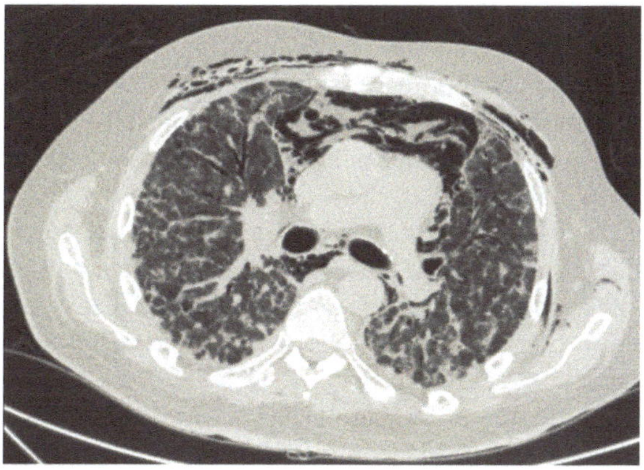

FIGURE 6.2 High-resolution computed tomography of the chest showing pneumomediastinum.

Treatment consisted of a combination of methylprednisolone, TAC, and polymyxin B hemoperfusion, subsequently continued with a plasmapheresis scheme followed by intravenous immunoglobulin, which led to a gradual improvement of this severe condition. Two months later the patient was much improved clinically and HRCT findings were near normal. The patient was discharged with a FVC of 42% and a therapeutic schedule including TAC and steroid therapy. At 6 months follow-up, the FVC had increased to 64%, and 1 year later, to 85%. Five years later, TAC was switched to MMF due to a slight decrease in renal function.

Comment

Although several anti-MDA5-related phenotypes have been described, the one reported in the clinical vignette is the most severe [147]. Clinicians must bear in mind the possibility of anti-MDA5 syndrome in patients with rapidly progressive ILD, especially when skin lesions are present. Occasionally these lesions are difficult to detect, particularly when glucocorticoids have been administered. A recently published treatment scheme has been suggested by a panel of experts, which include the therapeutic approach herein reported [144]. More research is needed for better management of this catastrophic syndrome.

Antifibrotic treatment

The concept of chronic ILD with a progressive fibrosing phenotype (PF-ILD) has emerged in recent years to describe a clinical situation, common to several types of ILD, characterized by a progressive decline in pulmonary function in combination with worsening respiratory symptoms or increased extent of fibrosis on HRCT within 24 months [151]. Two antifibrotic drugs, pirfenidone and nintedanib, have proven useful for reducing the rate of FVC decline in patients with IPF, the paradigm of PF-ILD.

Histologically, IM-ILD is characterized by a variety of patterns, including NSIP, OP, and UIP. In many cases, especially those with UIP patterns, after a phase in which immunosuppressive treatment manages to stabilize lung involvement, the patient may begin to show progressive lung function deterioration, with a poor response to immunosuppressive treatment and progression of pulmonary fibrosis. This clinical course often culminates in end-stage lung disease and suggests that fibrotic and not autoimmune mechanisms are likely involved in the functional deterioration in late stages. Thus, a potential role of antifibrotic drugs is suggested in IM-ILD treatment.

To date, antifibrotic drug use has been evaluated in three clinical trials in connective tissue disease ILD (CTD-ILD). SENSICS, a phase-III, randomized, placebo-controlled, double-blind, parallel-group trial, evaluated the safety and efficacy of nintedanib versus placebo in 576 patients with scleroderma (288 in each group) [152]. A significantly lower decline in the adjusted annual FVC rate was observed in the treatment group (−52.4 mL in the nintedanib group vs. −3.3 mL in the placebo group, $P = .04$). The INBUILD study involved 663 patients with PF-ILD of different etiologies, including 25.6% of patients with various CTDs [153]. Over a 52-week treatment period, nintedanib was also superior to placebo in reducing the FVC decline (−80.8 mL vs. −187.8 mL, $P < .001$). Based on the findings from these clinical trials, nintedanib was approved by the FDA in March 2020 for the treatment of progressive fibrosing ILD, including CTD-ILD. In addition, nintedanib was licensed for use in patients with SSc-ILD by the FDA in September 2019 and the EMA in April 2020.

Finally, a single study was conducted in 30 patients with RP-ILD associated with CADM to evaluate the usefulness of pirfenidone added to conventional treatment [154]. This open-label, prospective study with matched retrospective controls, reported no significant differences in survival at 12 months (primary endpoint) between the groups. However, in the subgroup with subacute disease (disease duration 3−6 months), patients ($n = 10$) receiving pirfenidone had a significantly higher survival rate than patients ($n = 9$) receiving standard treatment (90% vs. 44.4% $P = .045$). The authors hypothesized that fibrosing mechanisms may have a more relevant role in the group of patients with subacute ILD. Two clinical trials are currently ongoing to evaluate the efficacy of pirfenidone in patients with DM−ILD (NCT02821689 and NCT03857854) [155,156].

Lung transplantation

LT is the only treatment proven to increase survival in patients with end-stage or refractory pulmonary disease [157]. The most extensively reported experience of LT in a single CTD has been for scleroderma [158,159], with several studies showing complication and survival rates similar to those of patients with IPF undergoing LT. Based on the positive results of LT in scleroderma patients and data from general epidemiologic studies, LT is now broadly considered a valid option to treat patients with end-stage CTD-ILD [160,161]. Nevertheless, as nonscleroderma CTD patients are usually grouped together in cohort studies, there is little information on possible specific challenges in LT management in each of these entities. In a study conducted by Courtwright et al., DM and PM accounted for 22% of 275 patients with nonscleroderma CTD who underwent LT from 2005 to 2016 [161]. The authors found no significant differences in survival, acute or chronic rejection, or extrapulmonary organ dysfunction between patients receiving LT for nonscleroderma CTD or for IPF. Similarly, in a large retrospective study on CTD-ILD, Takagishi et al. reported survival rates similar to those of IPF patients and a low rate of CTD post-LT flares in their subgroup of 34 patients with PM/DM [160]. An additional limited number of case reports and small series have reported similar results [162]. In contrast, in a cohort of 36 patients with CTD-ILD including 8 patients with PM/DM, Yang et al. reported a significantly lower cumulative survival rate in PM/DM-ILD patients than those with IPF, especially at 6 months (38% vs. 73%, $P = .04$). In addition, PM/DM-ILD patients had higher incidence of primary graft dysfunction ($P = .006$) and a lengthier intensive care unit stay ($P < .001$) than those with IPF. Specific information on transplantation in patients with anti-MDA5 is limited to a small number of case reports with variable results [163,164]. Much more information is needed on the impact that the specific problems of IM patients may have on the outcome of LT. Some of these potential challenges include the presence of subclinical cardiac involvement (myocarditis and conduction abnormalities), muscle weakness that can induce hypoventilation, gastroesophageal reflux disease, dysphagia, increased risk of malignancy, and risk of relapse of the underlying disease.

Overall, according to the limited evidence, LT can be considered a valid therapeutic option in IM-ILD patients with end-stage or refractory ILD. Potential candidates for LT should be referred early to a transplantation center for evaluation.

Management of specific comorbidities in ILD patients

Arthritis Arthritis is one of the main features of ASS, especially in patients with anti-Jo1 antibody. Arthritis appears mainly at disease onset and often adopts a symmetrical polyarticular pattern similar to that seen in RA. In contrast, an oligoarticular or asymmetric pattern is more typical in patients who develop arthritis as an ex-novo manifestation during follow-up. Positive testing to anti-cyclic citrullinated peptide (anti-CCP) and rheumatoid factor has been described in around 11% and 27% of ASS patients, respectively [27], suggesting (at least in the first case) a true overlap with RA. The therapeutic approach to arthritis in ILD-ASS patients can be challenging, as both conventional and biologic disease-modifying antirheumatic drugs (DMARDs) have been related to development of drug-related pulmonary toxicity, although the data are conflicting [165]. In ASS patients with active myositis and/or ILD at disease onset, concomitant arthritis rarely determines the initial therapeutic management. Joint involvement has a good response to medium-high doses of glucocorticoids, which are generally used as first-line treatment for these extra-articular manifestations. Patients often achieve rapid and sustained remission of joint activity, the latter thanks to the slow reduction in glucocorticoid dose in tapering schedules. With this approach, arthritis may not be a major clinical problem in some patients during follow-up. However, others experiment flares of arthritis following glucocorticoid tapering or even after months or years of clinical remission. This situation is favored by the fact that the conventional DMARDs most often used as glucocorticoid-sparing agents to treat myositis and ILD, such as AZT, MMF, and calcineurin inhibitors (CYC and TAC), have little or no effect against arthritis. In the absence of controlled studies, the therapeutic approach to arthritis in these ASS cases is based on empirical data from retrospective case series and case reports, and mimics strategies followed in other autoimmune diseases that combine arthritis and ILD, such as RA.

MTX could be a good option to treat arthritis in the absence of ILD. However, as MTX has been associated with occasional cases of acute or subacute hypersensitivity pneumonitis, a rare complication occurring in less than 0.3% of patients mainly during the first year of treatment, its use is generally eluded in patients with overt ILD who develop arthritis as a new manifestation. Conversely, in ASS patients with arthritis that have been treated with MTX for more than 1 year and develop ILD, there is no evidence to support discontinuation of MTX. Notwithstanding, tight monitoring of respiratory symptoms and lung function is recommended in these patients. As an alternative, leflunomide (LFN) can be a good option to treat arthritis in non-Asian patients with ASS. In the Asian population, LFN has been associated with de novo development or exacerbation of a preexisting ILD in around 1% of patients, whereas the frequency of these complications in Western countries is estimated to be less than 0.02% [166]. In refractory cases or if these treatments are not appropriate or not well tolerated, rituximab, abatacept, and tocilizumab, all of them highly effective against arthritis, can be considered as alternative options.

Clinical vignette 4

A 66-year-old woman was admitted to our hospital with progressive dyspnea without cough or fever, polyarthritis with involvement of large and small joints, and upper limb weakness. The respiratory symptoms had started 3 months earlier, at which time she was diagnosed with left basal pneumonia following chest radiography in the emergency department. She received antibiotic treatment for 10 days with little improvement. Due to the persistent symptoms and abnormal X-ray findings, the study was extended with chest CT, which showed bilateral basal infiltrates and hilar and mediastinal adenopathy. A new empirical antibiotic treatment was prescribed, but the patient did not improve. In the following days,

Clinical vignette 4—cont'd

she experienced an onset of stiffness, pain, and polyarticular swelling, together with muscle weakness predominantly proximal to the upper extremities. On admission, she showed bilateral basal crackles and symmetrical polyarthritis affecting the metacarpophalangeal, proximal interphalangeal, carpal, and knee joints, as well as hyperkeratotic lesions on the fingers, suggestive of mechanic's hands. Laboratory analyses disclosed elevated CK (1293 IU/L, NV<195 IU/L), ESR (81 mm/h), and CRP (2.6 mg/dL) values. Electromyography detected an inflammatory myogenic pattern in the proximal musculature of the four extremities, and muscle biopsy showed findings consistent with a diagnosis of polymyositis. Functional respiratory study showed a restrictive pattern with FVC values of 50.7%. DLCO was not performed for technical reasons. The autoantibody study was positive for anti-Jo1 and anti-Ro52 antibodies at high titers and a diagnosis of ASS was established. Anti-CCP and rheumatoid factor were negative.

The patient started treatment with TAC and prednisone at 60 mg/day for 1 month with subsequently taper, with a good clinical evolution. In the following weeks, CK levels and muscle strength normalized, dyspnea significantly improved, and arthritis completely remitted. Functional respiratory testing performed in the following months showed an improvement of functional parameters, with FVC at 66.6% and a DLCO 61%.

Five months after discharge, while on treatment with TAC 3 mg/12h and prednisone 7.5 mg/24h, the patient consulted again for recurrent polyarthritis with a distribution similar to the initial symptoms. The prednisone dose was temporarily increased and, given the patient's interstitial lung involvement, treatment with LFN 20 mg/day was started. In the following weeks, there was a significant improvement in joint symptoms, but the patient developed moderate-severe diarrhea as an LFN side effect, which led to a reduction in the LFN dose to 10 mg/day. Due to persistent joint activity in the following months, biological treatment with subcutaneous abatacept 125 mg/weekly was started, and LFN was discontinued. With this treatment, the patient achieved sustained arthritis remission in the following weeks. Serial PFT continued to show stable values in the following months.

Comment

This case is illustrative of how arthritis can be a clinically relevant manifestation of ASS, requiring specific treatment for its management. In our experience, LFN has been effective to control joint manifestations in many ASS patients. LFN is a generally well-tolerated drug that can be considered safe in patients with ILD. As was mentioned above, LFN-associated pulmonary toxicity in Caucasian patients is extremely rare. Its use ahead of MTX is justified to avoid potential confounding factors, such as MTX-associated hypersensitive pneumonitis, which could influence follow-up assessment of an ongoing ILD. Our patient, after an initially good joint response to LFN, began to present with daily watery diarrhea, a relatively common and usually mild side effect (1%—10%) associated with this drug, which significantly affected her quality of life and initially led to a dose reduction and later drug withdrawal. Subcutaneous abatacept was then started, with good tolerance and efficacy. The patient achieved sustained joint remission after 5 weeks of treatment.

Continued

Clinical vignette 4—cont'd

Abatacept seems to have a good safety profile in RA patients with ILD, and its use has not been related with deteriorated respiratory function in this population [165]. Moreover, some studies suggest a potential positive effect of abatacept on ILD, although controlled trials are needed to support this statement. In addition, abatacept seems to have a better safety profile than other biological DMARDs used in RA, and has been associated with a lower rate of severe infections, especially those affecting the respiratory system, in comparison to anti-TNFα [167]. Rituximab has been widely used in RA treatment and is also considered a safe therapy in patients with ILD [165]. Several retrospective and observational series support its use to treat severe refractory ILD in ASS patients [138–140]. However, rituximab is associated with a high rate of infections and hypogammaglobulinemia [140,168]. Our patient had achieved stable lung function after glucocorticoids and TAC, and we preferred to reserve rituximab in case of ILD progression. Tocilizumab could be another alternative safety option, although data on its use in RA-ILD is anecdotical and conflicting [165]. Finally, the use of anti-TNFα is not recommended as it has been associated to new onset or exacerbation of RA-ILD [165].

Pulmonary hypertension PH, defined as an increase in mean pulmonary arterial pressure ≥20 mmHg at rest as assessed by right heart catheterization, is not a rare complication of ASS [6]. In a retrospective study, Hervier et al. reported a catheterization-confirmed 7.9% prevalence of PH [6]. This value is similar to data reported in patients with other CTDs such as systemic lupus erythematosus [169], but it is slightly lower than that described in SSc [170]. PH can be caused by various pathophysiological mechanisms, which should differentiate to provide appropriate treatment according to each underlying condition. In contrast to other CTDs, PH in ASS seems to be mainly secondary to ILD (Group 3 of the clinical classification of PH), whereas primary vasculopathy of the small pulmonary arteries (Group 1 pulmonary arterial hypertension, defined as PH in the absence of other causes of precapillary PH such as ILD or chronic thromboembolic PH, among others) is, for instance, the most frequent PH form in SSc. However, indirect evidence suggests probable primary pulmonary vascular involvement in the development of PH in ASS patients. Most patients with PH and ILD have severe PH that is considered disproportionate to the degree of interstitial involvement. In addition, a high percentage of these patients have an FVC/DLCO ratio >1.8, a parameter proposed as a marker of pulmonary vascular disease in SSc [6].

PH has been associated with a poorer prognosis and lower survival rates in ASS patients. Therefore, PH screening could be considered a recommended practice in these patients. Transthoracic echocardiography is the most used screening test for PH. It could be performed at baseline and periodically thereafter, especially in patients with severe dyspnea with no compatible HRCT findings or with a DLCO drop out of proportion to the FVC drop. When elevated pulmonary artery systolic pressure is estimated on echocardiography, right heart catheterization is needed to confirm the PH diagnosis.

Treatment of PH in ASS patients follows the general principles of PH management. Immunosuppressive treatment of ILD is indicated to stop progression of the underlying condition. Supplementary oxygen and diuretic therapy are mainstays of PH-ILD treatment in patients with hypoxemia (at rest, or during exercise or sleep) and fluid retention from PH-related right ventricular failure. The potential benefit of drugs specifically directed to reduce pulmonary arterial hypertension, such as prostacyclin pathway agonists, endothelin receptor antagonists, phosphodiesterase inhibitors, or nitric oxide-cGMP enhancers, is controversial and usually limited to patients in WHO functional class III or IV. However, considering that PH in some ASS patients can be ocassionally unrelated to their lung disease, these treatments could be used in selected cases in the setting of center with expertise in PH management.

Other treatments considerations

Vaccination for influenza and pneumococcal pneumonia is recommended in all patients with ILD-IM, and mandatory for the recent pandemic SARS-CoV-2 virus. Bone density assessment and osteoporosis prevention should be initiated in any patient on glucocorticoid treatment. Prophylaxis for *Pneumocystis jirovecii* pneumonia should be considered in patients receiving more than 20 mg of prednisone or equivalent, and in those on a combination of glucocorticoids (equivalent to 10 mg of prednisone or more) and a second agent.

The lung in mixed connective tissue disease

MCTD, initially described by Sharp et al., is considered a well-defined autoimmune systemic disease with proper diagnostic criteria and a good immunology biomarker, the anti-RNP antibodies [171]. Few studies have investigated the prevalence of ILD in MCTD. The recently published Norwegian cohort is one of the most reliable studies, reporting an ILD prevalence of 41% in MCTD [172–175]. Not only ILD is not rare in patients with MCTD but it is also associated with high mortality, depending on the percentage of affected lung on HRCT. Thus, the greater the HRCT lung involvement, the lesser the cumulative survival rate, which may decrease to 60% at 10 years when lung involvement is higher than 10% [172].

The main factors implicated in lower 5 to 10 year survival include male sex, lung function status at disease onset, and the immunological profile, with high levels of anti-RNP antibodies or presence of anti-Ro52 antibodies as biomarkers of a worse prognosis [172,176,177]. Raynaud phenomenon has also been linked to ILD in MCTD patients [178,179]. Analysis of pathological findings is scarce. Only one study has focused on the lung pathology, and analysis of 16 patients found NISP in all cases, with different grades of fibrosis [173].

There are no studies specifically addressing therapy in MCTD patients with ILD, but it seems logical to use an early intervention, mainly MMF administration, following the studies in systemic sclerosis and retrospective data on this drug in MCTD patients. Calcineurin inhibitors (CYC or TAC) or rituximab may also be good options, even in absence of scientific evidence [180].

PH is a potential manifestation of lung involvement in MCTD even without ILD. Clinicians must consider this scenario when dyspnea appears in the absence of ILD, characteristically with a reduced DLCO, normal FVC, and no features of ILD on HRCT. The first recommended step is echocardiography and if necessary, right heart catheterization to confirm the presence of PH (mean pulmonary arterial pressure [PAP] >20 mm Hg). This is important because in addition to their immunosuppressive therapy, classical PH therapy, such as endothelin receptor antagonists, phosphodiesterase inhibitors, or other specific agents, may considerably improve the clinical status of these patients [181].

Dyspnea at rest, exertional dyspnea, and auscultation of bibasilar crackles may be the first manifestation of ILD. These findings should prompt completion of the study with PFT (FVC and DLCO), HRCT, and echocardiography to rule out PH. Of note, MCTD patients with arthritis, pleuritis, myositis, and other clinical features may develop some type of dyspnea that could be attributed to ILD, and failing that, to possible PH.

Clinical vignette 5

A 17-year-old woman was referred to our outpatient clinic for a decrease in lung function (FVC 58%, DLCO 51%) over the previous 2 years. She had been diagnosed with juvenile MCTD at the age of 9 years based on arthritis, Raynaud phenomenon, dysphagia, and ILD (first FVC in 2010, 69%, DLCO was not performed; HRCT with ground glass areas and honeycombing in the lower lobes, Fig. 6.3). Hypergammaglobulinemia and high anti-RNP antibody levels and negative testing for other antigenic specificities supported the diagnosis of MCTD. Fine crackles were auscultated at both lung bases. Creatine kinase was normal, and there was no muscle weakness or kidney involvement. The patient received treatment with low-dose glucocorticoids and TAC from the onset, with an initial evident clinical and functional improvement (FVC three years later, 76.6%, DLCO value unavailable) that subsequently diminished, which was why the patient was referred to our unit.

At the age of 20 years, with the last FVC value at 59% while under TAC treatment, she stopped attending her regular appointments at our outpatient clinic and spontaneously discontinued any type of medication. She returned 5 years later. At this point, her FVC had improved relative to the value at 20 years (FVC 72%, DLCO 52%). We decided to repeat the HRCT study (Fig. 6.4) to obtain a

Clinical vignette 5—cont'd

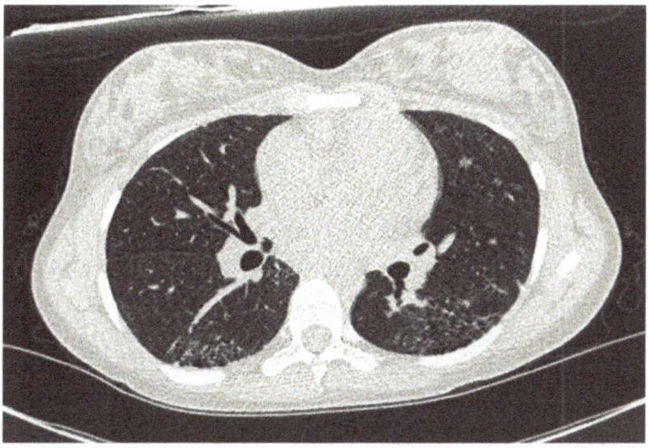

FIGURE 6.3 High resolution computed tomography scan shows ground glass areas and honeycombing in the lower lobes.

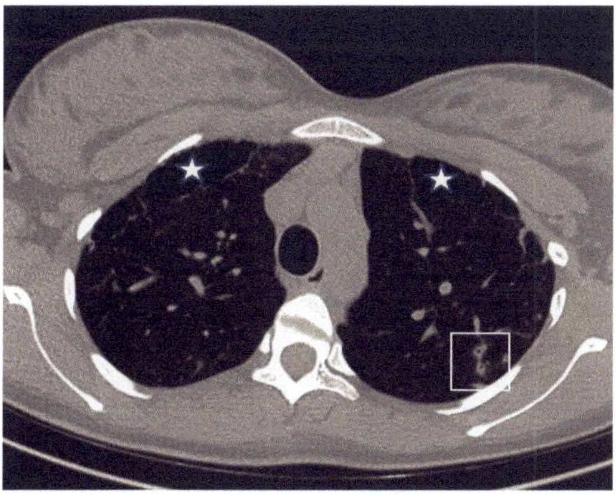

FIGURE 6.4 High-resolution computed tomography of the chest depicts several poorly circumscribed, cavitating nodules (an example outlined in white). Residual cystic lesions and emphysematous changes are also present, indicated by stars).

more comprehensive evaluation and design an appropriate therapy, which she was not currently receiving. In addition to the known ILD, which had not changed, HRCT findings included the presence of pseudo-nodules with cavitation, suggesting an infectious-inflammatory cause. While waiting for fibrobronchoscopy assessment, the results from a broad autoimmune profile reported positive testing for antineutrophil cytoplasmic antibodies (ANCA) with myeloperoxidase (anti-MPO) specificity (in addition to positive testing for anti-RNP antibodies). Kidney biopsy performed to investigate microscopic hematuria and impaired kidney function disclosed a pauci-immune glomerulonephritis with cellular crescents and

Continued

Clinical vignette 5—cont'd

fibrinoid necrosis. She was diagnosed with microscopic polyangiitis and received therapy with cyclophosphamide pulses and rituximab. One year after starting this regimen the patient was doing well, and the lung involvement was stable, with FVC at 75%.

Comment

Some messages can be drawn from this clinical vignette. First, we must keep in mind that MCTD can appear in childhood as a juvenile form, and that development of ILD over time in this age group is not rare. A cross-sectional study in large cohort of 52 juvenile MCTD patients from Norway reported that 27% of cases could develop ILD after 16 years of follow-up, mainly as a mild disease without great progression [182]. Thus, ILD in juvenile forms seems to be more stable and have a better outcome over time, although longitudinal studies have not been reported. We cannot know whether ILD stabilization in the reported case occurred because of the immunosuppressive therapy. For 5 years she received no therapy and FVC remained stable. Nevertheless, a situation in which FVC decreases over time and progressive ILD is documented on HRCT would logically prompt establishment of immunosuppressive treatment. Glucocorticoids and steroid-sparing agents such as calcineurin inhibitors (TAC or CYC) are our preferred choice, but MMF or rituximab are also good options. There is no evidence-based data to support one approach or another. In the case reported here, the current therapy is rituximab for microscopic polyangiitis. In time we will see the outcome of this therapeutic strategy.

A second, and not inconsequential message, is that patients with MCTD can develop ANCA-associated vasculitis in addition to characteristic features of lupus, RA, or myositis. To our knowledge, 11 such cases have been reported to date [183]. Physicians must keep in mind this association and carry out ANCA analysis or even lung biopsy if the patient's radiologic features change from those seen in ILD (UIP or NSIP) to a nodular or cavitating pattern. Early diagnosis of ANCA-associated vasculitis involving lung or kidney is of paramount relevance to institute appropriate therapy.

References

[1] Diamon B, Lipsky E. Autoimmunity and autoimune diseases. Harrison's principles of internal medicine. 20th ed. McGraw Hill; 2018.

[2] Jeganathan N, Sathananthan M. Connective tissue disease-related interstitial lung disease: prevalence, patterns, predictors, prognosis, and treatment. Lung 2020;198:735–59. https://doi.org/10.1007/s00408-020-00383-w.

[3] Kuwana M, Gil-Vila A, Selva-O'Callaghan A. Role of autoantibodies in the diagnosis and prognosis of interstitial lung disease in autoimmune rheumatic disorders. Ther Adv Musculoskelet Dis 2021;13. https://doi.org/10.1177/1759720X211032457.

[4] Selva-O'Callaghan A, Pinal-Fernandez I, Trallero-Araguás E, Milisenda JC, Grau-Junyent JM, Mammen AL. Classification and management of adult inflammatory myopathies. Lancet Neurol 2018;17:816–28. https://doi.org/10.1016/S1474-4422(18)30254-0.

[5] Barba T, Mainbourg S, Nasser M, Lega J-C, Cottin V. Lung diseases in inflammatory myopathies. Semin Respir Crit Care Med 2019;40:255–70. https://doi.org/10.1055/s-0039-1685187.

[6] Hervier B, Meyer A, Dieval C, Uzunhan Y, Devilliers H, Launay D, et al. Pulmonary hypertension in antisynthetase syndrome: prevalence, aetiology and survival. Eur Respir J 2013;42:1271–82. https://doi.org/10.1183/09031936.00156312.

[7] Li Y, Wang P, Li L, Wang F, Liu Y. Increased risk of venous thromboembolism associated with polymyositis and dermatomyositis: a meta-analysis. Therapeut Clin Risk Manag 2018;14:157–65. https://doi.org/10.2147/TCRM.S157085.

[8] Selva-O'Callaghan A, Fernández-Luque A, Martínez-Gómez X, Labirua-Iturburu A, Vilardell-Tarrés M. Venous thromboembolism in patients with dermatomyositis and polymyositis. Clin Exp Rheumatol 2011;29:846–9.

[9] Selva-O'Callaghan A, Sanchez-Sitjes L, Muñoz-Gall X, Mijares-Boeckh-Behrens T, Solans-Laque R, Angel Bosch-Gil J, et al. Respiratory failure due to muscle weakness in inflammatory myopathies: maintenance therapy with home mechanical ventilation. Rheumatology 2000;39:914–6. https://doi.org/10.1093/rheumatology/39.8.914.

[10] Selva-O'Callaghan A, Sampol G, Romero O, Lloberes P, Trallero-Araguás E, Vilardell-Tarrés M. Obstructive sleep apnea in patients with inflammatory myopathies. Muscle Nerve 2009;39:144–9. https://doi.org/10.1002/mus.21204.

[11] Aboussouan LS. Sleep-disordered breathing in neuromuscular disease. Am J Respir Crit Care Med 2015;191:979–89. https://doi.org/10.1164/rccm.201412-2224CI.

[12] Mellies U, Ragette R, Schwake C, Baethmann M, Voit T, Teschler H. Sleep-disordered breathing and respiratory failure in acid maltase deficiency. Neurology 2001;57:1290–5. https://doi.org/10.1212/wnl.57.7.1290.

[13] Runte M, Spiesshoefer J, Heidbreder A, Dreher M, Young P, Brix T, et al. Sleep-related breathing disorders in facioscapulohumeral dystrophy. Sleep Breath 2019;23:899–906. https://doi.org/10.1007/s11325-019-01843-1.

[14] Subramony SH, Wymer JP, Pinto BS, Wang ET. Sleep disorders in myotonic dystrophies. Muscle Nerve 2020;62:309–20. https://doi.org/10.1002/mus.26866.

[15] Rodríguez Cruz PM, Needham M, Hollingsworth P, Mastaglia FL, Hillman DR. Sleep disordered breathing and subclinical impairment of respiratory function are common in sporadic inclusion body myositis. Neuromuscul Disord 2014;24:1036–41. https://doi.org/10.1016/j.nmd.2014.08.003.

[16] Lakhanpal S, Lie JT, Conn DL, Martin WJ. Pulmonary disease in polymyositis/dermatomyositis: a clinicopathological analysis of 65 autopsy cases. Ann Rheum Dis 1987;46:23–9. https://doi.org/10.1136/ard.46.1.23.

[17] Teixeira A, Cherin P, Demoule A, Levy-Soussan M, Straus C, Verin E, et al. Diaphragmatic dysfunction in patients with idiopathic inflammatory myopathies. Neuromuscul Disord 2005;15:32–9. https://doi.org/10.1016/j.nmd.2004.09.006.

[18] Selva-O'Callaghan A, Labrador-Horrillo M, Muñoz-Gall X, Martínez-Gomez X, Majó-Masferrer J, Solans-Laque R, et al. Polymyositis/dermatomyositis-associated lung disease: analysis of a series of 81 patients. Lupus 2005;14:534–42. https://doi.org/10.1191/0961203305lu2158oa.

[19] Chong WH, Saha B, Jones DM, Beegle S. Respiratory failure secondary to diaphragmatic paralysis from acute exacerbation of dermatomyositis. Am J Med Sci 2021;361:659–65. https://doi.org/10.1016/j.amjms.2020.06.029.

[20] Astudillo LM, Carreiro M, Sailler L, Dingremont CF, Arlet PM. Hypercapnic coma due to diaphragmatic involvement in a patient with dermatomyositis. Clin Exp Rheumatol 2001;19:456–8.

[21] Lega J-C, Reynaud Q, Belot A, Fabien N, Durieu I, Cottin V. Idiopathic inflammatory myopathies and the lung. Eur Respir Rev 2015;24:216–38. https://doi.org/10.1183/16000617.00002015.

[22] Wells A, Devaraj A, Renzoni EA, Denton CP. Multidisciplinary evaluation in patients with lung disease associated with connective tissue disease. Semin Respir Crit Care Med 2019;40:184–93. https://doi.org/10.1055/s-0039-1684020.

[23] Zou J, Guo Q, Chi J, Wu H, Bao C. HRCT score and serum ferritin level are factors associated to the 1-year mortality of acute interstitial lung disease in clinically amyopathic dermatomyositis patients. Clin Rheumatol 2015;34:707–14. https://doi.org/10.1007/s10067-015-2866-5.

[24] Fujiki Y, Kotani T, Isoda K, Ishida T, Shoda T, Yoshida S, et al. Evaluation of clinical prognostic factors for interstitial pneumonia in anti-MDA5 antibody-positive dermatomyositis patients. Mod Rheumatol 2018;28:133–40. https://doi.org/10.1080/14397595.2017.1318468.

[25] Khanna D, Mittoo S, Aggarwal R, Proudman SM, Dalbeth N, Matteson EL, et al. Connective tissue disease-associated interstitial lung diseases (CTD-ILD) - report from OMERACT CTD-ILD working group. J Rheumatol 2015;42:2168–71. https://doi.org/10.3899/jrheum.141182.

[26] McHugh NJ, Tansley SL. Autoantibodies in myositis. Nat Rev Rheumatol 2018;14:290–302. https://doi.org/10.1038/nrrheum.2018.56.

[27] Cavagna L, Trallero-Araguás E, Meloni F, Cavazzana I, Rojas-Serrano J, Feist E, et al. Influence of antisynthetase antibodies specificities on antisynthetase syndrome clinical spectrum time course. J Clin Med 2019;8:E2013. https://doi.org/10.3390/jcm8112013.

[28] Moghadam-Kia S, Oddis CV, Sato S, Kuwana M, Aggarwal R. Antimelanoma differentiation-associated gene 5 antibody: expanding the clinical spectrum in North American patients with dermatomyositis. J Rheumatol 2017;44:319–25. https://doi.org/10.3899/jrheum.160682.

[29] Chen Z, Cao M, Plana MN, Liang J, Cai H, Kuwana M, et al. Utility of anti-melanoma differentiation-associated gene 5 antibody measurement in identifying patients with dermatomyositis and a high risk for developing rapidly progressive interstitial lung disease: a review of the literature and a meta-analysis. Arthritis Care Res 2013;65:1316–24. https://doi.org/10.1002/acr.21985.

[30] Peterson LK, Jaskowski TD, La'ulu SL, Tebo AE. Antibodies to small ubiquitin-like modifier activating enzyme are associated with a diagnosis of dermatomyositis: results from an unselected cohort. Immunol Res 2018;66:431–6. https://doi.org/10.1007/s12026-018-9006-7.

[31] Albayda J, Mecoli C, Casciola-Rosen L, Danoff SK, Lin CT, Hines D, et al. A North American cohort of anti-SAE dermatomyositis: clinical phenotype, testing, and review of cases. ACR Open Rheumatol 2021;3:287–94. https://doi.org/10.1002/acr2.11247.

[32] Betteridge ZE, Gunawardena H, Chinoy H, North J, Ollier WER, Cooper RG, et al. Clinical and human leucocyte antigen class II haplotype associations of autoantibodies to small ubiquitin-like modifier enzyme, a dermatomyositis-specific autoantigen target, in UK

Caucasian adult-onset myositis. Ann Rheum Dis 2009;68:1621–5. https://doi.org/10.1136/ard.2008.097162.

[33] Tarricone E, Ghirardello A, Rampudda M, Bassi N, Punzi L, Doria A. Anti-SAE antibodies in autoimmune myositis: identification by unlabelled protein immunoprecipitation in an Italian patient cohort. J Immunol Methods 2012;384:128–34. https://doi.org/10.1016/j.jim.2012.07.019.

[34] Vuillard C, Pineton de Chambrun M, de Prost N, Guérin C, Schmidt M, Dargent A, et al. Clinical features and outcome of patients with acute respiratory failure revealing anti-synthetase or anti-MDA-5 dermato-pulmonary syndrome: a French multicenter retrospective study. Ann Intensive Care 2018;8:87. https://doi.org/10.1186/s13613-018-0433-3.

[35] Tillie-Leblond I, Wislez M, Valeyre D, Crestani B, Rabbat A, Israel-Biet D, et al. Interstitial lung disease and anti-Jo-1 antibodies: difference between acute and gradual onset. Thorax 2008;63:53–9. https://doi.org/10.1136/thx.2006.069237.

[36] Trallero-Araguás E, Grau-Junyent JM, Labirua-Iturburu A, García-Hernández FJ, Monteagudo-Jiménez M, Fraile-Rodriguez G, et al. Clinical manifestations and long-term outcome of anti-Jo1 antisynthetase patients in a large cohort of Spanish patients from the GEAS-IIM group. Semin Arthritis Rheum 2016;46:225–31. https://doi.org/10.1016/j.semarthrit.2016.03.011.

[37] Muro Y, Sugiura K, Akiyama M. Low prevalence of anti-small ubiquitin-like modifier activating enzyme antibodies in dermatomyositis patients. Autoimmunity 2013;46:279–84. https://doi.org/10.3109/08916934.2012.755958.

[38] Fujimoto M, Matsushita T, Hamaguchi Y, Kaji K, Asano Y, Ogawa F, et al. Autoantibodies to small ubiquitin-like modifier activating enzymes in Japanese patients with dermatomyositis: comparison with a UK Caucasian cohort. Ann Rheum Dis 2013;72:151–3. https://doi.org/10.1136/annrheumdis-2012-201736.

[39] Marie I, Lahaxe L, Benveniste O, Delavigne K, Adoue D, Mouthon L, et al. Long-term outcome of patients with polymyositis/dermatomyositis and anti-PM-Scl antibody. Br J Dermatol 2010;162:337–44. https://doi.org/10.1111/j.1365-2133.2009.09484.x.

[40] Mahler M, Raijmakers R. Novel aspects of autoantibodies to the PM/Scl complex: clinical, genetic and diagnostic insights. Autoimmun Rev 2007;6:432–7. https://doi.org/10.1016/j.autrev.2007.01.013.

[41] Selva-O'Callaghan A, Labrador-Horrillo M, Solans-Laque R, Simeon-Aznar CP, Martínez-Gómez X, Vilardell-Tarrés M. Myositis-specific and myositis-associated antibodies in a series of eighty-eight Mediterranean patients with idiopathic inflammatory myopathy. Arthritis Rheum 2006;55:791–8. https://doi.org/10.1002/art.22237.

[42] Yang H, Li W, Tian X, Wang G, Shu X, Peng Q, et al. Immune-mediated necrotizing myopathies and interstitial lung disease are predominant characteristics in anti-Ku positive patients with idiopathic inflammatory myopathies. Ann Rheum Dis 2020. https://doi.org/10.1136/annrheumdis-2020-217096.

[43] Schulte-Pelkum J, Fritzler M, Mahler M. Latest update on the Ro/SS-A autoantibody system. Autoimmun Rev 2009;8:632–7. https://doi.org/10.1016/j.autrev.2009.02.010.

[44] Rutjes SA, Vree Egberts WT, Jongen P, Van Den Hoogen F, Pruijn GJ, Van Venrooij WJ. Anti-Ro52 antibodies frequently co-occur with anti-Jo-1 antibodies in sera from patients with idiopathic inflammatory myopathy. Clin Exp Immunol 1997;109:32–40. https://doi.org/10.1046/j.1365-2249.1997.4081308.x.

[45] Xu A, Ye Y, Fu Q, Lian X, Chen S, Guo Q, et al. Prognostic values of anti-Ro52 antibodies in anti-MDA5-positive clinically amyopathic dermatomyositis associated with interstitial

lung disease. Rheumatology 2021;60:3343–51. https://doi.org/10.1093/rheumatology/keaa786.

[46] Bauhammer J, Blank N, Max R, Lorenz H-M, Wagner U, Krause D, et al. Rituximab in the treatment of Jo1 antibody-associated antisynthetase syndrome: anti-Ro52 positivity as a marker for severity and treatment response. J Rheumatol 2016;43:1566–74. https://doi.org/10.3899/jrheum.150844.

[47] Marie I, Hatron PY, Dominique S, Cherin P, Mouthon L, Menard J-F, et al. Short-term and long-term outcome of anti-Jo1-positive patients with anti-Ro52 antibody. Semin Arthritis Rheum 2012;41:890–9. https://doi.org/10.1016/j.semarthrit.2011.09.008.

[48] Chen F, Zuo Y, Li S, Shi J, Wang G, Shu X. Clinical characteristics of dermatomyositis patients with isolated anti-Ro-52 antibody associated rapid progressive interstitial lung disease: data from the largest single Chinese center. Respir Med 2019;155:127–32. https://doi.org/10.1016/j.rmed.2019.07.020.

[49] Fathi M, Lundberg IE. Interstitial lung disease in polymyositis and dermatomyositis. Curr Opin Rheumatol 2005;17:701–6. https://doi.org/10.1097/01.bor.0000179949.65895.53.

[50] Marguerie C, Bunn CC, Beynon HL, Bernstein RM, Hughes JM, So AK, et al. Polymyositis, pulmonary fibrosis and autoantibodies to aminoacyl-tRNA synthetase enzymes. Q J Med 1990;77:1019–38. https://doi.org/10.1093/qjmed/77.1.1019.

[51] Betteridge Z, McHugh N. Myositis-specific autoantibodies: an important tool to support diagnosis of myositis. J Intern Med 2016;280:8–23. https://doi.org/10.1111/joim.12451.

[52] Hamaguchi Y, Fujimoto M, Matsushita T, Kaji K, Komura K, Hasegawa M, et al. Common and distinct clinical features in adult patients with anti-aminoacyl-tRNA synthetase antibodies: heterogeneity within the syndrome. PLoS One 2013;8:e60442. https://doi.org/10.1371/journal.pone.0060442.

[53] Stenzel W, Preuße C, Allenbach Y, Pehl D, Junckerstorff R, Heppner FL, et al. Nuclear actin aggregation is a hallmark of anti-synthetase syndrome-induced dysimmune myopathy. Neurology 2015;84:1346–54. https://doi.org/10.1212/WNL.0000000000001422.

[54] Mescam-Mancini L, Allenbach Y, Hervier B, Devilliers H, Mariampillay K, Dubourg O, et al. Anti-Jo-1 antibody-positive patients show a characteristic necrotizing perifascicular myositis. Brain 2015;138:2485–92. https://doi.org/10.1093/brain/awv192.

[55] Uruha A, Nishikawa A, Tsuburaya RS, Hamanaka K, Kuwana M, Watanabe Y, et al. Sarcoplasmic MxA expression: a valuable marker of dermatomyositis. Neurology 2017;88:493–500. https://doi.org/10.1212/WNL.0000000000003568.

[56] Hervier B, Benveniste O. Clinical heterogeneity and outcomes of antisynthetase syndrome. Curr Rheumatol Rep 2013;15:349. https://doi.org/10.1007/s11926-013-0349-8.

[57] Hervier B, Devilliers H, Stanciu R, Meyer A, Uzunhan Y, Masseau A, et al. Hierarchical cluster and survival analyses of antisynthetase syndrome: phenotype and outcome are correlated with anti-tRNA synthetase antibody specificity. Autoimmun Rev 2012;12:210–7. https://doi.org/10.1016/j.autrev.2012.06.006.

[58] Marie I, Josse S, Decaux O, Diot E, Landron C, Roblot P, et al. Clinical manifestations and outcome of anti-PL7 positive patients with antisynthetase syndrome. Eur J Intern Med 2013;24:474–9. https://doi.org/10.1016/j.ejim.2013.01.002.

[59] Marie I, Josse S, Decaux O, Dominique S, Diot E, Landron C, et al. Comparison of long-term outcome between anti-Jo1- and anti-PL7/PL12 positive patients with antisynthetase syndrome. Autoimmun Rev 2012;11:739–45. https://doi.org/10.1016/j.autrev.2012.01.006.

[60] Casal-Dominguez M, Pinal-Fernandez I, Mego M, Accarino A, Jubany L, Azpiroz F, et al. High-resolution manometry in patients with idiopathic inflammatory myopathy: elevated

prevalence of esophageal involvement and differences according to autoantibody status and clinical subset. Muscle Nerve 2017;56:386–92. https://doi.org/10.1002/mus.25507.

[61] Dieval C, Deligny C, Meyer A, Cluzel P, Champtiaux N, Lefevre G, et al. Myocarditis in patients with antisynthetase syndrome: prevalence, presentation, and outcomes. Medicine 2015;94:e798. https://doi.org/10.1097/MD.0000000000000798.

[62] Labirua-Iturburu A, Selva-O'Callaghan A, Vincze M, Dankó K, Vencovsky J, Fisher B, et al. Anti-PL-7 (anti-threonyl-tRNA synthetase) antisynthetase syndrome: clinical manifestations in a series of patients from a European multicenter study (EUMYONET) and review of the literature. Medicine 2012;91:206–11. https://doi.org/10.1097/MD.0b013e318260977c.

[63] Castañeda-Pomeda M, Prieto-González S, Grau JM. Antisynthetase syndrome and malignancy: our experience. J Clin Rheumatol 2011;17:458. https://doi.org/10.1097/RHU.0b013e31823b1878.

[64] Legault D, McDermott J, Crous-Tsanaclis AM, Boire G. Cancer-associated myositis in the presence of anti-Jo1 autoantibodies and the antisynthetase syndrome. J Rheumatol 2008;35:169–71.

[65] Rozelle A, Trieu S, Chung L. Malignancy in the setting of the anti-synthetase syndrome. J Clin Rheumatol 2008;14:285–8. https://doi.org/10.1097/RHU.0b013e31817d116f.

[66] Lu X, Yang H, Shu X, Chen F, Zhang Y, Zhang S, et al. Factors predicting malignancy in patients with polymyositis and dermatomyostis: a systematic review and meta-analysis. PLoS One 2014;9:e94128. https://doi.org/10.1371/journal.pone.0094128.

[67] Oldroyd AGS, Allard AB, Callen JP, Chinoy H, Chung L, Fiorentino D, et al. A systematic review and meta-analysis to inform cancer screening guidelines in idiopathic inflammatory myopathies. Rheumatology 2021;60:2615–28. https://doi.org/10.1093/rheumatology/keab166.

[68] Sebastiani M, Triantafyllias K, Manfredi A, González-Gay MA, Palmou-Fontana N, Cassone G, et al. Nailfold capillaroscopy characteristics of antisynthetase syndrome and possible clinical associations: results of a multicenter international study. J Rheumatol 2019;46:279–84. https://doi.org/10.3899/jrheum.180355.

[69] Connors GR, Christopher-Stine L, Oddis CV, Danoff SK. Interstitial lung disease associated with the idiopathic inflammatory myopathies: what progress has been made in the past 35 years? Chest 2010;138:1464–74. https://doi.org/10.1378/chest.10-0180.

[70] Solomon J, Swigris JJ, Brown KK. Myositis-related interstitial lung disease and antisynthetase syndrome. J Bras Pneumol 2011;37:100–9. https://doi.org/10.1590/s1806-37132011000100015.

[71] Hamaguchi Y, Kuwana M, Takehara K. Comparison of anti-OJ antibody detection assays between an immunoprecipitation assay and line blot assay. Mod Rheumatol 2017;27:551–2. https://doi.org/10.1080/14397595.2016.1213947.

[72] Cavazzana I, Fredi M, Ceribelli A, Mordenti C, Ferrari F, Carabellese N, et al. Testing for myositis specific autoantibodies: comparison between line blot and immunoprecipitation assays in 57 myositis sera. J Immunol Methods 2016;433:1–5. https://doi.org/10.1016/j.jim.2016.02.017.

[73] Targoff IN, Trieu EP, Miller FW. Reaction of anti-OJ autoantibodies with components of the multi-enzyme complex of aminoacyl-tRNA synthetases in addition to isoleucyl-tRNA synthetase. J Clin Invest 1993;91:2556–64. https://doi.org/10.1172/JCI116493.

[74] Vulsteke J-B, Satoh M, Malyavantham K, Bossuyt X, De Langhe E, Mahler M. Anti-OJ autoantibodies: rare or underdetected? Autoimmun Rev 2019;18:658–64. https://doi.org/10.1016/j.autrev.2019.05.002.

[75] Shi J, Li S, Yang H, Zhang Y, Peng Q, Lu X, et al. Clinical profiles and prognosis of patients with distinct antisynthetase autoantibodies. J Rheumatol 2017;44:1051–7. https://doi.org/10.3899/jrheum.161480.

[76] Marie I, Josse S, Hatron PY, Dominique S, Hachulla E, Janvresse A, et al. Interstitial lung disease in anti-Jo-1 patients with antisynthetase syndrome. Arthritis Care Res 2013;65:800–8. https://doi.org/10.1002/acr.21895.

[77] Debray M-P, Borie R, Revel M-P, Naccache J-M, Khalil A, Toper C, et al. Interstitial lung disease in anti-synthetase syndrome: initial and follow-up CT findings. Eur J Radiol 2015;84:516–23. https://doi.org/10.1016/j.ejrad.2014.11.026.

[78] Waseda Y, Johkoh T, Egashira R, Sumikawa H, Saeki K, Watanabe S, et al. Antisynthetase syndrome: pulmonary computed tomography findings of adult patients with antibodies to aminoacyl-tRNA synthetases. Eur J Radiol 2016;85:1421–6. https://doi.org/10.1016/j.ejrad.2016.05.012.

[79] Tanizawa K, Handa T, Nakashima R, Kubo T, Hosono Y, Aihara K, et al. The prognostic value of HRCT in myositis-associated interstitial lung disease. Respir Med 2013;107:745–52. https://doi.org/10.1016/j.rmed.2013.01.014.

[80] Watanabe K, Handa T, Tanizawa K, Hosono Y, Taguchi Y, Noma S, et al. Detection of antisynthetase syndrome in patients with idiopathic interstitial pneumonias. Respir Med 2011;105:1238–47. https://doi.org/10.1016/j.rmed.2011.03.022.

[81] He L, Ge Y, Li S, Huang K, Liu X, Chen F, et al. Clinical role of bronchoalveolar lavage in dermatomyositis-associated interstitial lung disease. Rheumatology 2021:keab586. https://doi.org/10.1093/rheumatology/keab586.

[82] Sato S, Hirakata M, Kuwana M, Suwa A, Inada S, Mimori T, et al. Autoantibodies to a 140-kd polypeptide, CADM-140, in Japanese patients with clinically amyopathic dermatomyositis. Arthritis Rheum 2005;52:1571–6. https://doi.org/10.1002/art.21023.

[83] Labrador-Horrillo M, Martinez MA, Selva-O'Callaghan A, Trallero-Araguas E, Balada E, Vilardell-Tarres M, et al. Anti-MDA5 antibodies in a large Mediterranean population of adults with dermatomyositis. J Immunol Res 2014;2014:290797. https://doi.org/10.1155/2014/290797.

[84] Hoa S, Troyanov Y, Fritzler MJ, Targoff IN, Chartrand S, Mansour AM, et al. Describing and expanding the clinical phenotype of anti-MDA5-associated rapidly progressive interstitial lung disease: case series of nine Canadian patients and literature review. Scand J Rheumatol 2018;47:210–24. https://doi.org/10.1080/03009742.2017.1334814.

[85] Nakashima R, Imura Y, Kobayashi S, Yukawa N, Yoshifuji H, Nojima T, et al. The RIG-I-like receptor IFIH1/MDA5 is a dermatomyositis-specific autoantigen identified by the anti-CADM-140 antibody. Rheumatology 2010;49:433–40. https://doi.org/10.1093/rheumatology/kep375.

[86] Takeuchi O, Akira S. MDA5/RIG-I and virus recognition. Curr Opin Immunol 2008;20:17–22. https://doi.org/10.1016/j.coi.2008.01.002.

[87] Fiorentino D, Chung L, Zwerner J, Rosen A, Casciola-Rosen L. The mucocutaneous and systemic phenotype of dermatomyositis patients with antibodies to MDA5 (CADM-140): a retrospective study. J Am Acad Dermatol 2011;65:25–34. https://doi.org/10.1016/j.jaad.2010.09.016.

[88] Hall JC, Casciola-Rosen L, Samedy L-A, Werner J, Owoyemi K, Danoff SK, et al. Anti-melanoma differentiation-associated protein 5-associated dermatomyositis: expanding the clinical spectrum. Arthritis Care Res 2013;65:1307–15. https://doi.org/10.1002/acr.21992.

[89] Kobayashi I, Okura Y, Yamada M, Kawamura N, Kuwana M, Ariga T. Anti-melanoma differentiation-associated gene 5 antibody is a diagnostic and predictive marker for

interstitial lung diseases associated with juvenile dermatomyositis. J Pediatr 2011;158:675–7. https://doi.org/10.1016/j.jpeds.2010.11.033.

[90] Tansley SL, Betteridge ZE, Gunawardena H, Jacques TS, Owens CM, Pilkington C, et al. Anti-MDA5 autoantibodies in juvenile dermatomyositis identify a distinct clinical phenotype: a prospective cohort study. Arthritis Res Ther 2014;16:R138. https://doi.org/10.1186/ar4600.

[91] Moghadam-Kia S, Oddis CV, Aggarwal R. Anti-MDA5 antibody spectrum in western world. Curr Rheumatol Rep 2018;20:78. https://doi.org/10.1007/s11926-018-0798-1.

[92] Muro Y, Sugiura K, Akiyama M. Cutaneous manifestations in dermatomyositis: key clinical and serological features-a comprehensive review. Clin Rev Allergy Immunol 2016;51:293–302. https://doi.org/10.1007/s12016-015-8496-5.

[93] Allenbach Y, Uzunhan Y, Toquet S, Leroux G, Gallay L, Marquet A, et al. Different phenotypes in dermatomyositis associated with anti-MDA5 antibody: study of 121 cases. Neurology 2020;95:e70–8. https://doi.org/10.1212/WNL.0000000000009727.

[94] Bohan A, Peter JB. Polymyositis and dermatomyositis (first of two parts). N Engl J Med 1975;292:344–7. https://doi.org/10.1056/NEJM197502132920706.

[95] Hoogendijk JE, Amato AA, Lecky BR, Choy EH, Lundberg IE, Rose MR, et al. 119th ENMC international workshop: trial design in adult idiopathic inflammatory myopathies, with the exception of inclusion body myositis, 10–12 October 2003, Naarden, The Netherlands. Neuromuscul Disord 2004;14:337–45. https://doi.org/10.1016/j.nmd.2004.02.006.

[96] Lundberg IE, Tjärnlund A, Bottai M, Werth VP, Pilkington C, Visser de M, et al. European league against rheumatism/American College of Rheumatology classification criteria for adult and juvenile idiopathic inflammatory myopathies and their major subgroups. Ann Rheum Dis 2017;76:1955–64. https://doi.org/10.1136/annrheumdis-2017-211468.

[97] Koga T, Fujikawa K, Horai Y, Okada A, Kawashiri S-Y, Iwamoto N, et al. The diagnostic utility of anti-melanoma differentiation-associated gene 5 antibody testing for predicting the prognosis of Japanese patients with DM. Rheumatology 2012;51:1278–84. https://doi.org/10.1093/rheumatology/ker518.

[98] Sakamoto N, Ishimoto H, Nakashima S, Yura H, Miyamura T, Okuno D, et al. Clinical features of anti-MDA5 antibody-positive rapidly progressive interstitial lung disease without signs of dermatomyositis. Intern Med 2019;58:837–41. https://doi.org/10.2169/internalmedicine.1516-18.

[99] Huang K, Vinik O, Shojania K, Yeung J, Shupak R, Nimmo M, et al. Clinical spectrum and therapeutics in Canadian patients with anti-melanoma differentiation-associated gene 5 (MDA5)-positive dermatomyositis: a case-based review. Rheumatol Int 2019;39:1971–81. https://doi.org/10.1007/s00296-019-04398-2.

[100] Hozumi H, Fujisawa T, Nakashima R, Johkoh T, Sumikawa H, Murakami A, et al. Comprehensive assessment of myositis-specific autoantibodies in polymyositis/dermatomyositis-associated interstitial lung disease. Respir Med 2016;121:91–9. https://doi.org/10.1016/j.rmed.2016.10.019.

[101] Zuo Y, Ye L, Liu M, Li S, Liu W, Chen F, et al. Clinical significance of radiological patterns of HRCT and their association with macrophage activation in dermatomyositis. Rheumatology 2020;59:2829–37. https://doi.org/10.1093/rheumatology/keaa034.

[102] Chino H, Sekine A, Baba T, Kitamura H, Iwasawa T, Okudela K, et al. Interstitial lung disease with anti-melanoma differentiation-associated protein 5 antibody: rapidly progressive perilobular opacity. Intern Med 2019;58:2605–13. https://doi.org/10.2169/internalmedicine.2328-18.

[103] Wu W, Xu W, Sun W, Zhang D, Zhao J, Luo Q, et al. Forced vital capacity predicts the survival of interstitial lung disease in anti-MDA5 positive dermatomyositis: a multi-centre cohort study. Rheumatology 2021:keab305. https://doi.org/10.1093/rheumatology/keab305.

[104] Wu W, Guo L, Fu Y, Wang K, Zhang D, Xu W, et al. Interstitial lung disease in anti-MDA5 positive dermatomyositis. Clin Rev Allergy Immunol 2021;60:293–304. https://doi.org/10.1007/s12016-020-08822-5.

[105] Matsushita T, Mizumaki K, Kano M, Yagi N, Tennichi M, Takeuchi A, et al. Anti-melanoma differentiation-associated protein 5 antibody level is a novel tool for monitoring disease activity in rapidly progressive interstitial lung disease with dermatomyositis. Br J Dermatol 2017;176:395–402. https://doi.org/10.1111/bjd.14882.

[106] Gono T, Sato S, Kawaguchi Y, Kuwana M, Hanaoka M, Katsumata Y, et al. Anti-MDA5 antibody, ferritin and IL-18 are useful for the evaluation of response to treatment in interstitial lung disease with anti-MDA5 antibody-positive dermatomyositis. Rheumatology 2012;51:1563–70. https://doi.org/10.1093/rheumatology/kes102.

[107] Serum KL-6 level is a prognostic marker in patients with anti-MDA5 antibody-positive dermatomyositis associated with interstitial lung disease. J Clin Lab Anal 2019;33. https://pubmed.ncbi.nlm.nih.gov/31301087/.

[108] Lian X, Zou J, Guo Q, Chen S, Lu L, Wang R, et al. Mortality risk prediction in amyopathic dermatomyositis associated with interstitial lung disease: the FLAIR model. Chest 2020;158:1535–45. https://doi.org/10.1016/j.chest.2020.04.057.

[109] Li Y, Li Y, Wu J, Miao M, Gao X, Cai W, et al. Predictors of poor outcome of anti-MDA5-associated rapidly progressive interstitial lung disease in a Chinese cohort with dermatomyositis. J Immunol Res 2020;2020:2024869. https://doi.org/10.1155/2020/2024869.

[110] Shimizu T, Koga T, Furukawa K, Horai Y, Fujikawa K, Okada A, et al. IL-15 is a biomarker involved in the development of rapidly progressive interstitial lung disease complicated with polymyositis/dermatomyositis. J Intern Med 2021;289:206–20. https://doi.org/10.1111/joim.13154.

[111] Yamaguchi K, Yamaguchi A, Kashiwagi C, Sawada Y, Taguchi K, Umetsu K, et al. Differential clinical features of patients with clinically amyopathic dermatomyositis who have circulating anti-MDA5 autoantibodies with or without myositis-associated autoantibodies. Respir Med 2018;140:1–5. https://doi.org/10.1016/j.rmed.2018.05.010.

[112] Yang Q, Li T, Zhang X, Lyu K, Wu S, Chen Y, et al. Initial predictors for short-term prognosis in anti-melanoma differentiation-associated protein-5 positive patients. Orphanet J Rare Dis 2021;16:58. https://doi.org/10.1186/s13023-021-01705-8.

[113] Jablonska S, Blaszyk M. Scleromyositis (scleroderma/polimyositis overlap) is an entity. J Eur Acad Dermatol Venereol 2004;18:265–6. https://doi.org/10.1111/j.1468-3083.2004.00869.x.

[114] Oddis CV, Okano Y, Rudert WA, Trucco M, Duquesnoy RJ, Medsger TA. Serum autoantibody to the nucleolar antigen PM-Scl. Clinical and immunogenetic associations. Arthritis Rheum 1992;35:1211–7. https://doi.org/10.1002/art.1780351014.

[115] Lega J-C, Cottin V, Fabien N, Thivolet-Béjui F, Cordier J-F. Interstitial lung disease associated with anti-PM/Scl or anti-aminoacyl-tRNA synthetase autoantibodies: a similar condition? J Rheumatol 2010;37:1000–9. https://doi.org/10.3899/jrheum.090652.

[116] Rothwell S, Chinoy H, Lamb JA, Miller FW, Rider LG, Wedderburn LR, et al. Focused HLA analysis in Caucasians with myositis identifies significant associations with autoantibody subgroups. Ann Rheum Dis 2019;78:996–1002. https://doi.org/10.1136/annrheumdis-2019-215046.

[117] Guillen-Del Castillo A, Pilar Simeón-Aznar C, Fonollosa-Pla V, Alonso-Vila S, Reverte-Vinaixa MM, Muñoz X, et al. Good outcome of interstitial lung disease in patients with scleroderma associated to anti-PM/Scl antibody. Semin Arthritis Rheum 2014;44:331–7. https://doi.org/10.1016/j.semarthrit.2014.07.002.

[118] Ussavarungsi K, Nugent K, Gerke AK, Krasowski MD, Tuetken RS, Lenert PS. Interstitial lung disease associated with anti-PM-Scl antibody: a single center experience. Autoimmun Rev 2019;18:102355. https://doi.org/10.1016/j.autrev.2019.102355.

[119] De Lorenzo R, Pinal-Fernandez I, Huang W, Albayda J, Tiniakou E, Johnson C, et al. Muscular and extramuscular clinical features of patients with anti-PM/Scl autoantibodies. Neurology 2018;90:e2068–76. https://doi.org/10.1212/WNL.0000000000005638.

[120] D'Aoust J, Hudson M, Tatibouet S, Wick J, Canadian Scleroderma Research Group, Mahler M, et al. Clinical and serologic correlates of anti-PM/Scl antibodies in systemic sclerosis: a multicenter study of 763 patients. Arthritis Rheumatol 2014;66:1608–15. https://doi.org/10.1002/art.38428.

[121] Lazzaroni M-G, Marasco E, Campochiaro C, DeVries-Bouwstra J, Gonzalez-Perez M-I, Rojas-Serrano J, et al. The clinical phenotype of Systemic Sclerosis patients with anti-PM/Scl antibodies: results from the EUSTAR cohort. Rheumatology 2021:keab152. https://doi.org/10.1093/rheumatology/keab152.

[122] Yang X, Wei D, Liu M, Wu B, Zhang J, Xu H, et al. Survival and outcomes after lung transplantation for connective tissue disease-associated interstitial lung diseases. Clin Rheumatol 2021;40:3789–95. https://doi.org/10.1007/S10067-021-05704-9.

[123] Remuzgo-Martínez S, Atienza-Mateo B, Ocejo-Vinyals JG, Pulito-Cueto V, Prieto-Peña D, Genre F, et al. HLA association with the susceptibility to anti-synthetase syndrome. Jt Bone Spine 2021;88:105115. https://doi.org/10.1016/j.jbspin.2020.105115.

[124] Kang EH, Go DJ, Mimori T, Lee SJ, Kwon HM, Park JW, et al. Novel susceptibility alleles in HLA region for myositis and myositis specific autoantibodies in Korean patients. Semin Arthritis Rheum 2019;49:283–7. https://doi.org/10.1016/j.semarthrit.2019.03.005.

[125] Furuya T, Hakoda M, Tsuchiya N, Kotake S, Ichikawa N, Nanke Y, et al. Immunogenetic features in 120 Japanese patients with idiopathic inflammatory myopathy. J Rheumatol 2004;31:1768–74.

[126] Gallay L, Gayed C, Hervier B. Antisynthetase syndrome pathogenesis: knowledge and uncertainties. Curr Opin Rheumatol 2018;30:664–73. https://doi.org/10.1097/BOR.0000000000000555.

[127] Casciola-Rosen L, Nagaraju K, Plotz P, Wang K, Levine S, Gabrielson E, et al. Enhanced autoantigen expression in regenerating muscle cells in idiopathic inflammatory myopathy. J Exp Med 2005;201:591–601. https://doi.org/10.1084/jem.20041367.

[128] Chen Z, Wang Y, Kuwana M, Xu X, Hu W, Feng X, et al. HLA-DRB1 alleles as genetic risk factors for the development of anti-MDA5 antibodies in patients with dermatomyositis. J Rheumatol 2017;44:1389–93. https://doi.org/10.3899/jrheum.170165.

[129] Gono T, Kawaguchi Y, Kuwana M, Sugiura T, Furuya T, Takagi K, et al. Brief report: association of HLA-DRB1*0101/*0405 with susceptibility to anti-melanoma differentiation-associated gene 5 antibody-positive dermatomyositis in the Japanese population. Arthritis Rheum 2012;64:3736–40. https://doi.org/10.1002/art.34657.

[130] Barba T, Fort R, Cottin V, Provencher S, Durieu I, Jardel S, et al. Treatment of idiopathic inflammatory myositis associated interstitial lung disease: a systematic review and meta-analysis. Autoimmun Rev 2019;18:113–22. https://doi.org/10.1016/j.autrev.2018.07.013.

[131] Nakazawa M, Kaneko Y, Takeuchi T. Risk factors for the recurrence of interstitial lung disease in patients with polymyositis and dermatomyositis: a retrospective cohort study. Clin Rheumatol 2018;37:765–71. https://doi.org/10.1007/s10067-017-3854-8.

[132] Takada K, Kishi J, Miyasaka N. Step-up versus primary intensive approach to the treatment of interstitial pneumonia associated with dermatomyositis/polymyositis: a retrospective study. Mod Rheumatol 2007;17:123–30. https://doi.org/10.1007/s10165-007-0553-3.

[133] Mira-Avendano IC, Parambil JG, Yadav R, Arrossi V, Xu M, Chapman JT, et al. A retrospective review of clinical features and treatment outcomes in steroid-resistant interstitial lung disease from polymyositis/dermatomyositis. Respir Med 2013;107:890–6. https://doi.org/10.1016/j.rmed.2013.02.015.

[134] Hanaoka H, Iida H, Kiyokawa T, Takakuwa Y, Kawahata K. Mycophenolate mofetil treatment with or without a calcineurin inhibitor in resistant inflammatory myopathy. Clin Rheumatol 2019;38:585–90. https://doi.org/10.1007/s10067-018-4294-9.

[135] Huapaya JA, Silhan L, Pinal-Fernandez I, Casal-Dominguez M, Johnson C, Albayda J, et al. Long-term treatment with azathioprine and mycophenolate mofetil for myositis-related interstitial lung disease. Chest 2019;156:896–906. https://doi.org/10.1016/j.chest.2019.05.023.

[136] Calcineurin inhibitor for the treatment of myositis-associated interstitial lung disease: comparison between cyclosporine and tacrolimus. ACR Meeting Abstracts. n.d. https://acrabstracts.org/abstract/calcineurin-inhibitor-for-the-treatment-of-myositis-associated-interstitial-lung-disease-comparison-between-cyclosporine-and-tacrolimus/. [accessed 8 September 2021].

[137] Ge Y, Peng Q, Zhang S, Zhou H, Lu X, Wang G. Cyclophosphamide treatment for idiopathic inflammatory myopathies and related interstitial lung disease: a systematic review. Clin Rheumatol 2015;34:99–105. https://doi.org/10.1007/s10067-014-2803-z.

[138] Marie I, Dominique S, Janvresse A, Levesque H, Menard J-F. Rituximab therapy for refractory interstitial lung disease related to antisynthetase syndrome. Respir Med 2012;106:581–7. https://doi.org/10.1016/j.rmed.2012.01.001.

[139] Andersson H, Sem M, Lund MB, Aaløkken TM, Günther A, Walle-Hansen R, et al. Long-term experience with rituximab in anti-synthetase syndrome-related interstitial lung disease. Rheumatology 2015;54:1420–8. https://doi.org/10.1093/rheumatology/kev004.

[140] Doyle TJ, Dhillon N, Madan R, Cabral F, Fletcher EA, Koontz DC, et al. Rituximab in the treatment of interstitial lung disease associated with antisynthetase syndrome: a multicenter retrospective case review. J Rheumatol 2018;45:841–50. https://doi.org/10.3899/jrheum.170541.

[141] Langlois V, Gillibert A, Uzunhan Y, Chabi M-L, Hachulla E, Landon-Cardinal O, et al. Rituximab and cyclophosphamide in antisynthetase syndrome-related interstitial lung disease: an observational retrospective study. J Rheumatol 2020;47:1678–86. https://doi.org/10.3899/jrheum.190505.

[142] Kurasawa K, Arai S, Namiki Y, Tanaka A, Takamura Y, Owada T, et al. Tofacitinib for refractory interstitial lung diseases in anti-melanoma differentiation-associated 5 gene antibody-positive dermatomyositis. Rheumatology 2018;57:2114–9. https://doi.org/10.1093/rheumatology/key188.

[143] Chen Z, Wang X, Ye S. Tofacitinib in amyopathic dermatomyositis-associated interstitial lung disease. N Engl J Med 2019;381:291–3. https://doi.org/10.1056/NEJMc1900045.

[144] Romero-Bueno F, Diaz Del Campo P, Trallero-Araguás E, Ruiz-Rodríguez JC, Castellvi I, Rodriguez-Nieto MJ, et al. Recommendations for the treatment of anti-melanoma differentiation-associated gene 5-positive dermatomyositis-associated rapidly progressive

interstitial lung disease. Semin Arthritis Rheum 2020;50:776–90. https://doi.org/10.1016/j.semarthrit.2020.03.007.

[145] Tsuji H, Nakashima R, Hosono Y, Imura Y, Yagita M, Yoshifuji H, et al. Multicenter prospective study of the efficacy and safety of combined immunosuppressive therapy with high-dose glucocorticoid, tacrolimus, and cyclophosphamide in interstitial lung diseases accompanied by anti-melanoma differentiation-associated gene 5-positive dermatomyositis. Arthritis Rheumatol 2020;72:488–98. https://doi.org/10.1002/art.41105.

[146] Muro Y, Sugiura K, Akiyama M. Limitations of a single-point evaluation of anti-MDA5 antibody, ferritin, and IL-18 in predicting the prognosis of interstitial lung disease with anti-MDA5 antibody-positive dermatomyositis. Clin Rheumatol 2013;32:395–8. https://doi.org/10.1007/s10067-012-2142-x.

[147] Silveira MG, Selva-O'Callaghan A, Ramos-Terrades N, Arredondo-Agudelo KV, Labrador-Horrillo M, Bravo-Masgoret C. Anti-MDA5 dermatomyositis and progressive interstitial pneumonia. QJM 2016;109:49–50. https://doi.org/10.1093/qjmed/hcv068.

[148] Okabayashi H, Ichiyasu H, Hirooka S, Akaike K, Kojima K, Jodai T, et al. Clinical effects of direct hemoperfusion using a polymyxin B-immobilized fiber column in clinically amyopathic dermatomyositis-associated rapidly progressive interstitial pneumonias. BMC Pulm Med 2017;17:134. https://doi.org/10.1186/s12890-017-0479-2.

[149] Teruya A, Kawamura K, Ichikado K, Sato S, Yasuda Y, Yoshioka M. Successful polymyxin B hemoperfusion treatment associated with serial reduction of serum anti-CADM-140/MDA5 antibody levels in rapidly progressive interstitial lung disease with amyopathic dermatomyositis. Chest 2013;144:1934–6. https://doi.org/10.1378/chest.13-0186.

[150] Endo Y, Koga T, Suzuki T, Hara K, Ishida M, Fujita Y, et al. Successful treatment of plasma exchange for rapidly progressive interstitial lung disease with anti-MDA5 antibody-positive dermatomyositis: a case report. Medicine 2018;97:e0436. https://doi.org/10.1097/MD.0000000000010436.

[151] Makino S. Progressive fibrosing interstitial lung diseases: a new concept and indication of nintedanib. Mod Rheumatol 2021;31:13–9. https://doi.org/10.1080/14397595.2020.1826665.

[152] Distler O, Highland KB, Gahlemann M, Azuma A, Fischer A, Mayes MD, et al. Nintedanib for systemic sclerosis-associated interstitial lung disease. N Engl J Med 2019;380:2518–28. https://doi.org/10.1056/NEJMoa1903076.

[153] Flaherty KR, Wells AU, Cottin V, Devaraj A, Walsh SLF, Inoue Y, et al. Nintedanib in progressive fibrosing interstitial lung diseases. N Engl J Med 2019;381:1718–27. https://doi.org/10.1056/NEJMoa1908681.

[154] Li T, Guo L, Chen Z, Gu L, Sun F, Tan X, et al. Pirfenidone in patients with rapidly progressive interstitial lung disease associated with clinically amyopathic dermatomyositis. Sci Rep 2016;6:33226. https://doi.org/10.1038/srep33226.

[155] Search of: NCT02821689 - List results - ClinicalTrials.gov. n.d. https://clinicaltrials.gov/ct2/results?cond=&term=NCT02821689&cntry=&state=&city=&dist=. [accessed 5 September 2021].

[156] Search of: NCT03857854 - List results - ClinicalTrials.gov n.d. https://clinicaltrials.gov/ct2/results?cond=&term=NCT03857854&cntry=&state=&city=&dist=. [accessed 5 September 2021].

[157] Hosenpud JD, Bennett LE, Keck BM, Edwards EB, Novick RJ. Effect of diagnosis on survival benefit of lung transplantation for end-stage lung disease. Lancet 1998;351:24–7. https://doi.org/10.1016/S0140-6736(97)06405-2.

[158] Fernández-Codina A, Berastegui C, Pinal-Fernández I, Silveira MG, López-Meseguer M, Monforte V, et al. Lung transplantation in systemic sclerosis: a single center cohort study. Joint Bone Spine 2018;85:79–84. https://doi.org/10.1016/j.jbspin.2017.03.012.

[159] Chan EY, Goodarzi A, Sinha N, Nguyen DT, Youssef JG, Suarez EE, et al. Long-term survival in bilateral lung transplantation for scleroderma-related lung disease. Ann Thorac Surg 2018;105:893–900. https://doi.org/10.1016/j.athoracsur.2017.09.038.

[160] Takagishi T, Ostrowski R, Alex C, Rychlik K, Pelletiere K, Tehrani R. Survival and extrapulmonary course of connective tissue disease after lung transplantation. J Clin Rheumatol 2012;18:283–9. https://doi.org/10.1097/RHU.0b013e3182676089.

[161] Courtwright AM, El-Chemaly S, Dellaripa PF, Goldberg HJ. Survival and outcomes after lung transplantation for non-scleroderma connective tissue-related interstitial lung disease. J Heart Lung Transplant 2017;36:763–9. https://doi.org/10.1016/j.healun.2016.12.013.

[162] Ameye H, Ruttens D, Benveniste O, Verleden GM, Wuyts WA. Is lung transplantation a valuable therapeutic option for patients with pulmonary polymyositis? Experiences from the Leuven transplant cohort. Transplant Proc 2014;46:3147–53. https://doi.org/10.1016/j.transproceed.2014.09.163.

[163] Leclair V, Labirua-Iturburu A, Lundberg IE. Successful lung transplantation in a case of rapidly progressive interstitial lung disease associated with antimelanoma differentiation-associated gene 5 antibodies. J Rheumatol 2018;45:581–3. https://doi.org/10.3899/jrheum.171047.

[164] Pacot L, Pouchot J, De Prost N, Senant M, Tartour E, Le Pimpec-Barthes F, et al. Interstitial lung disease-complicated anti-MDA5 antibody in clinically amyopathic dermatomyositis patients: report of two cases with distinct clinical features. Front Med 2020;7:77. https://doi.org/10.3389/fmed.2020.00077.

[165] Cassone G, Manfredi A, Vacchi C, Luppi F, Coppi F, Salvarani C, et al. Treatment of rheumatoid arthritis-associated interstitial lung disease: lights and shadows. J Clin Med 2020;9:E1082. https://doi.org/10.3390/jcm9041082.

[166] Sawada T, Inokuma S, Sato T, Otsuka T, Saeki Y, Takeuchi T, et al. Leflunomide-induced interstitial lung disease: prevalence and risk factors in Japanese patients with rheumatoid arthritis. Rheumatology 2009;48:1069–72. https://doi.org/10.1093/rheumatology/kep052.

[167] Chen SK, Liao KP, Liu J, Kim SC. Risk of hospitalized infection and initiation of abatacept versus tumor necrosis factor inhibitors among patients with rheumatoid arthritis: a propensity score-matched cohort study. Arthritis Care Res 2020;72:9–17. https://doi.org/10.1002/acr.23824.

[168] Barmettler S, Ong M-S, Farmer JR, Choi H, Walter J. Association of immunoglobulin levels, infectious risk, and mortality with rituximab and hypogammaglobulinemia. JAMA Netw Open 2018;1:e184169. https://doi.org/10.1001/jamanetworkopen.2018.4169.

[169] Pan TL, Thumboo J, Boey ML. Primary and secondary pulmonary hypertension in systemic lupus erythematosus. Lupus 2000;9:338–42. https://doi.org/10.1191/096120300678828361.

[170] Hachulla E, Gressin V, Guillevin L, Carpentier P, Diot E, Sibilia J, et al. Early detection of pulmonary arterial hypertension in systemic sclerosis: a French nationwide prospective multicenter study. Arthritis Rheum 2005;52:3792–800. https://doi.org/10.1002/art.21433.

[171] Sharp GC, Irvin WS, Tan EM, Gould RG, Holman HR. Mixed connective tissue disease–an apparently distinct rheumatic disease syndrome associated with a specific antibody to an extractable nuclear antigen (ENA). Am J Med 1972;52:148–59. https://doi.org/10.1016/0002-9343(72)90064-2.

[172] Reiseter S, Gunnarsson R, Mogens Aaløkken T, Lund MB, Mynarek G, Corander J, et al. Progression and mortality of interstitial lung disease in mixed connective tissue disease: a long-term observational nationwide cohort study. Rheumatology 2018;57:255–62. https://doi.org/10.1093/rheumatology/kex077.
[173] Hajas A, Szodoray P, Nakken B, Gaal J, Zöld E, Laczik R, et al. Clinical course, prognosis, and causes of death in mixed connective tissue disease. J Rheumatol 2013;40:1134–42. https://doi.org/10.3899/jrheum.121272.
[174] Bodolay E, Szekanecz Z, Dévényi K, Galuska L, Csípo I, Vègh J, et al. Evaluation of interstitial lung disease in mixed connective tissue disease (MCTD). Rheumatology 2005;44:656–61. https://doi.org/10.1093/rheumatology/keh575.
[175] Saito Y, Terada M, Takada T, Ishida T, Moriyama H, Ooi H, et al. Pulmonary involvement in mixed connective tissue disease: comparison with other collagen vascular diseases using high resolution CT. J Comput Assist Tomogr 2002;26:349–57. https://doi.org/10.1097/00004728-200205000-00006.
[176] Lhote R, Grenier P, Haroche J, Miyara M, Boussouar S, Mathian A, et al. Characterization of interstitial lung disease associated with anti-ribonucleoprotein antibodies. J Clin Rheumatol 2020;26:327–33. https://doi.org/10.1097/RHU.0000000000001127.
[177] Gunnarsson R, El-Hage F, Aaløkken TM, Reiseter S, Lund MB, Garen T, et al. Associations between anti-Ro52 antibodies and lung fibrosis in mixed connective tissue disease. Rheumatology 2016;55:103–8. https://doi.org/10.1093/rheumatology/kev300.
[178] Narula N, Narula T, Mira-Avendano I, Wang B, Abril A. Interstitial lung disease in patients with mixed connective tissue disease: pilot study on predictors of lung involvement. Clin Exp Rheumatol 2018;36:648–51.
[179] Celińska-Löwenhoff M, Pastuszczak M, Pełka K, Stec-Polak M, Wojas-Pelc A, Musiał J. Associations between nailfold capillaroscopy findings and interstitial lung disease in patients with mixed connective tissue disease. Arch Med Sci 2020;16:297–301. https://doi.org/10.5114/aoms.2018.81129.
[180] Chaigne B, Scirè CA, Talarico R, Alexander T, Amoura Z, Avcin T, et al. Mixed connective tissue disease: state of the art on clinical practice guidelines. RMD Open 2018;4:e000783. https://doi.org/10.1136/rmdopen-2018-000783.
[181] Kato M, Sugimoto A, Atsumi T. Diagnostic and prognostic markers and treatment of connective tissue disease-associated pulmonary arterial hypertension: current recommendations and recent advances. Expet Rev Clin Immunol 2020;16:993–1004. https://doi.org/10.1080/1744666X.2021.1825940.
[182] Hetlevik SO, Flatø B, Aaløkken TM, Lund MB, Reiseter S, Mynarek GK, et al. Pulmonary manifestations and progression of lung disease in juvenile-onset mixed connective tissue disease. J Rheumatol 2019;46:93–100. https://doi.org/10.3899/jrheum.180019.
[183] Ando M, Goto A, Yamasue M, Usagawa Y, Oka H, Shigenaga T, et al. Pulmonary-limited granulomatosis with polyangiitis coexisting with mixed connective tissue disease. Tohoku J Exp Med 2017;242:109–14. https://doi.org/10.1620/tjem.242.109.

Chapter 7

Lung involvement in ANCA-associated vasculitis

Sebastian Unizony[1] and Andy Abril[2,*]
[1]*Division of Rheumatology, Allergy and Immunology, The Edward A. Fox Chair in Medicine, Massachusetts General Hospital, Medicine Harvard Medical School, Boston, MA, United States;*
[2]*Division of Rheumatology, Mayo Clinic, Jacksonville, FL, United States*
[*]*Corresponding author at: abril.Andy@mayo.edu.*

Introduction

ANCA-associated vasculitis (AAV) can present with a wide range of pulmonary manifestations including pulmonary nodules, diffuse alveolar hemorrhage (DAH), interstitial lung disease (ILD), nonspecific parenchymal lung opacities, pleural effusion, large airway lesions, asthma, and pulmonary embolism [1–4]. The incidence of pulmonary involvement is higher in patients with granulomatosis with polyangiitis (GPA) and eosinophilic granulomatosis with polyangiitis (EGPA) (85%–90%) than in patients with microscopic polyangiitis (MPA) (25%–60%) [5–8]. Whereas some manifestations may occur in all three types of AAV (e.g., DAH, nonspecific infiltrates and pleural effusion), other manifestations are relatively specific to each AAV type (e.g., asthma in EGPA and tracheobronchial lesions in GPA) [2]. The clinical impact of lung involvement in AAV may range from asymptomatic findings to acute respiratory failure (e.g., DAH) with poor prognosis despite aggressive immunosuppression. Pulmonary involvement at disease onset is associated with more severe disease and represents a risk factor for long-term disease- and treatment-related damage [9]. This chapter reviews the most relevant pulmonary manifestations that occur in patients with AAV.

Pulmonary manifestations shared among all types of AAV

Diffuse alveolar hemorrhage

DAH is a life-threatening complication that can be seen in 25%–60% of patients with MPA, 20%–30% of patients with GPA and 4% of patients with

The Lung in Autoimmune Diseases. https://doi.org/10.1016/B978-0-323-91083-5.00007-4

EGPA [1,10]. Patients with DAH are usually acutely ill and present with hemoptysis and dyspnea [10]. Work up reveals hypoxemia, anemia due to acute blood loss, and rapidly changing alveolar opacities on chest X-ray. Computed tomography (CT) findings may range from lobular or lobar areas of ground glass opacity, when there is subtotal alveolar blood filling, to frank consolidation in well-established cases (Fig. 7.1). Noteworthy, hemoptysis is lacking in one third of the cases and chest X-rays can be initially normal in up to 50% of the patients [11].

Early bronchoscopy with bronchoalveolar lavage (BAL) is generally required to make the diagnosis of DAH and rule out infection [1]. In patients with active intra-alveolar bleeding, BAL retrieves a bright red fluid, and sequential aliquots from the same location demonstrate rising red blood cell counts [11]. In patients who are not actively bleeding at the time of bronchoscopy, DAH is suggested by the presence of more than 20% of hemosiderin-labeled macrophages in the BAL fluid [1].

In selected cases, a surgical lung biopsy (e.g., video-assisted thoracoscpic surgery [VATS]) is needed to confirm the presence of DAH. The histopathology in these cases demonstrates pauci-immune vasculitis with fibrinoid necrosis involving the microcirculation of the alveolar septa (i.e., capillaritis) along with red blood cell extravasation into the interstitial and alveolar spaces [1,12]. Surgical lung biopsies are often not possible due to increased risk of complications in the setting of severe acute lung injury.

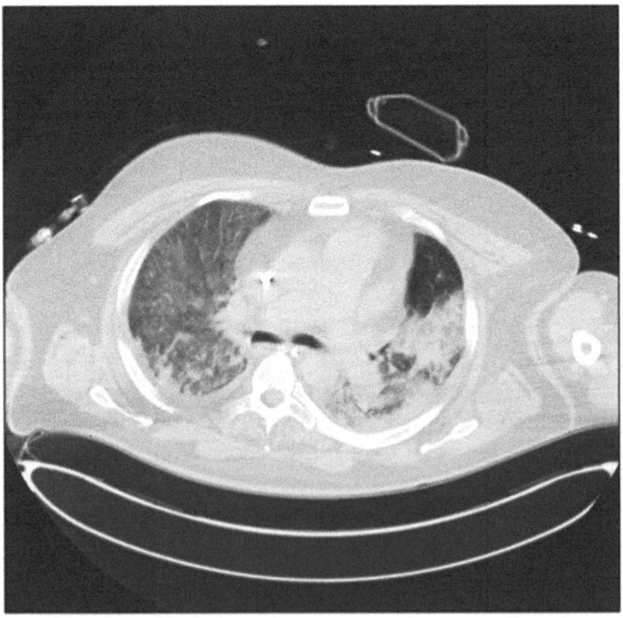

FIGURE 7.1 Diffuse alveolar hemorrhage in a patient with microscopic polyangiitis.

In a sizable percent of cases, DAH leads to acute respiratory failure requiring intubation and mechanical ventilation. Studies have shown that hypoxemia, increased C-reactive protein (CRP) levels, and high number of neutrophils on the BAL fluid at presentation reflect the severity of this condition, and help predict the risk of respiratory failure [13].

In patients with known AAV, DAH must be differentiated from other causes of hemoptysis. These may include bland pulmonary hemorrhage (e.g., coagulopathy, increased left-side heart pressure [e.g., mitral stenosis], pulmonary veno-occlusive disease and pulmonary hemosiderosis) and bleeding that can occur with infection, drug reactions, toxic inhalations, and radiation therapy [1,11]. In patients with GPA in particular, hemoptysis may occur when a lung nodule erodes a bronchial artery or can develop in the presence of tracheobronchial disease [2]. In patients in which the diagnosis of AAV has not yet been established, other causes of immune-mediated DAH including other primary vasculitides (e.g., cryoglobulinemic vasculitis and IgA-mediated vasculitis), secondary vasculitides (e.g., systemic lupus erythematosus-associated vasculitis), antiglomerular basement membrane disease (i.e., Good-Pasture's syndrome), and antiphospholipid syndrome should also be considered [11].

Interstitial lung disease

ILD may develop in 7%–45% of patients with AAV according to different studies [14–17]. This lung manifestation, which typically antedates or starts concomitantly with the onset of vasculitis [15,18], seems to be much more frequent in patients with MPO-ANCA than in patients with PR3-ANCA [17,19,20]. Therefore, patients with the clinicopathological phenotype of MPA develop ILD more often than those with the one of GPA [17,21]. A recent North American study, however, has shown a higher incidence of ILD in patients with GPA than previously reported in Japanese and European studies [22].

Clinical and radiographic characteristics of ILD in patients with AAV are similar to those in patients with interstitial pneumonia with autoimmune features (IPAF) [19]. Patients are usually males and the age of onset is between 58 and 70 years [20,21,23]. Signs and symptoms include dyspnea on exertion, chronic cough, and fine expiratory rales on auscultation [24]. In mild cases, patients are asymptomatic. Pulmonary function tests demonstrate decreased forced vital capacity, normal Tiffeneau-Pinelli index, and decreased carbon monoxide diffusing capacity (DCLO) [21,23]. The most common CT patterns reported in these patients have been usual interstitial pneumonia (UIP)-like including honeycombing, chronic hypersensitivity pneumonitis-like and nonspecific interstitial pneumonia (NSIP) [17,20–24], which predominantly involve the lower lobes [23] (Fig. 7.2).

The pathogenesis of ILD in patients with ANCA-associated vasculitis is poorly understood. Possible mechanisms include repetitive subclinical alveolar

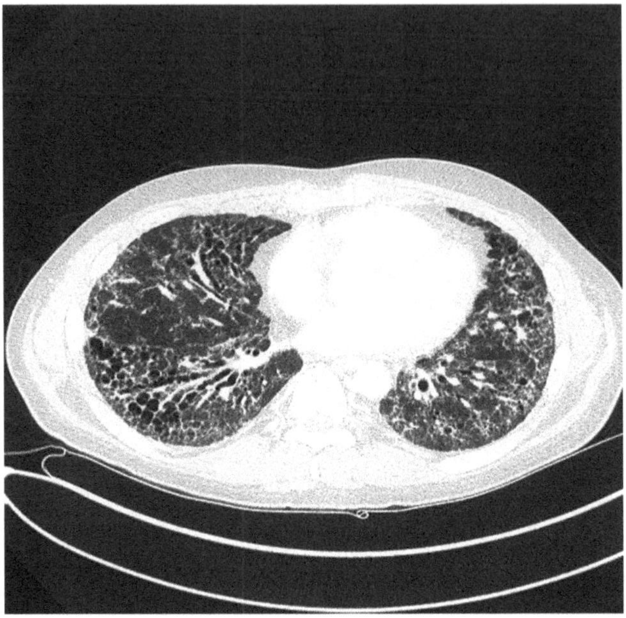

FIGURE 7.2 Interstitial lung disease in a patient with microscopic polyangiitis and positive MPO ANCA.

hemorrhage leading to fibrosis (similarly to the mechanism proposed for ILD in idiopathic pulmonary hemosiderosis) [25–28], and tissue repair and fibrosis following the resolution of capillaritis. Some research suggest that ANCA-stimulated neutrophils may be key players in AAV-related ILD by releasing reactive oxygen species and promoting fibroblast activity [29], while other investigators propose a causative role for eosinophils [19,30]. Histopathologically, AAV-ILD lesions resemble idiopathic pulmonary fibrosis (UIP), but tend to be more "cellular" and commonly exhibit inflammatory cell infiltration, lymphoid aggregates, bronchiolitis, and organizing pneumonia [23,31]. Often times, however, AAV-ILD biopsy findings are indistinguishable from idiopathic pulmonary fibrosis lesions [23]. Of note, classic vasculitic or granulomatous changes are rarely found in lung specimens of AAV patients with ILD [12].

Nonspecific pulmonary opacities

Nonspecific pulmonary opacities may be seen in all types of AAV. In patients with EGPA, areas of consolidation or ground glass opacity are a common CT finding, present in over 90% of the cases [32]. In addition, in patients with this type of AAV, it is not infrequent to observe transient, nonsegmental, patchy migratory infiltrates due to eosinophilic pneumonia, which may be present even before the onset of the vasculitic manifestations. These glucocorticoid-responsive infiltrates can be unilateral or bilateral without preference for any specific lung zones, and may be asymptomatic or cause nonspecific symptoms like cough and chest discomfort [17,33–35]. Because these infiltrates tend to disappear over a period of days to weeks (with or without treatment) and then new infiltrates develop in other areas of the lung, they have been referred to as "fleeting" pulmonary infiltrates. These migratory lesions are not pathognomonic of EGPA and can be seen in other conditions such as infection and antiglomerular basement membrane disease.

In GPA and MPA, the presence of nonspecific areas of bilateral consolidation and ground glass opacity with perihilar predominance and relative subpleural sparing may be indicative of the presence of DAH [36]. In patients with GPA, some of these lesions may later cavitate. A recent study of 74 patients with AAV showed that nonspecific patterns of ground glass opacities and consolidation were more frequently seen in patients with MPA or EGPA, whereas nodules were the most common lung lesion seen in patients with GPA [37].

Pleural effusion

Pleural effusion, usually exudative and bilateral, can be seen in 12%–20% of patients with EGPA, GPA, and MPA [38]. Pleural thickening, nonspecific pleural irregularities, nodules, or pneumothorax may be present rarely [17,39]. Pleural fluid in patients with EGPA is typically eosinophilic [34,40], while effusions have a lymphocytic predominance in GPA and MPA patients. Recent studies have shown that pleural effusions are slightly more common in patients with MPO-ANCA than with PR3-ANCA [38].

Pulmonary embolism

Several studies have reported an increased incidence of venous thromboembolism including pulmonary embolism in patients with AAV, particularly during active disease [3,41–43]. A large retrospective cohort study of AAV subtypes found venous thromboembolism incidences of 8.2% among patients with EGPA, 8% among patients with GPA, and 7.6% among patients with MPA [43]. The pathophysiology of thrombotic events in AAV is not well understood, but several risk factors have been identified including higher Birmingham vasculitis activity score (BVAS), elevated CRP levels, renal involvement, hypoalbuminemia, advanced age, male sex, and increased body mass index [43,44]. Some reports have suggested that complementary PR3-ANCA-mediated antiplasmin activity may drive hypercoagulability in some AAV patients [45]. However, a recent meta-analysis ($N = 4422$) described increased risk of venous thromboembolism in patients with MPO-ANCA while patients with PR3-ANCA showed decreased incidence of this complication [44].

Pulmonary manifestations primarily seen in GPA and EGPA

Pulmonary nodules

Approximately 50% of the patients with GPA and 15% of the patients with EGPA develop lung parenchymal nodules, which are identified by chest X-ray or CT [1]. These patients may be asymptomatic or present with cough, chest pain due to pleural irritation, dyspnea, or hemoptysis [2,46]. Lung nodules tend to be multiple and bilateral, and they locate in subpleural more than peribronchial areas [47] (Fig. 7.3). Occasionally, solitary lesions can be seen. In addition, in patients with GPA, nodules may coalesce into larger masses or even cavitate [47]. At times, areas of organizing pneumonia could develop around a nodule giving the tomographic appearance of a halo [47].

At diagnosis or during the course of the disease, a surgical lung biopsy (e.g., VATS) may be required to confirm the diagnosis of AAV and/or to rule other conditions that can present with lung nodules such as malignancy and infection including tuberculosis and mycosis (e.g., histoplasmosis, coccidioidomycosis, bastomycosis, nocardiosis, and aspergillosis) [1,2]. Histologically, GPA nodules demonstrate neutrophilic debris forming microabscesses in areas of vascular fibrinoid necrosis, which are surrounded by histiocytes that tend to arrange in a palisading pattern [12]. Microabscesses may coalesce into more extensive areas of necrosis referred to as "geographic necrosis" [12]. Lesions eventually acquire granulomatous features that may range from poorly form to well-established granulomas containing $CD4^+$ T cells, histiocytes, scattered

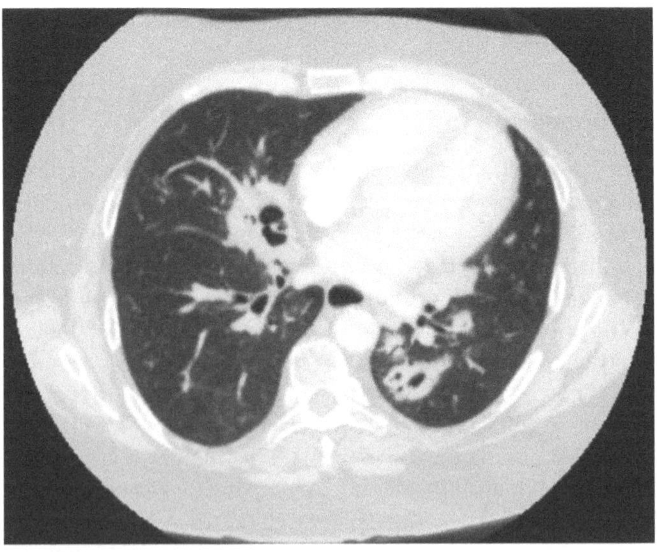

FIGURE 7.3 CT of the chest in a patient with GPA demonstrating bilateral cavitary and non-cavitary nodules. *Image courtesy of Dr. John H. Stone.*

neutrophils, multinucleated giant cells, and B cells [2,12]. EGPA nodules share some of the features seen in GPA nodules, but EGPA lesions also exhibit increased numbers of eosinophils. Besides necrotizing granulomatous inflammation, lung biopsies in patients with AAV presenting with nodules may show other characteristic histologic findings including necrotizing angiitis of small- and medium-sized blood vessels (GPA and EGPA) and nonspecific interstitial eosinophilic infiltrates (EGPA) [2,12].

Pulmonary manifestations primarily seen in GPA

Large-airway involvement

Lower airway involvement is seen in 15%–55% of patients with GPA [1]. Inflammation may occur anywhere in the laryngeo-tracheobronchial tree, but the location most commonly affected is the subglottic area [2]. Patients with this type of clinical manifestations are more likely to be female, younger, PR3-ANCA positive, and have ear-nose-throat (ENT) disease (including saddle-nose deformities), but less likely to have glomerulonephritis [48]. Of note, large airway disease can be the only active feature at the time of relapse in systemic GPA [48], and in a subset of GPA patients, the disease is limited to the upper and lower respiratory tract (i.e., limited GPA) [49], which may become a diagnostic challenge.

Vasculitis and granulomatous inflammation may lead to damage including mucosal ulceration and airway stenosis. When the process involves the cartilaginous structures of the airway, tracheomalacia or bronchomalacia may develop [1]. Clinical manifestations may include stridor, dyspnea, cough, hoarseness, and hemoptysis. When airways of smaller caliber are involved, wheezing can be appreciated. Pulmonary function test with inspiratory and expiratory volume flow loops and dynamic expiratory CT are noninvasive tests frequently employed for the workup of these patients [1,48]. Diagnostic confirmation usually requires direct bronchoscopic inspection of the airways with biopsy, which in the majority of the cases reveals nonspecific inflammation and damage (e.g., fibrosis) [1].

Pulmonary manifestations primarily seen in EGPA

Asthma

EGPA is unique among AAV given the importance of eosinophilia and eosinophilic infiltrates in the tissues for the pathogenesis and clinical presentation of this disease. Moreover, ANCA (usually MPO-ANCA) are only positive in 30%–40% of the patients [50]. Asthma, which is present in 91%–100% of patients, is one of the most characteristic features of EGPA [2]. Obstructive airway disease is often severe and may precede the formal diagnosis of EGPA for several years [4]. A French cohort study found that asthma became more severe and glucocorticoid dependent in the months prececeding the onset of vasculitis, and remained generally severe throughout the course of the disease even after the vasculitic manifestations (e.g., glomerulonephritis) were controlled [40]. Data from the Mayo clinic showed that patients with EGPA who are present with severe rhinosinusitis, pulmonary infiltrates, increased body weight, and uncontrolled asthma, had a higher probability to experience long-term severe and difficult to treat asthma even in the absence of active vasculitis [51]. This study suggested the possibility that eosinophil-induced chronic airway damage leading to refractory asthma maybe already established by the time of EGPA diagnosis in some patients [51]. Therapeutic studies with the interleukin (IL)-5 inhibitor mepolizumab showed significant improvement of the ENT and asthma symptoms, but the pulmonary function tests remained unchanged, supporting the hypothesis of permanent airway damage [52]. Other groups have reported that many patients with systemic vasculitis controlled with glucocorticoids and immunosuppressive therapy continue to experience asthma exacerbations upon tapering the daily glucocorticoid dose below 15−10 mg of prednisone or equivalent [53]. Even though asthma is a critical component of EGPA, expert consensus suggest that a transient and fully reversible exacerbation of asthma or upper respiratory symptoms especially if an infectious trigger is identified, does not necessarily represent a relapse of EGPA, although it will require therapy [54]. Conditions such as idiopathic chronic eosinophilic pneumonia, allergic bronchopulmonary aspergillosis, and hypereosinophilic syndrome may present with clinical manifestations that may mimic EGPA, including asthma, eosinophilia, sinusitis, and pulmonary infiltrate. Therefore, these entities should be considered and ruled out as the possibility of EGPA is entertained [54].

Treatment of lung involvement in ANCA-associated vasculitis

The current treatment paradigm for patients with GPA and MPA, including those with lung manifestations (e.g., nodules, DAH, and large airway involvement), entails a relatively short induction of remission phase to control the inflammatory activity of the disease followed by a longer, lower intensity remission maintenance phase to prevent disease relapse [2,55].

The first line regimens for the purpose of induction of remission include a combination of high doses of glucocorticoids (e.g., prednisone 1 mg/kg/day) with either rituximab (1000 mg intravenously two weeks apart or four weekly infusions of 375 mg/m^2) or 3−6 months of oral cyclophosphamide (1.5−2 mg/kg/day) [56−59]. Remission maintenance is usually accomplished with a glucocorticoid taper with aim for discontinuation and either rituximab (500−1000 mg) infusions every 4−6 months [60,61] or azathioprine 2−3 mg/kg/day [58]. In selected clinical scenarios (e.g., nonsevere disease) or in patients with contra-indications or limited access to first line immunosuppressants, second line agents including methotrexate and mycophenolate mofetil may be used [62–66]. Recently, encouraging results have been obtained with the complement component 5a (C5a) receptor inhibitor avacopan, which demonstrated long-term remission maintenance for up to 52 weeks in the absence of glucocorticoids in GPA and MPA patients receiving standard of care with rituximab or cyclophosphamide followed by azathioprine [67]. Nevertheless, how avacopan may impact the different lung and airway manifestations seen in AAV patients is currently unknown.

Compared to GPA and MPA, the treatment of EGPA is less well defined. However, when EGPA patients develop vasculitic manifestations, similar guidelines are followed with variable rates of success [68–73]. More recently, a randomized controlled study demonstrated efficacy of IL-5 blockade with mepolizumab in EGPA patients with relapsing or refractory disease not able to wean off glucocorticoids regardless of the type of clinical manifestations (e.g., vasculitic vs. nonvasculitic); patients who received mepolizumab had more weeks on remission and a larger number patients receiving it entered remission compared to placebo. Nevertheless, there was still high percentage of patients that received mepolizumab (47%) who did not achieve remission. Patients who received mepolizumab also required a lower daily dose of glucocorticoids at weeks 48–50 compared to placebo [52]. Unfortunately, even after the vasculitic component of EGPA is controlled, refractory asthma, often poorly responsive to treatment may remain, presenting an important challenge for the management of these patients [51,52].

Besides adequate supportive care, which may often require mechanical ventilation, patients with AAV-associated DAH need prompt and aggressive treatment with high doses of glucocorticoids and immunosuppressants such as rituximab and/or cyclophosphamide following the general guidelines of treatment of organ- or life-threatening AAV (e.g., rapidly progressive glomerulonephritis) [2,13,55,57,74,75]. Given the severity of DAH, patients should receive high doses of intravenous glucocorticoids (e.g., 3–5 pulses of 1000 mg of methylprednisolone) followed by 1 mg per Kg of prednisone or equivalent glucocorticoid. For several years, plasma exchange has been recommended for critically ill patients with AAV and DAH [55], but a recent randomized controlled study did not show additional benefits of adding plasma exchange to a regimen of glucocorticoids plus immunosuppressants in terms of death and progression to end-stage renal disease [76]. Unfortunately, the prognosis of DAH remains poor with mortality rates as high as 25%–50% [10,13].

The prognosis of patients with AAV-related ILD seems to be worse than the one of patients with connective tissue disease (CTD)-associated ILD, but better than the prognosis of patients with idiopathic pulmonary fibrosis [19,22,24]. Unfortunately, at the moment there is scant evidence-based data to guide the treatment of AAV-related ILD, so the conventional treatment of AAV is usually followed with variable results reported in the literature

[17,20,31,77]. Patients commonly receive induction treatment with high dosages of glucocorticoids and either rituximab or cyclophosphamide, followed by maintenance therapy with agents such as rituximab, azathioprine, or mycophenolate mofetil [17,20]. Like with other causes of ILD (e.g., rheumatoid arthritis), some authors recommend avoiding the use of methotrexate in AAV patients with ILD given the risk of methotrexate-induced pneumonitis, which could deteriorate the clinical status of these patients further and act as a confounder in case of ILD progression. In individuals with positive ANCA and ILD but no other vasculitis-related manifestations, treatment according to the guidelines of idiopathic pulmonary fibrosis could be considered until more information is available [17,78]. An open label study is currently evaluating the efficacy and safety of the antifibrotic agent pirfenidone in patients with ILD and positive MPO-ANCA (PIRFENIVAS; ClinicalTrials.gov Identifier: NCT03385668).

Subglottic and tracheobronchial inflammation may lead to airway stenosis and malacia, and should be considered a serious manifestation of GPA. Induction of remission in these cases also includes high doses of glucocorticoids and either rituximab or cyclophosphamide [55]. However, methotrexate could be an alternative in selected patients with no evidence of other serious organ involvement [62]. In specific cases or when systemic immunosuppressive treatments are ineffective, direct intralesional injections of glucocorticoids can improve stenotic lesions. In addition, some patients with fixed, damage-related stenosis may require surgical interventions including laser ablation, cryotherapy, expansion probes, microsurgical lysis, and reconstructive surgery [1,79]. Occasionally, tracheostomy is needed [79]. At times, it may be difficult to differentiate between active airway inflammation and postinflammatory damage, especially in patients with negative ANCA tests and no other clinical manifestation of disease activity. That determination is crucial because intensification of immunosuppression in patients with damage-related symptomatology will be futile and likely lead to side effects including infection. Furthermore, bronchiomalacia and endobronchial stenosis may be complicated with recurrent postobstructive pneumonia and bronchiectasis [2] that will also have to be differentiated form GPA activity given the important treatment implications of that distinction (e.g., antibiotics vs. immunosuppression).

Conclusions

The spectrum of lung manifestations in AAV is broad and may include parenchymal, pleural, airway, and vascular involvement. While some lung manifestations may have asymptomatic or mildly symptomatic courses (e.g., nodules, effusion, or fleeting pulmonary infiltrates), other manifestations may have catastrophic consequences (e.g., DAH) making early detection and aggressive treatment essential. Growing evidence indicates that ILD can be a complication of AAV, but further research is needed to better understand how to treat this problem. Finally, asthma is refractory in some patients with EGPA even in the absence of active vasculitis, which highlights an important therapeutic unmet need for this patient population to prevent excessive glucocorticoid exposure and toxicity. In summary, ANCA-associated vasculitis may present with different types of pulmonary involvement, and clinicians, especially rheumatologists and pulmonologists, should be aware of the broad potential clinical and imaging manifestations, and an important take home message would be the importance of a multidisciplinary approach for the optimal diagnosis and management patients which should involve rheumatologists, pulmonologists, and radiologists.

References

[1] Sacoto G, Boukhlal S, Specks U, Flores-Suarez LF, Cornec D. Lung involvement in ANCA-associated vasculitis. Presse Med 2020;49(3):104039.

[2] Unizony SH, Stone JH. Antineutrophil cytoplasmic antibody-associated vasculitis. In: Hochberg MC, Silman AJ, Smolen JS, Weinblatt ME, Weisman MH, editors. Rheumatology. 6th ed., vol. 1. Mosby-Elsevier; 2015. p. 1310–21.

[3] Merkel PA, Lo GH, Holbrook JT, Tibbs AK, Allen NB, Davis Jr JC, Hoffman GS, McCune WJ, St Clair EW, Specks U, et al. Brief communication: high incidence of venous thrombotic events among patients with Wegener granulomatosis: the Wegener's Clinical Occurrence of Thrombosis (WeCLOT) Study. Ann Intern Med 2005;142(8):620–6.

[4] Abril A. Churg-strauss syndrome: an update. Curr Rheumatol Rep 2011;13(6):489–95.

[5] Gómez-Puerta JA, Hernández-Rodríguez J, López-Soto A, Bosch X. Antineutrophil cytoplasmic antibody-associated vasculitides and respiratory disease. Chest 2009;136(4):1101–11.

[6] Hoffman GS, Kerr GS, Leavitt RY, Hallahan CW, Lebovics RS, Travis WD, Rottem M, Fauci AS. Wegener granulomatosis: an analysis of 158 patients. Ann Intern Med 1992;116(6):488–98.

[7] Guillevin L, Durand-Gasselin B, Cevallos R, Gayraud M, Lhote F, Callard P, Amouroux J, Casassus P, Jarrousse B. Microscopic polyangiitis: clinical and laboratory findings in eighty-five patients. Arthritis Rheum 1999;42(3):421–30.

[8] Lanham JG, Elkon KB, Pusey CD, Hughes GR. Systemic vasculitis with asthma and eosinophilia: a clinical approach to the Churg-Strauss syndrome. Medicine 1984;63(2):65–81.

[9] Hassan TM, Hassan AS, Igoe A, Logan M, Gunaratnam C, McElvaney NG, O'Neill SJ. Lung involvement at presentation predicts disease activity and permanent organ damage at 6, 12 and 24 months follow - up in ANCA - associated vasculitis. BMC Immunol 2014;15:20.

[10] West S, Arulkumaran N, Ind PW, Pusey CD. Diffuse alveolar haemorrhage in ANCA-associated vasculitis. Intern Med 2013;52(1):5–13.

[11] Nasser M, Cottin V. Alveolar hemorrhage in vasculitis (primary and secondary). Semin Respir Crit Care Med 2018;39(4):482–93.

[12] Travis WD, Hoffman GS, Leavitt RY, Pass HI, Fauci AS. Surgical pathology of the lung in Wegener's granulomatosis. Rcview of 87 open lung biopsies from 67 patients. Am J Surg Pathol 1991;15(4):315–33.

[13] Cartin-Ceba R, Diaz-Caballero L, Al-Qadi MO, Tryfon S, Fervenza FC, Ytterberg SR, Specks U. Diffuse alveolar hemorrhage secondary to antineutrophil cytoplasmic antibody-associated vasculitis: predictors of respiratory failure and clinical outcomes. Arthritis Rheum 2016;68(6):1467−76.

[14] Ando Y, Okada F, Matsumoto S, Mori H. Thoracic manifestation of myeloperoxidase-antineutrophil cytoplasmic antibody (MPO-ANCA)-related disease. CT findings in 51 patients. J Comput Assist Tomogr 2004;28(5):710−6.

[15] Tzelepis GE, Kokosi M, Tzioufas A, Toya SP, Boki KA, Zormpala A, Moutsopoulos HM. Prevalence and outcome of pulmonary fibrosis in microscopic polyangiitis. Eur Respir J 2010;36(1):116−21.

[16] Arulkumaran N, Periselneris N, Gaskin G, Strickland N, Ind PW, Pusey CD, Salama AD. Interstitial lung disease and ANCA-associated vasculitis: a retrospective observational cohort study. Rheumatology 2011;50(11):2035−43.

[17] Sebastiani M, Manfredi A, Vacchi C, Cassone G, Faverio P, Cavazza A, Sverzellati N, Salvarani C, Luppi F. Epidemiology and management of interstitial lung disease in ANCA-associated vasculitis. Clin Exp Rheumatol 2020;38(Suppl. 124(2)):221−31.

[18] Hervier B, Pagnoux C, Agard C, Haroche J, Amoura Z, Guillevin L, Hamidou MA, French Vasculitis Study G. Pulmonary fibrosis associated with ANCA-positive vasculitides. Retrospective study of 12 cases and review of the literature. Ann Rheum Dis 2009;68(3):404−7.

[19] Alba MA, Flores-Suarez LF, Henderson AG, Xiao H, Hu P, Nachman PH, Falk RJ, Charles Jennette J. Interstital lung disease in ANCA vasculitis. Autoimmun Rev 2017;16(7):722−9.

[20] Comarmond C, Crestani B, Tazi A, Hervier B, Adam-Marchand S, Nunes H, Cohen-Aubart F, Wislez M, Cadranel J, Housset B, et al. Pulmonary fibrosis in antineutrophil cytoplasmic antibodies (ANCA)-associated vasculitis: a series of 49 patients and review of the literature. Medicine 2014;93(24):340−9.

[21] Foulon G, Delaval P, Valeyre D, Wallaert B, Debray MP, Brauner M, Nicaise P, Cadranel J, Cottin V, Tazi A, et al. ANCA-associated lung fibrosis: analysis of 17 patients. Respir Med 2008;102(10):1392−8.

[22] Kwon M, Lee AS, Mira-Avendano I, Rojas CA, Grage R, Abril A. Interstitial lung disease in antineutrophil cytoplasmic antibody-associated vasculitis patients: comparison with idiopathic pulmonary fibrosis. J Clin Rheumatol 2020. https://doi.org/10.1097/RHU.0000000000001357.

[23] Baqir M, Yi EE, Colby TV, Cox CW, Ryu JH, Specks U. Radiologic and pathologic characteristics of myeloperoxidase-antineutrophil cytoplasmic antibody-associated interstitial lung disease: a retrospective analysis. Sarcoidosis Vasc Diffuse Lung Dis 2019;36(3):195−201.

[24] Homma S, Matsushita H, Nakata K. Pulmonary fibrosis in myeloperoxidase antineutrophil cytoplasmic antibody-associated vasculitides. Respirology 2004;9(2):190−6.

[25] Buschman DL, Ballard R. Progressive massive fibrosis associated with idiopathic pulmonary hemosiderosis. Chest 1993;104(1):293−5.

[26] Corrin B, Jagusch M, Dewar A, Tungekar MF, Davies DR, Warner JO, Turner-Warwick M, Empey D. Fine structural changes in idiopathic pulmonary haemosiderosis. J Pathol 1987;153(3):249−56.

[27] Schnabel A, Reuter M, Csernok E, Richter C, Gross WL. Subclinical alveolar bleeding in pulmonary vasculitides: correlation with indices of disease activity. Eur Respir J 1999;14(1):118−24.

[28] Birnbaum J, Danoff S, Askin FB, Stone JH. Microscopic polyangiitis presenting as a "pulmonary-muscle" syndrome: is subclinical alveolar hemorrhage the mechanism of pulmonary fibrosis? Arthritis Rheum 2007;56(6):2065–71.

[29] Yoshida M, Yamada M, Sudo Y, Kojima T, Tomiyasu T, Yoshikawa N, Oda T, Yamada M. Myeloperoxidase anti-neutrophil cytoplasmic antibody affinity is associated with the formation of neutrophil extracellular traps in the kidney and vasculitis activity in myeloperoxidase anti-neutrophil cytoplasmic antibody-associated microscopic polyangiitis. Nephrology 2016;21(7):624–9.

[30] Peterson MW, Monick M, Hunninghake GW. Prognostic role of eosinophils in pulmonary fibrosis. Chest 1987;92(1):51–6.

[31] Hosoda C, Baba T, Hagiwara E, Ito H, Matsuo N, Kitamura H, Iwasawa T, Okudela K, Takemura T, Ogura T. Clinical features of usual interstitial pneumonia with anti-neutrophil cytoplasmic antibody in comparison with idiopathic pulmonary fibrosis. Respirology 2016;21(5):920–6.

[32] Silva CI, Muller NL, Fujimoto K, Johkoh T, Ajzen SA, Churg A. Churg-Strauss syndrome: high resolution CT and pathologic findings. J Thorac Imag 2005;20(2):74–80.

[33] Choi YH, Im JG, Han BK, Kim JH, Lee KY, Myoung NH. Thoracic manifestation of Churg-Strauss syndrome: radiologic and clinical findings. Chest 2000;117(1):117–24.

[34] Nguyen Y, Guillevin L. Eosinophilic granulomatosis with polyangiitis (Churg-Strauss). Semin Respir Crit Care Med 2018;39(4):471–81.

[35] Chung MP, Yi CA, Lee HY, Han J, Lee KS. Imaging of pulmonary vasculitis. Radiology 2010;255(2):322–41.

[36] Feragalli B, Mantini C, Sperandeo M, Galluzzo M, Belcaro G, Tartaro A, Cotroneo AR. The lung in systemic vasculitis: radiological patterns and differential diagnosis. Br J Radiol 2016;89(1061):20150992.

[37] Park HJ, Jung SM, Song JJ, Park YB, Song JS, Lee SW. Comparison of radiological and histological findings of lung parenchyma in patients with antineutrophil cytoplasmic antibody-associated vasculitis. Yonsei Med J 2019;60(5):454–60.

[38] Mohammad AJ, Mortensen KH, Babar J, Smith R, Jones RB, Nakagomi D, Sivasothy P, Jayne DRW. Pulmonary involvement in antineutrophil cytoplasmic antibodies (ANCA)-associated vasculitis: the influence of ANCA subtype. J Rheumatol 2017;44(10):1458–67.

[39] Sheehan RE, Flint JD, Muller NL. Computed tomography features of the thoracic manifestations of Wegener granulomatosis. J Thorac Imag 2003;18(1):34–41.

[40] Cottin V, Bel E, Bottero P, Dalhoff K, Humbert M, Lazor R, Sinico RA, Sivasothy P, Wechsler ME, Groh M, et al. Respiratory manifestations of eosinophilic granulomatosis with polyangiitis (Churg-Strauss). Eur Respir J 2016;48(5):1429–41.

[41] Stassen PM, Derks RP, Kallenberg CG, Stegeman CA. Venous thromboembolism in ANCA-associated vasculitis–incidence and risk factors. Rheumatology 2008;47(4):530–4.

[42] Zoller B, Li X, Sundquist J, Sundquist K. Risk of pulmonary embolism in patients with autoimmune disorders: a nationwide follow-up study from Sweden. Lancet 2012;379(9812):244–9.

[43] Allenbach Y, Seror R, Pagnoux C, Teixeira L, Guilpain P, Guillevin L, French Vasculitis Study G. High frequency of venous thromboembolic events in Churg-Strauss syndrome, Wegener's granulomatosis and microscopic polyangiitis but not polyarteritis nodosa: a systematic retrospective study on 1130 patients. Ann Rheum Dis 2009;68(4):564–7.

[44] Hansrivijit P, Trongtorsak A, Gadhiya KP, Lnu K, Dimech CT, Thongprayoon C, Cheungpasitporn W, Lecker SH. Incidence and risk factors of venous thromboembolism in ANCA-associated vasculitis: a metaanalysis and metaregression. Clin Rheumatol 2021;40(7):2843–53.

[45] Bautz DJ, Preston GA, Lionaki S, Hewins P, Wolberg AS, Yang JJ, Hogan SL, Chin H, Moll S, Jennette JC, et al. Antibodies with dual reactivity to plasminogen and complementary PR3 in PR3-ANCA vasculitis. J Am Soc Nephrol 2008;19(12):2421–9.

[46] Anderson G, Coles ET, Crane M, Douglas AC, Gibbs AR, Geddes DM, Peel ET, Wood JB. Wegener's granuloma. A series of 265 British cases seen between 1975 and 1985. A report by a sub-committee of the British Thoracic Society Research Committee. Q J Med 1992;83(302):427–38.

[47] Mahmoud S, Ghosh S, Farver C, Lempel J, Azok J, Renapurkar RD. Pulmonary vasculitis: spectrum of imaging appearances. Radiol Clin N Am 2016;54(6):1097–118.

[48] Quinn KA, Gelbard A, Sibley C, Sirajuddin A, Ferrada MA, Chen M, Cuthbertson D, Carette S, Khalidi NA, Koening CL, et al. Subglottic stenosis and endobronchial disease in granulomatosis with polyangiitis. Rheumatology 2019;58(12):2203–11.

[49] Zimba O, Doskaliuk B, Yatsyshyn R, Bahrii M, Hrytsevych M. Challenges in diagnosis of limited granulomatosis with polyangiitis. Rheumatol Int 2021;41(7):1337–45.

[50] Comarmond C, Pagnoux C, Khellaf M, Cordier JF, Hamidou M, Viallard JF, Maurier F, Jouneau S, Bienvenu B, Puechal X, et al. Eosinophilic granulomatosis with polyangiitis (Churg-Strauss): clinical characteristics and long-term followup of the 383 patients enrolled in the French Vasculitis Study Group cohort. Arthritis Rheum 2013;65(1):270–81.

[51] Berti A, Cornec D, Casal Moura M, Smyth RJ, Dagna L, Specks U, Keogh KA. Eosinophilic granulomatosis with polyangiitis: clinical predictors of long-term asthma severity. Chest 2020;157(5):1086–99.

[52] Wechsler ME, Akuthota P, Jayne D, Khoury P, Klion A, Langford CA, Merkel PA, Moosig F, Specks U, Cid MC, et al. Mepolizumab or placebo for eosinophilic granulomatosis with polyangiitis. N Engl J Med 2017;376(20):1921–32.

[53] Latorre M, Baldini C, Seccia V, Pepe P, Novelli F, Celi A, Bacci E, Cianchetti S, Dente FL, Bombardieri S, et al. Asthma control and airway inflammation in patients with eosinophilic granulomatosis with polyangiitis. J Allergy Clin Immunol Pract 2016;4(3):512–9.

[54] Groh M, Pagnoux C, Baldini C, Bel E, Bottero P, Cottin V, Dalhoff K, Dunogue B, Gross W, Holle J, et al. Eosinophilic granulomatosis with polyangiitis (Churg-Strauss) (EGPA) Consensus Task Force recommendations for evaluation and management. Eur J Intern Med 2015;26(7):545–53.

[55] Yates M, Watts RA, Bajema IM, Cid MC, Crestani B, Hauser T, Hellmich B, JU H, Laudien M, Little MA, et al. EULAR/ERA-EDTA recommendations for the management of ANCA-associated vasculitis. Ann Rheum Dis 2016;75(9):1583–94.

[56] Jones RB, Tervaert JW, Hauser T, Luqmani R, Morgan MD, Peh CA, Savage CO, Segelmark M, Tesar V, van Paassen P, et al. Rituximab versus cyclophosphamide in ANCA-associated renal vasculitis. N Engl J Med 2010;363(3):211–20.

[57] Stone JH, Merkel PA, Spiera R, Seo P, Langford CA, Hoffman GS, Kallenberg CG, St Clair EW, Turkiewicz A, Tchao NK, et al. Rituximab versus cyclophosphamide for ANCA-associated vasculitis. N Engl J Med 2010;363(3):221–32.

[58] Jayne D, Rasmussen N, Andrassy K, Bacon P, Tervaert JW, Dadoniene J, Ekstrand A, Gaskin G, Gregorini G, de Groot K, et al. A randomized trial of maintenance therapy for vasculitis associated with antineutrophil cytoplasmic autoantibodies. N Engl J Med 2003;349(1):36–44.

[59] Smith RM, Jones RB, Specks U, Bond S, Nodale M, Aljayyousi R, Andrews J, Bruchfeld A, Camilleri B, Carette S, et al. Rituximab as therapy to induce remission after relapse in ANCA-associated vasculitis. Ann Rheum Dis 2020;79(9):1243–9.

[60] Guillevin L, Pagnoux C, Karras A, Khouatra C, Aumaitre O, Cohen P, Maurier F, Decaux O, Ninet J, Gobert P, et al. Rituximab versus azathioprine for maintenance in ANCA-associated vasculitis. N Engl J Med 2014;371(19):1771–80.

[61] Smith R, Jayne D, Merkel P. LB004A randomized, controlled trial of rituximab versus azathioprine after induction of remission with rituximab for patients with ANCA-associated vasculitis and relapsing disease. Nephrol Dial Transplant 2020;35(Suppl. 3).

[62] De Groot K, Rasmussen N, Bacon PA, Tervaert JW, Feighery C, Gregorini G, Gross WL, Luqmani R, Jayne DR. Randomized trial of cyclophosphamide versus methotrexate for induction of remission in early systemic antineutrophil cytoplasmic antibody-associated vasculitis. Arthritis Rheum 2005;52(8):2461–9.

[63] Pagnoux C, Mahr A, Hamidou MA, Boffa JJ, Ruivard M, Ducroix JP, Kyndt X, Lifermann F, Papo T, Lambert M, et al. Azathioprine or methotrexate maintenance for ANCA-associated vasculitis. N Engl J Med 2008;359(26):2790–803.

[64] Jones RB, Hiemstra TF, Ballarin J, Blockmans DE, Brogan P, Bruchfeld A, Cid MC, Dahlsveen K, de Zoysa J, Espigol-Frigole G, et al. Mycophenolate mofetil versus cyclophosphamide for remission induction in ANCA-associated vasculitis: a randomised, non-inferiority trial. Ann Rheum Dis 2019;78(3):399–405.

[65] Hiemstra TF, Walsh M, Mahr A, Savage CO, de Groot K, Harper L, Hauser T, Neumann I, Tesar V, Wissing KM, et al. Mycophenolate mofetil vs azathioprine for remission maintenance in antineutrophil cytoplasmic antibody-associated vasculitis: a randomized controlled trial. J Am Med Assoc 2010;304(21):2381–8.

[66] Draibe J, Poveda R, Fulladosa X, Vidaller A, Zulberti C, Goma M, Pujol R, Ripoll E, Torras J, Grinyo JM. Use of mycophenolate in ANCA-associated renal vasculitis: 13 years of experience at a university hospital. Nephrol Dial Transplant 2015;30(Suppl. 1):i132–137.

[67] Jayne DRW, Merkel PA, Schall TJ, Bekker P, Group AS. Avacopan for the treatment of ANCA-associated vasculitis. N Engl J Med 2021;384(7):599–609.

[68] Cohen P, Pagnoux C, Mahr A, Arene JP, Mouthon L, Le Guern V, Andre MH, Gayraud M, Jayne D, Blockmans D, et al. Churg-Strauss syndrome with poor-prognosis factors: a prospective multicenter trial comparing glucocorticoids and six or twelve cyclophosphamide pulses in forty-eight patients. Arthritis Rheum 2007;57(4):686–93.

[69] Gayraud M, Guillevin L, Cohen P, Lhote F, Cacoub P, Deblois P, Godeau B, Ruel M, Vidal E, Piontud M, et al. Treatment of good-prognosis polyarteritis nodosa and Churg-Strauss syndrome: comparison of steroids and oral or pulse cyclophosphamide in 25 patients. French Cooperative Study Group for Vasculitides. Br J Rheumatol 1997;36(12):1290–7.

[70] Teixeira V, Mohammad AJ, Jones RB, Smith R, Jayne D. Efficacy and safety of rituximab in the treatment of eosinophilic granulomatosis with polyangiitis. RMD Open 2019;5(1):e000905.

[71] Metzler C, Hellmich B, Gause A, Gross WL, de Groot K. Churg Strauss syndrome–successful induction of remission with methotrexate and unexpected high cardiac and pulmonary relapse ratio during maintenance treatment. Clin Exp Rheumatol 2004;22(6 Suppl. 36):S52–61.

[72] Assaf C, Mewis G, Orfanos CE, Geilen CC. Churg-Strauss syndrome: successful treatment with mycophenolate mofetil. Br J Dermatol 2004;150(3):598–600.

[73] Puechal X, Pagnoux C, Baron G, Quemeneur T, Neel A, Agard C, Lifermann F, Liozon E, Ruivard M, Godmer P, et al. Adding azathioprine to remission-induction glucocorticoids for eosinophilic granulomatosis with polyangiitis (Churg-Strauss), microscopic polyangiitis, or polyarteritis nodosa without poor prognosis factors: a randomized, controlled trial. Arthritis Rheum 2017;69(11):2175–86.

[74] Cortazar FB, Muhsin SA, Pendergraft 3rd WF, Wallace ZS, Dunbar C, Laliberte K, Niles JL. Combination therapy with rituximab and cyclophosphamide for remission induction in ANCA vasculitis. Kidney Int Rep 2018;3(2):394–402.

[75] Lionaki S, Fragoulis GE, Venetsanopoulou A, Vlachoyiannopoulos P, Boletis JN, Tzioufas AG. Cyclophosphamide followed by rituximab for aggressive multiple-relapsing antineutrophil cytoplasmic antibody-associated vasculitis. Clin Exp Rheumatol 2017;35(Suppl. 103(1)):155–64.

[76] Walsh M, Merkel PA, Peh CA, Szpirt WM, Puechal X, Fujimoto S, Hawley CM, Khalidi N, Flossmann O, Wald R, et al. Plasma exchange and glucocorticoids in severe ANCA-associated vasculitis. N Engl J Med 2020;382(7):622–31.

[77] Nozu T, Kondo M, Suzuki K, Tamaoki J, Nagai A. A comparison of the clinical features of ANCA-positive and ANCA-negative idiopathic pulmonary fibrosis patients. Respiration 2009;77(4):407–15.

[78] Raghu G, Rochwerg B, Zhang Y, Garcia CA, Azuma A, Behr J, Brozek JL, Collard HR, Cunningham W, Homma S, et al. An official ATS/ERS/JRS/ALAT clinical practice guideline: treatment of idiopathic pulmonary fibrosis. An update of the 2011 clinical practice guideline. Am J Respir Crit Care Med 2015;192(2):e3–19.

[79] Taylor SC, Clayburgh DR, Rosenbaum JT, Schindler JS. Clinical manifestations and treatment of idiopathic and Wegener granulomatosis-associated subglottic stenosis. JAMA Otolaryngol Head Neck Surg 2013;139(1):76–81.

Chapter 8

The lung in autoimmune diseases: sarcoidosis

Robert P. Baughman* and Elyse E. Lower
Department of Medicine, University of Cincinnati Medical Center, Cincinnati, OH, United States
**Corresponding author at: baughmrp@ucmail.uc.edu.*

Introduction

Sarcoidosis is a multiorgan disease which affects the lung in more than 90% of cases [1]. The distinguishing feature of sarcoidosis is the granuloma in affected organs [2]. The etiologic agent of sarcoidosis remains unknown, with several possible environmental agents including infections and inorganic materials [3,4]. The immunologic response of sarcoidosis has some features consistent with autoimmune diseases [5].

Pulmonary sarcoidosis affects different parts of the lung including the lymphatic system, parenchyma, and vasculature. In particular, lymph node involvement with or without parenchymal lung disease is a characteristic feature of the disease. In 1961, Scadding observed that the chest X-ray in most sarcoidosis patients followed one of four patterns, which he chose to call stages (Fig. 8.1) [6]. This has become the standard for assessing thoracic involvement and Fig. 8.2 summarizes the percentage of the different stages reported by various centers across the world [1,7–9]. For four groups, we have the chest X-ray stage at time of initial diagnosis [1,8,9] and for three groups the highest chest X-ray stage was reported [6,7]. Stage 4 findings were more commonly seen over time.

Lymphatic involvement

As shown in Fig. 8.2, sarcoidosis patients often have hilar and mediastinal adenopathy with or without parenchymal lung disease. Fig. 8.3 demonstrates a patient with significant adenopathy seen on plain chest X-ray (Fig. 8.3A) and mediastinal windows on computer tomography (CT) (Fig. 8.3B). On CT scan,

The Lung in Autoimmune Diseases. https://doi.org/10.1016/B978-0-323-91083-5.00011-6

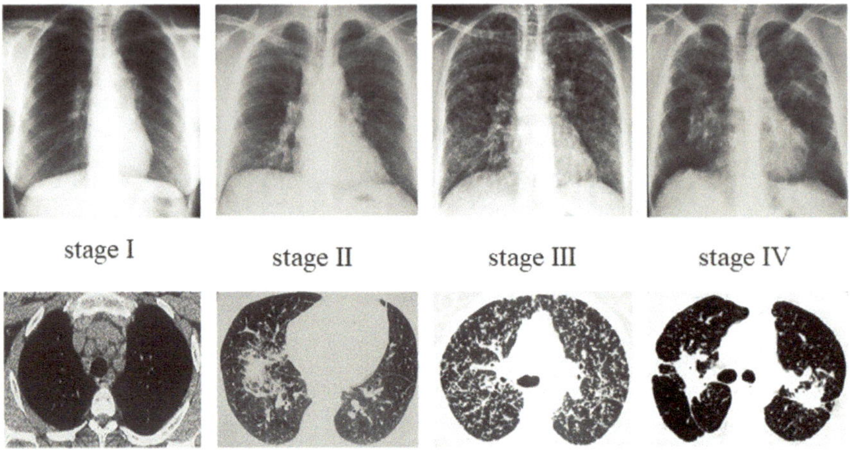

FIGURE 8.1 Chest X-ray and representative computer tomography images for the various stages as described by Scadding [6]. *Courtesy of Dr. Marjolein Drent.*

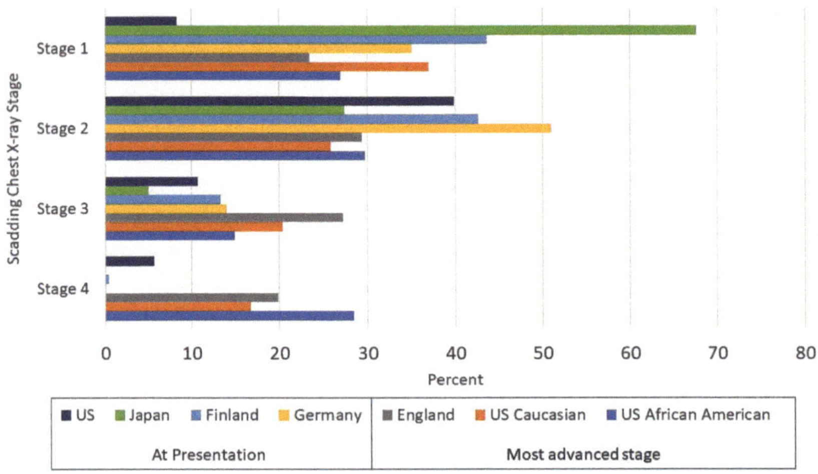

FIGURE 8.2 Percentage of chest X-ray stages [6] at time of presentation in the United States [1], Japan [8], Finland [8], and Germany [9] or the highest chest X-ray stage observed during follow-up for England [6], United States (US) Caucasians [7], and US African-Americans [7].

parenchymal nodules and bronchovascular thickening are also seen (Fig. 8.3C).

The common involvement of the lymphatics is one of the features which differentiates sarcoidosis from other interstitial lung diseases. It has been long appreciated that significant right paratracheal and bilateral hilar adenopathy in an asymptomatic patient is usually sarcoidosis [10,11]. A recent consensus panel felt that one did not have to pursue a pathologic sample in a patient with

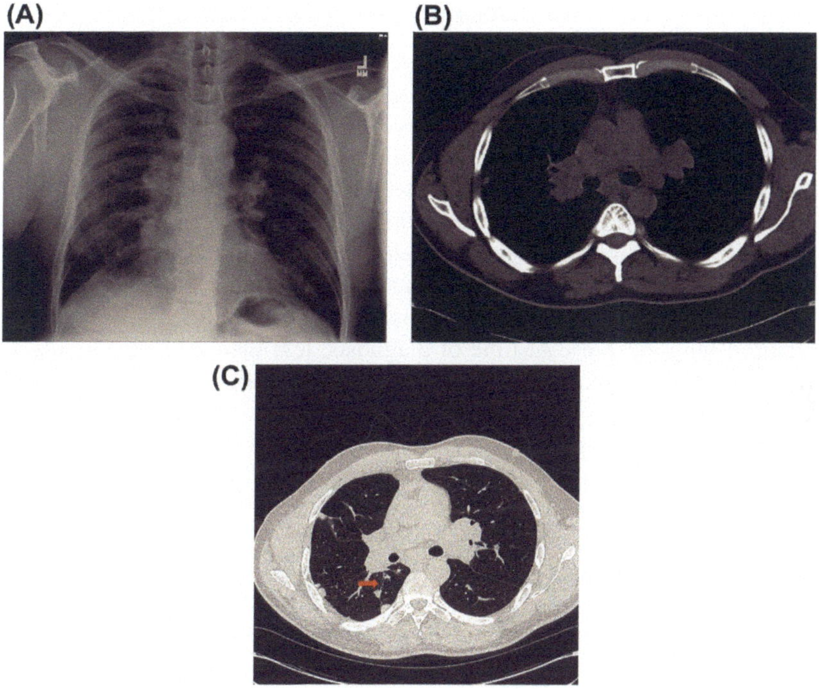

FIGURE 8.3 Bulky paratracheal and hilar adenopathy on chest X-ray (3A) and representative CT image (3B). Patient also had parenchymal nodules and bronchovascular thickening (3C).

mild to no symptoms with such adenopathy [2]. There were certain caveats about such a recommendation. The less symptomatic the patient, the more likely one is dealing with sarcoidosis. The larger and symmetrical the hilar adenopathy, the more confident one can be of the diagnosis of sarcoidosis [12]. It should be noted that endobronchial ultrasound (EBUS) is a readily available procedure with a high diagnostic yield in stage 1 or 2 sarcoidosis patients [13–15]. Because of lower cost and morbidity, EBUS is preferred over mediastinoscopy as the first step to establish a diagnosis [2].

Bronchovascular involvement is another feature seen in sarcoidosis [16,17]. It may be seen in other conditions such as lymphomatoid granulomatosis, lymphoma, and lymphangitic carcinoma [18,19]. Peribronchial nodules and fibrosis can be seen with hypersensitivity pneumonitis [20]. However, the high-resolution CT (HRCT) scan in chronic hypersensitivity usually shows upper lobe ground glass and air trapping in a pattern different from sarcoidosis and idiopathic pulmonary fibrosis [21]. The presence of bronchovascular disease in sarcoidosis is associated with presence of granulomas found with bronchial biopsy [22]. This explains the higher yield of transbronchial biopsy in sarcoidosis compared to other interstitial lung diseases.

Parenchymal lung involvement

Interstitial lung disease is a common feature of sarcoidosis. Scadding stages 2, 3, and 4 all represent interstitial lung disease and are seen in more than half of patients in most series (Fig. 8.2). Interstitial changes include small and large nodules, ground glass opacities, and fibrosis. Patients often have a mixed pattern including fibrosis and other interstitial lung involvement. Because of the mixed pattern, precise characterization of a patient in one stage or another can be difficult, with disagreement often seen between radiologists [23].

The parenchymal lung disease of sarcoidosis leads to both restriction and obstruction. In general, the extent of disease is fairly mild compared to other interstitial lung diseases. At time of diagnosis, less than 20% of patients will have a forced vital capacity (FVC) of less than 70% of predicted [1,9]. Fig. 8.4 shows the relationship between chest X-ray stage and FVC percent predicted for two studies [9,24]. From stages 1 to 3, there was a fall in the percentage of patients with normal lung function, but more than half of patients with stage 3 disease still had normal FVC percent predicted. For the United States patients, some patients were already at stage 4 at time of diagnosis. However, only a third of those presenting with stage 4 on chest X-ray had an FVC of less than 70% of predicted [24] (Fig. 8.4A).

As an interstitial lung disease, sarcoidosis can lead to reduction of lung volumes and diffusion of lung of carbon monoxide (DLCO) with no obstruction [25]. However, airway obstruction has been observed in a significant proportion of patients [26]. Fig. 8.5 shows the percent of patients with reduced FEV-1/FVC at time of diagnosis for two groups of patients [9,24]. For those from Germany, there was an increasing percentage of patients with reduced FEV-1/FVC with more advanced parenchymal disease. However, this was more striking for the United States population, where more than two thirds of patients with stage 4 disease had reduced FEV-1/FVC [24].

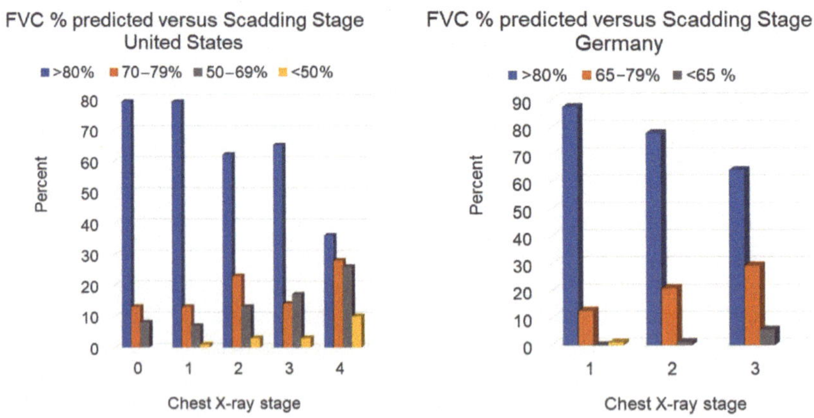

FIGURE 8.4 The percent predicted versus chest X-ray stage at time of diagnosis for those in United States [24] and Germany [9]. For those in Germany, no patients with stage 4 disease or normal chest X-ray were reported.

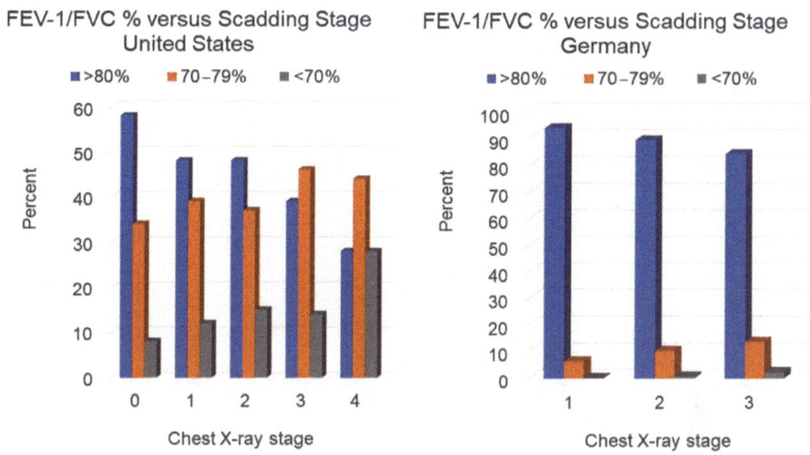

FIGURE 8.5 The FEV-1/FVC ratio versus chest X-ray stage at time of diagnosis for those in United States [24] and Germany [9]. For those in Germany, no patients with stage 4 disease or normal chest X-ray were reported.

Kouranos et al. reported on a large series of sarcoidosis patients seen at their referral clinic in London [27]. Of their 1110 patients, only 33% had normal lung function testing with 30% obstructive, 27% restrictive, and 10% mixed. The mixed pattern used standardized criteria of both reduced lung volume and FEV-1/FVC ratio [28]. Two thirds of the patients with this mixed pattern had stage 4 disease, significantly different from the other two patterns. In addition, those with a mixed pattern had a lower DLCO and higher mortality than the other two patterns. This mixed pattern appears to be related to airway distortion as a result of fibrosis (Fig. 8.6) [29]. When large airway obstruction occurs, it often involves more than one area [30]. Large airway

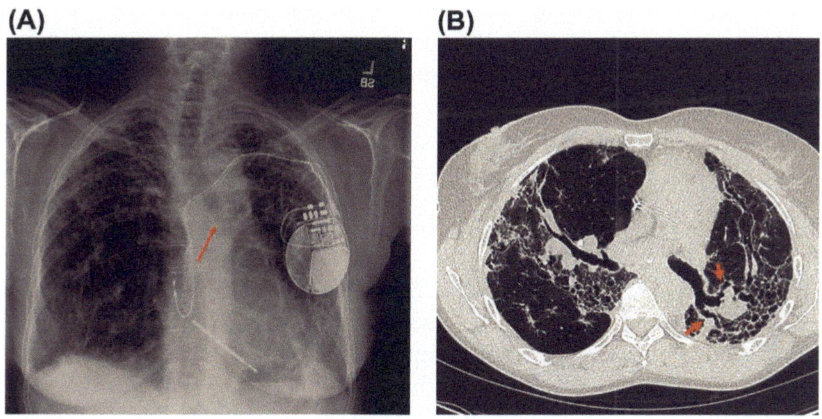

FIGURE 8.6 Posterior anterior chest X-ray (A) and representative CT image (B) of patient with fibrotic sarcoidosis and fixed airway obstruction due to airway distortion, especially in left lung (*arrows*).

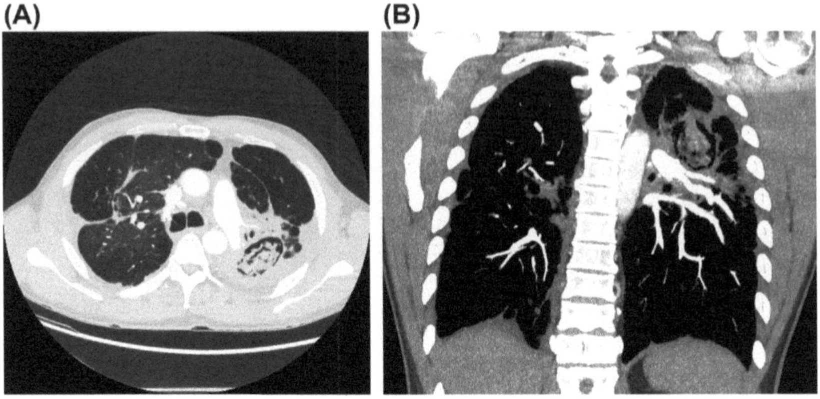

FIGURE 8.7 Sagital (A) and coronal (B) demonstrating mycetoma in left upper lobe of sarcoidosis patient who presented with massive bleeding.

obstruction may reverse with anti-inflammatory therapy if treatment is initiated within the first 6−12 months, but prolonged obstruction is usually unresponsive [30].

Upper lobe bronchiectasis is often seen in fibrotic sarcoidosis. Infection in the areas of bronchiectasis can lead to acute worsening of symptoms [31]. These acute events may occur several times a year and often respond to short course treatment with antibiotics and glucocorticoids [32]. In addition, the cavities associated with bronchiectasis may become infected with aspergillus or other fungi (Fig. 8.7). These mycetomas can be a cause of significant morbidity and some mortality [33,34]. While past studies found sarcoidosis patients with a mycetoma may die from massive hemoptysis [33,35], a recent study found that the presence of a mycetoma was not an independent risk factor for death in sarcoidosis [36]. This may have been due to widespread use of azoles in treating chronic aspergillus infection [37]. That study did find mycetomas were associated with pulmonary fibrosis and pulmonary hypertension, which are important predictors of mortality from pulmonary sarcoidosis.

Pulmonary vascular involvement

Sarcoidosis-associated pulmonary hypertension (SAPH) is found in 5%−20% of sarcoidosis patients [38−42]. Up to 50% of sarcoidosis patients with chronic dyspnea were found to have SAPH [43,44]. Sarcoidosis can lead to pulmonary hypertension due to several mechanisms [45]. These include compression of vasculature by adenopathy [46]. Over half of patients with SAPH have precapillary pulmonary hypertension [44]. This form of pulmonary hypertension may respond to therapy directed at reducing pulmonary vasculature resistance [47].

TABLE 8.1 Features associated with sarcoidosis associated pulmonary hypertension: presence of one or more features should lead to transthoracic Doppler echocardiography to estimate pulmonary hypertension probability.

- Being considered for lung transplantation
- Persistent dyspnea despite aggressive anti-inflammatory therapy
- Clinical signs of right heart failure
- Six minute walk distance of <300 m and/or desaturation of >5%
- >20% decrease in six minute walk distance over time without changes in spirometry testing
- High level of brain natriuretic peptide (BNP)
- Pulmonary fibrosis >20% of lung parenchyma
- Increased pulmonary artery to aorta ratio[a]
- Suspicion of pulmonary hypertension and/or right ventricular dysfunction on cardiac MRI
- Signs of pulmonary hypertension on CT scan of chest
- Worsening of NYHA-FC without modification of forced vital capacity
- >15% decrease in DLCO without modification of FVC

CT, computer tomography; *DLCO*, diffusion lung carbon monoxide; *FVC*, force vital capacity; *MRI*, magnetic resonance imaging; *NYHA-FC*, New York Heart Association functional class.
[a]*May be more accurate if corrected for body surface area (BSA).*

Screening for SAPH involves a stepwise process. The first step is identifying those patients who may have SAPH based on clinical features. Table 8.1 lists features suggesting pulmonary hypertension and warranting further testing. Using a Delphi method, a panel of sarcoidosis and pulmonary hypertension experts recommend that patients with one or more of these features should undergo transthoracic echocardiography.

Echocardiography is the next step of evaluation for pulmonary hypertension. Echocardiography may identify features suggesting pulmonary hypertension [48]. The echocardiogram often is able to determine the peak tricuspid regurgitant velocity. If the velocity is > 3.4 m/s, then PH is highly likely. If the velocity is between 2.9 and 3.4 m/s, there is an intermediate probability for PH. If other features of the echocardiogram suggest PH, then the probability is raised. If the flow rate is < 2.9 m/s, then PH is unlikely unless there are other features suggesting PH. Other features seen on echocardiography suggesting PH include right ventricle/left ventricle basal diameter ratio >1.0, flattening of the interventricular septum (left ventricular eccentry index >1.1 in systole and/or diastole), right ventricular outflow Doppler acceleration time <105 msec and/or mid systolic notching, early diastolic pulmonary regurgitation velocity >2.2 m/s, pulmonary artery diameter >25 mm, inferior cava diameter >21 mm with decreased inspiratory collapse (<50% with a sniff or <20% with quiet inspiration), and/or right atrial area (end-systole) > 18 cm^2 [48].

Right heat catheterization is felt to be the definitive procedure in evaluating pulmonary hypertension [48]. In addition to confirming an elevated mean pulmonary artery pressure, it also allows one to determine whether there is increased left ventricular filling pressure as the cause of pulmonary hypertension (postcapillary pulmonary hypertension). Postcapillary pulmonary hypertension usually responds to treatments to reduce left ventricular filling pressure (e.g., diuretics) and is associated with a better prognosis than precapillary pulmonary hypertension [44]. In addition, a right heart catheterization allows one to measure the cardiac output and hence calculate the pulmonary vascular resistance (PVR). Precapillary pulmonary hypertension is defined as a mean pulmonary artery pressure of >20 mm Hg, a pulmonary artery occluding pressure of <16, and a PVR of 3 or more [49].

Diagnosis of sarcoidosis

Sarcoidosis is a multiorgan disease with a variable clinical presentation. An American Thoracic Society task force proposed a clinical and pathologic pathway for diagnosis of sarcoidosis [2]. A modified version of this pathway is shown in Fig. 8.8. Clinical presentation is a crucial aspect of the diagnosis of disease. Table 8.2 lists several features encountered in sarcoidosis patients. For many of these features, presence indicates specific organ involvement [50]. In addition, there are some clinical features which are highly supportive of

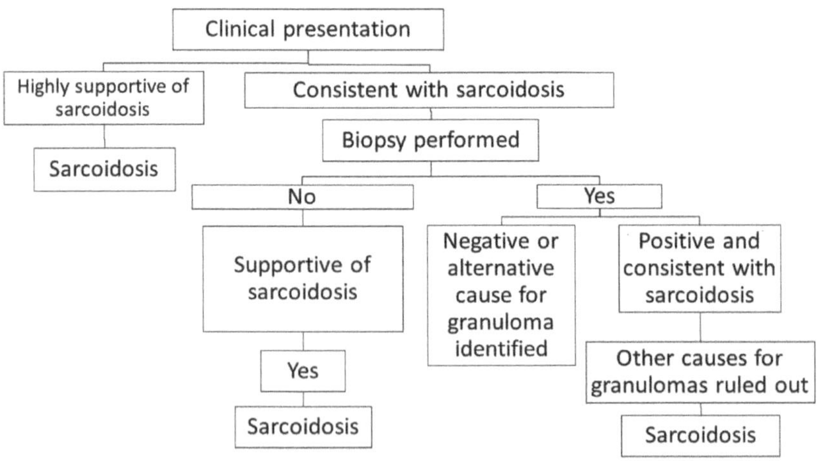

FIGURE 8.8 An approach to diagnosis of sarcoidosis incorporating clinical features with biopsy information when available. *Modified from Crouser ED, Maier LA, Wilson KC, Bonham CA, Morgenthau AS, Patterson KC, et al. Diagnosis and detection of sarcoidosis. An Official American Thoracic Society Clinical Practice Guideline. Am J Respir Crit Care Med 2020;201(8):e26–e51 and Judson MA, Costabel U, Drent M, Wells A, Maier L, Koth L, et al. The WASOG sarcoidosis organ assessment instrument: an update of a previous clinical tool. Sarcoidosis Vasc Diffuse Lung Dis 2014;31(1):19–27.*

TABLE 8.2 Clinical features supportive of diagnosis of sarcoidosis.

- Thoracic:
  - Bilateral hilar adenopathy[a]
  - Bilateral upper lobe infiltrates
  - Perilymphatic nodules on HRCT
  - Peribronchial thickening on HRCT
  - Lymphocytic alveolitis on BAL
- Skin:
  - Lupus pernio[a]
  - Erythema nodosum
  - Maculo-papular lesions
  - Papules within tattoo
- Ocular:
  - Uveitis
  - Pars planitis
  - Optic neuropathy
  - Mutton fat keratic precipitates
- Neurologic:
  - Seventh cranial nerve palsy
  - Lymphocytic meningitis
  - Gallium enhancing lesion on MRI
- Cardiac:
  - PET enhancement of myocardium
  - Gallium enhancement of myocardium
  - Ventricular arrhythmias
  - Cardiomyopathy
- Liver:
  - Increased alkaline phosphatase
  - Hepatosplenomegaly
- Abnormal calcium metabolism:
  - Hypercalcemia or hypercalciuria (with or without nephrolithiasis) with an increased 1,25-OH dihydroxy vitamin D level and reduced parathyroid hormone level
- Lofgren's syndrome[a]
  - Bilateral hilar adenopathy with erythema nodosum and/or periarticular swelling
- Heerfordt's syndrome[a]
  - Parotid swelling with uveitis

[a]*Highly supportive of diagnosis of sarcoidosis.*
Modified from Crouser ED, Maier LA, Wilson KC, Bonham CA, Morgenthau AS, Patterson KC, et al. Diagnosis and detection of sarcoidosis. An Official American Thoracic Society Clinical Practice Guideline. Am J Respir Crit Care Med 2020;201(8):e26–e51 and Judson MA, Costabel U, Drent M, Wells A, Maier L, Koth L, et al. The WASOG sarcoidosis organ assessment instrument: an update of a previous clinical tool. Sarcoidosis Vasc Diffuse Lung Dis 2014;31(1):19–27.

sarcoidosis, including bilateral hilar adenopathy, lupus pernio, and Lofgren's or Heerfordt's syndromes [2]. As shown in Fig. 8.8, presence of these highly supportive features may not require a biopsy for confirmation of the diagnosis.

Since sarcoidosis is a multiorgan disease, the detection of more than one organ involvement is common [1,7]. Recently, a sarcoidosis diagnostic score was developed [51]. The score assigns points to individual organ involvement detected on clinical and or pathologic criteria [50]. The higher the score, the more confident one was of the diagnosis of sarcoidosis. This scoring system has been proposed to improve the certainty of the diagnosis of sarcoidosis. However, one is never a 100% sure of the diagnosis of sarcoidosis.

The presence of a granuloma on pathologic specimen does not guarantee the diagnosis of sarcoidosis. Several other conditions are associated with granulomatous reactions, including tuberculosis, berylliosis, vasculitis, immunoglobulin deficiency, and cancer [2]. In many of these conditions, the granulomatous reaction is limited to one or two areas. However, some conditions such as immunoglobulin deficiency [52] and berylliosis [53] may look like sarcoidosis. Therefore, a detailed exposure history and quantitative immunoglobulin and other blood work should be considered in evaluating all potential sarcoidosis patients.

Treatment

Since there is no cure for sarcoidosis, the decision to treat sarcoidosis is guided by the patient's and clinician's concerns regarding fear of death or impairment of quality of life [54,55]. Table 8.3 indicates the various general categories for

TABLE 8.3 Treatment of pulmonary sarcoidosis.

Anti-inflammatory
- Prednisone
- Cytotoxics
  - Methotrexate
  - Azathioprine
  - Mycophenolate
  - Leflunomide
- Anti-TNF
  - Infliximab
  - Adalimumab
- Others
  - Rituximab
  - Repository corticotropin injection

Pulmonary hypertension
- Vasodilator therapy
  - Bosentan
  - Riociguat
  - Combination therapy

Fibrosis
- Nintenanib
- Pirfinedone

Infections
- Aspergilloma
- Bronchiectasis

Transplant

treating sarcoidosis, including anti-inflammatory therapy. The clinician may identify features associated with increased morbidity and/or mortality [56].

For advanced pulmonary sarcoidosis, three large series have been identified two major features associated with increased mortality: pulmonary fibrosis and pulmonary hypertension [57–59]. Fig. 8.9 demonstrates the hazards ratios for the presence of >20% pulmonary fibrosis on HRCT or pulmonary hypertension. A composite physiologic index (CPI) [60] score of greater than 40 was also predictive of increased mortality. Walsh et al. found that patients with a CPI score of >40, >20% pulmonary fibrosis on HRCT, or evidence of pulmonary of hypertension were at increased risk for dying at their center [59]. This was confirmed at the two other centers shown in Fig. 8.9. All these features were associated with increased mortality for all three studies and most were independent factors in the multiregression models each studied performed.

Pulmonary fibrosis in sarcoidosis is presumed to be the result of chronic inflammation. Anti-inflammatory therapy can arrest or even improve lung function in the majority of sarcoidosis patients with pulmonary fibrosis (stage 4 disease) [61]. In one study, over 90% of stage 4 sarcoidosis patients still had evidence of active granulomatous disease by PET scanning [62]. Since a positive PET scan predicts response to anti-inflammatory therapy [63–66], these patients should be considered for treatment.

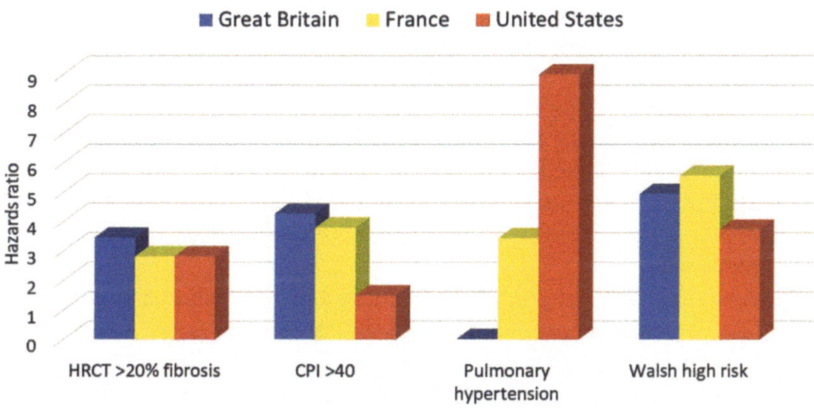

FIGURE 8.9 Calculated hazards ratio for mortality in advanced pulmonary sarcoidosis from centers in Great Britain [59], France [57], and the United States [58]. Increased risk for mortality was seen for the presence of >20% pulmonary fibrosis on high-resolution computer tomography (HRCT) or evidence of pulmonary hypertension. A composite physiologic index (CPI) [60] score of greater than 40 was also predictive of increased mortality. Walsh's high risk patients had a CPI score of >40, >20% pulmonary fibrosis on HRCT, or evidence of pulmonary of hypertension [59]. All these features were associated with increased mortality in all three studies and most were independent factors in the multiregression models each studied performed.

A recent European Respiratory Society (ERS) guideline based on Grades of Recommendation, Assessment, Development, and Evaluation (GRADE) techniques [67] has been published [54]. For patients with pulmonary disease at high risk for significant morbidity or mortality, initial therapy with glucocorticoids was a strong recommendation based on several clinical trials [68–71]. For patients who do not respond or have significant toxicity with glucocorticoids, methotrexate treatment was a conditional recommendation based on current studies [72–74]. Treatment with other cytotoxic agents such as azathioprine [73], mycophenolate [75], and leflunomide [76,77] are often used as an alternative to methotrexate [78]. Patients who still have progressive disease should be considered for biologic agents [78]. Infliximab was given a conditional recommendation based on randomized placebo controlled trials [79,80]. Over time, the majority of sarcoidosis patients treated with infliximab have to discontinue treatment despite persistent disease [81]. The ERS panel will commonly use adalimumab in those patients' intolerant to infliximab [54,82]. Other agents to be considered on a case by case basis include rituximab [81,83], Janus kinase (JAK) inhibitors [84,85], and repository corticotropin injection (RCI) [64,86].

In a survey of 1842 sarcoidosis patients across the world, impairment of quality of life and functionality were the most important reasons to consider therapy [87]. For patients with intermediate risk, but likely to have impaired quality of life, the task force gave a conditional recommendation of glucocorticoids as the first systemic therapy [54]. For patients who fail to respond or encounter toxicity with glucocorticoids, the current practice of the committee members was to use methotrexate, azathioprine, mycophenolate, or leflunomide. The use of infliximab or adalimumab was used for those who failed these first two steps of treatment. Again, other agents to be considered on a case by case basis include rituximab, JAK inhibitors, and RCI [64,86].

Significant pulmonary fibrosis is associated with increased mortality in sarcoidosis [57,58]. Nintenanib has been approved for the treatment of progressive pulmonary fibrosis, including that due to sarcoidosis [88]. Pirfenidone may also play a role in slowing the progressive fibrosis seen in some patients with sarcoidosis.

For SAPH, several drugs have been studied in open label, nonrandomized trials [45]. Sixteen weeks of bosentan led to improvement in pulmonary artery pressure compared to placebo [47]. However, there was no improvement in six minute walk at the end of the 16 weeks. A one year double blind placebo controlled trial of riociguat for SAPH found that riociguat led to improvement in the majority of treated patients, while many of the placebo-treated patients were worse by the end of the study. Overall, there was a 94 m difference in the change in six minute walk difference between the two groups [89]. The use of combination therapy is common in the management of World Health Organization group 1 patients. In SAPH, combination therapy based on individual patient response led to improvement in six minute walk distance in some patients [90,91].

In evaluating a patient with advanced sarcoidosis, one needs to consider the possibility of more than one feature leading to symptoms. Fig. 8.10 demonstrates one approach to advanced pulmonary sarcoidosis. A key initial step is to assess inflammation, usually with a PET scan. In Fig. 8.11, the significant upper lobe fibrosis was seen on CT scan (Fig. 8.11A), and this area contained significant activity demonstrated by PET scan (Fig. 8.11B). For patients with evidence of inflammation by either positive PET scan or worsening pulmonary function or chest imaging, treatment with anti-inflammatory therapy may

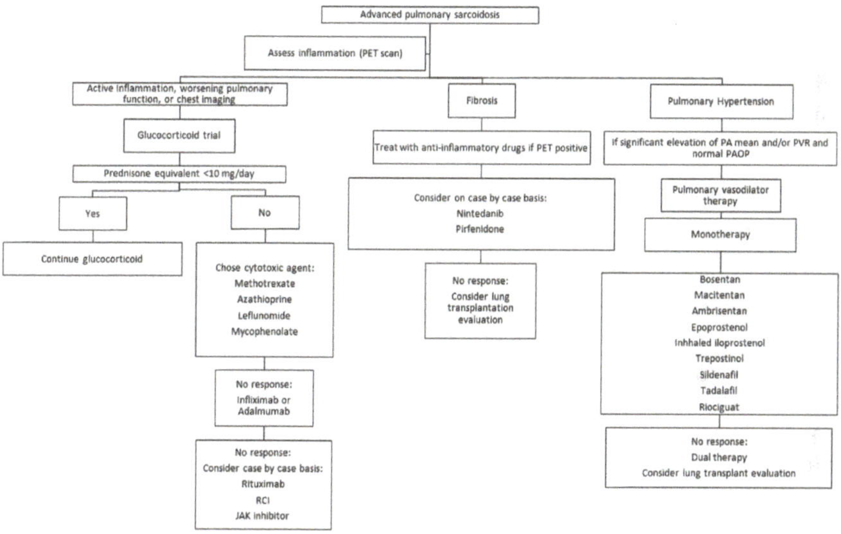

FIGURE 8.10 Approach to management of advanced sarcoidosis. The PET scan helps to determine whether there is ongoing inflammation present. Presence of fibrosis and pulmonary hypertension are diagnosed by CT scan and right heart catheterization respectively. *JAK*, Janus kinase; *PA mean*, mean pulmonary artery pressure; *PCW*, pulmonary occluding pressure; *PET*, positron emission tomography; *PVR*, pulmonary vascular resistance; *RCI*, repository corticotropin injection.

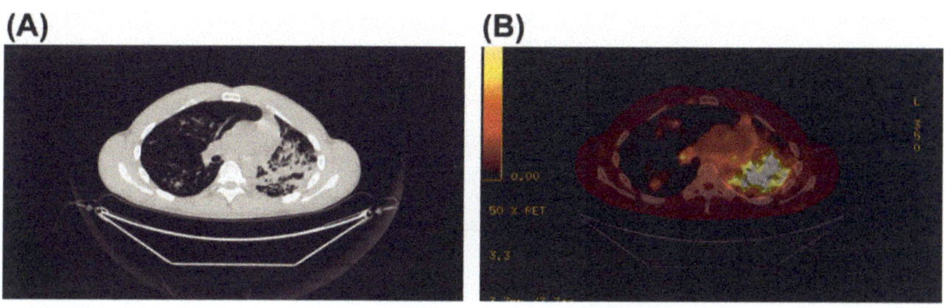

FIGURE 8.11 CT and PET scan images of a patient with significant upper lobe fibrosis seen on CT scan (Fig. 8.10A) and within the fibrotic area is increased activity on PET scan (Fig. 8.10B).

improve pulmonary function. As detailed above, glucocorticoids remain the first choice [54]. Further treatment depends on how well glucocorticoid therapy is tolerated. The figure also details the approach to treating pulmonary fibrosis and pulmonary hypertension.

Lung transplantation remains an option for those patients who fail systemic therapy. While transplantation has been successful in advanced pulmonary sarcoidosis [92,93], sarcoidosis patients listed for lung transplantation seem to have a worse outcome than those listed for other reasons [94]. This may be due to various factors, including the high rate of pulmonary hypertension and advanced fibrosis of these patients at the time of listing [92,94,95]. The risk of dying prior to transplant may be reduced by treating the pulmonary hypertension. A recent study found that pulmonary hypertension was not an independent predictor of mortality of advanced sarcoidosis awaiting lung transplantation [95].

Conclusion

Pulmonary involvement is the most common manifestation of sarcoidosis. Sarcoidosis can involve various components of the lung, including lymphatics, interstitium, and vasculature. Sarcoidosis also affects other parts of the body. Diagnosis depends on combining the information from clinical presentation with the results of analysis of tissue samples when available. Anti-inflammatory therapy remains the most important first step in treating sarcoidosis. However, treatment of other aspects of the disease should always be considered, especially in those with advance disease.

Take home messages

1. Over half of sarcoidosis patients requiring systemic therapy have chronic disease.
2. Methotrexate and other cytotoxic drugs have been shown to be effective steroid sparing for these chronic patients.
3. Infliximab is the most effective third line treatment of advanced pulmonary sarcoidosis.
4. Pulmonary hypertension is an important complication of advanced sarcoidosis.

References

[1] Baughman RP, Teirstein AS, Judson MA, Rossman MD, Yeager HJ, Bresnitz EA, et al. Clinical characteristics of patients in a case control study of sarcoidosis. Am J Respir Crit Care Med 2001;164:1885–9.

[2] Crouser ED, Maier LA, Wilson KC, Bonham CA, Morgenthau AS, Patterson KC, et al. Diagnosis and detection of sarcoidosis. An Official American Thoracic Society Clinical Practice Guideline. Am J Respir Crit Care Med 2020;201(8):e26–51.

[3] Oswald-Richter KA, Drake WP. The etiologic role of infectious antigens in sarcoidosis pathogenesis. Semin Respir Crit Care Med 2010;31(4):375–9.

[4] Izbicki G, Chavko R, Banauch GI, Weiden MD, Berger KI, Aldrich TK, et al. World Trade Center "sarcoid-like" granulomatous pulmonary disease in New York City Fire Department rescue workers. Chest 2007;131(5):1414–23.

[5] Kaiser Y, Eklund A, Grunewald J. Moving target - shifting the focus to pulmonary sarcoidosis as an autoimmune spectrum disorder. Eur Respir J 2019:13993003.

[6] Scadding JG. Prognosis of intrathoracic sarcoidosis in England. Br Med J 1961;4:1165–72.

[7] Judson MA, Boan AD, Lackland DT. The clinical course of sarcoidosis: presentation, diagnosis, and treatment in a large white and black cohort in the United States. Sarcoidosis Vasc Diffuse Lung Dis 2012;29(2):119–27.

[8] Pietinalho A, Ohmichi M, Lofroos AB, Hiraga Y, Selroos O. The prognosis of sarcoidosis in Finland and Hokkaido, Japan. A comparative five-year study of biopsy-proven cases. Sarcoidosis Vasc Diffuse Lung Dis 2000;17:158–66.

[9] Loddenkemper R, Kloppenborg A, Schoenfeld N, Grosser H, Costabel U. Clinical findings in 715 patients with newly detected pulmonary sarcoidosis—results of a cooperative study in former West Germany and Switzerland. WATL Study Group. Wissenschaftliche Arbeitsgemeinschaft fur die Therapie von Lungenkrankheitan. Sarcoidosis Vasc Diffuse Lung Dis 1998;15(2):178–82.

[10] Winterbauer RH, Belic N, Moores KD. A clinical interpretation of bilateral hilar adenopathy. Ann Intern Med 1973;78:65–71.

[11] Reich JM, Brouns MC, O'Connor EA, Edwards MJ. Mediastinoscopy in patients with presumptive stage I sarcoidosis: a risk/benefit, cost/benefit analysis. Chest 1998;113(1):147–53.

[12] Niimi H, Kang EY, Kwong JS, Carignan S, Muller NL. CT of chronic infiltrative lung disease: prevalence of mediastinal lymphadenopathy. J Comput Assist Tomogr 1996;20(2):305–8.

[13] Benzaquen S, Aragaki-Nakahodo AA. Bronchoscopic modalities to diagnose sarcoidosis. Curr Opin Pulm Med 2017;23(5):433–8.

[14] Agarwal R, Srinivasan A, Aggarwal AN, Gupta D. Efficacy and safety of convex probe EBUS-TBNA in sarcoidosis: a systematic review and meta-analysis. Respir Med 2012;106(6):883–92.

[15] Trisolini R, Lazzari AL, Tinelli C, De SA, Scotti V, Patelli M. Endobronchial ultrasound-guided transbronchial needle aspiration for diagnosis of sarcoidosis in clinically unselected study populations. Respirology 2015;20(2):226–34.

[16] Utpat K, Sasikumar C, Desai U, Joshi JM. Sarcoidosis at the Pulmonary Medicine Department of a tertiary care hospital in Mumbai. Our experience and the new modified criteria clinical radiological physiological (TNMC CRP) score for sarcoidosis: a novel proposition to assess the functional status. Monaldi Arch Chest Dis 2021;91(1):10.

[17] Nishimura K, Itoh H, Kitaichi M, Nagai S, Izumi T. Pulmonary sarcoidosis: correlation of CT and histopathologic findings. Radiology 1993;189(1):105–9.

[18] Rezvani S, Tominna M, Al-Katib S, Smith MD, Cousineau C, Al-Katib A. Lymphomatoid granulomatosis in a patient with chronic lymphocytic leukemia and rapidly progressing peribronchovascular pulmonary infiltrates. Case Rep Pulmonol 2019;2019:9870494. https://doi.org/10.1155/2019/9870494. eCollection@2019.:9870494.

[19] Honda O, Johkoh T, Ichikado K, Yoshida S, Mihara N, Higashi M, et al. Comparison of high resolution CT findings of sarcoidosis, lymphoma, and lymphangitic carcinoma: is there any difference of involved interstitium? J Comput Assist Tomogr 1999;23(3):374–9.

[20] Adler BD, Padley SP, MÜller NL, Remy-Jardin M, Remy J. Chronic hypersensitivity pneumonitis: high-resolution CT and radiographic features in 16 patients. Radiology 1992;185(1):91–5.

[21] Zompatori M, CalabrÃ E, Chetta A, Chiari G, Marangio E, Olivieri D. Chronic hypersensitivity pneumonitis or idiopathic pulmonary fibrosis? Diagnostic role of high resolution computed tomography (HRCT). Radiol Med 2003;106(3):135–46.

[22] Shorr AF, Torrington KG, Hnatiuk OW. Endobronchial biopsy for sarcoidosis: a prospective study. Chest 2001;120(1):109–14.

[23] Baughman RP, Shipley R, Desai S, Drent M, Judson MA, Costabel U, et al. Changes in chest roentgenogram of sarcoidosis patients during a clinical trial of infliximab therapy: comparison of different methods of evaluation. Chest 2009;136:526–35.

[24] Yeager H, Rossman MD, Baughman RP, Teirstein AS, Judson MA, Rabin DL, et al. Pulmonary and psychosocial findings at enrollment in the ACCESS study. Sarcoidosis Vasc Diffuse Lung Dis 2005;22(2):147–53.

[25] Boros PW, Enright PL, Quanjer PH, Borsboom GJ, Wesolowski SP, Hyatt RE. Impaired lung compliance and DL,CO but no restrictive ventilatory defect in sarcoidosis. Eur Respir J 2010;36(6):1315–22.

[26] Sharma OP, Johnson R. Airway obstruction in sarcoidosis. A study of 123 nonsmoking black American patients with sarcoidosis. Chest 1988;94(2):343–6.

[27] Kouranos V, Ward S, Kokosi MA, Castillo D, Chua F, Judge EP, et al. Mixed ventilatory defects in pulmonary sarcoidosis: prevalence and clinical features. Chest 2020;20:10.

[28] Pellegrino R, Viegi G, Brusasco V, Crapo RO, Burgos F, Casaburi R, et al. Interpretative strategies for lung function tests. Eur Respir J 2005;26(5):948–68.

[29] Naccache JM, Lavole A, Nunes H, Lamberto C, Letoumelin P, Brauner M, et al. High-resolution computed tomographic imaging of airways in sarcoidosis patients with airflow obstruction. J Comput Assist Tomogr 2008;32(6):905–12.

[30] Chambellan A, Turbie P, Nunes H, Brauner M, Battesti JP, Valeyre D. Endoluminal stenosis of proximal bronchi in sarcoidosis: bronchoscopy, function, and evolution. Chest 2005;127(2):472–81.

[31] Panselinas E, Judson MA. Acute pulmonary exacerbations of sarcoidosis. Chest 2012;142(4):827–36.

[32] Baughman RP, Lower EE. Frequency of acute worsening events in fibrotic pulmonary sarcoidosis patients. Respir Med 2013;107:2009–13.

[33] Denning DW, Pleuvry A, Cole DC. Global burden of chronic pulmonary aspergillosis complicating sarcoidosis. Eur Respir J 2013;41(3):621–6.

[34] Pena TA, Soubani AO, Samavati L. Aspergillus lung disease in patients with sarcoidosis: a case series and review of the literature. Lung 2011;189(2):167–72.

[35] Tomlinson JR, Sahn SA. Aspergilloma in sarcoid and tuberculosis. Chest 1987;92(3):505–8.

[36] Uzunhan Y, Nunes H, Jeny F, Lacroix M, Brun S, Brillet PY, et al. Chronic pulmonary aspergillosis complicating sarcoidosis. Eur Respir J 2017;49(6):1602396.

[37] Agarwal R, Vishwanath G, Aggarwal AN, Garg M, Gupta D, Chakrabarti A. Itraconazole in chronic cavitary pulmonary aspergillosis: a randomised controlled trial and systematic review of literature. Mycoses 2013;56(5):559–70.

[38] Tiosano S, Versini M, Dar AL, Spitzer L, Yavne Y, Watad A, et al. The long-term prognostic significance of sarcoidosis-associated pulmonary hypertension - a cohort study. Clin Immunol 2019;199:57–61.

[39] Keir GJ, Walsh SL, Gatzoulis MA, Marino PS, Dimopoulos K, Alonso R, et al. Treatment of sarcoidosis-associated pulmonary hypertension: a single centre retrospective experience using targeted therapies. Sarcoidosis Vasc Diffuse Lung Dis 2014;31(2):82–90.

[40] Bourbonnais JM, Samavati L. Clinical predictors of pulmonary hypertension in sarcoidosis. Eur Respir J 2008;32(2):296–302.

[41] Handa T, Nagai S, Miki S, Fushimi Y, Ohta K, Mishima M, et al. Incidence of pulmonary hypertension and its clinical relevance in patients with sarcoidosis. Chest 2006;129(5):1246–52.

[42] Huitema MP, Bakker ALM, Mager JJ, Rensing BJWM, Smits F, Snijder RJ, et al. Prevalence of pulmonary hypertension in pulmonary sarcoidosis: the first large European prospective study. Eur Respir J 2019;54(4):1900897.

[43] Sulica R, Teirstein AS, Kakarla S, Nemani N, Behnegar A, Padilla ML. Distinctive clinical, radiographic, and functional characteristics of patients with sarcoidosis-related pulmonary hypertension. Chest 2005;128(3):1483–9.

[44] Baughman RP, Engel PJ, Taylor L, Lower EE. Survival in sarcoidosis associated pulmonary hypertension: the importance of hemodynamic evaluation. Chest 2010;138:1078–85.

[45] Shlobin OA, Baughman RP. Sarcoidosis-associated pulmonary hypertension. Semin Respir Crit Care Med 2017;38(4):450–62.

[46] Hasegawa K, Ohno S, Takada M, Ogino H, Shiotsu S, Takumi C, et al. Sarcoidosis complicated with major pulmonary artery obstruction and stenosis. Intern Med 2012;51(19):2775–80.

[47] Baughman RP, Culver DA, Cordova FC, Padilla M, Gibson KF, Lower EE, et al. Bosentan for sarcoidosis associated pulmonary hypertension: a double-blind placebo controlled randomized trial. Chest 2014;145:810–7.

[48] Galie N, Humbert M, Vachiery JL, Gibbs S, Lang I, Torbicki A, et al. 2015 ESC/ERS guidelines for the diagnosis and treatment of pulmonary hypertension: the joint task force for the diagnosis and treatment of pulmonary hypertension of the European Society of Cardiology (ESC) and the European Respiratory Society (ERS): endorsed by: Association for European Paediatric and Congenital Cardiology (AEPC), International Society for Heart and Lung Transplantation (ISHLT). Eur Respir J 2015;46(4):903–75.

[49] Humbert M, Guignabert C, Bonnet S, DorfmÃ¼ller P, Klinger JR, Nicolls MR, et al. Pathology and pathobiology of pulmonary hypertension: state of the art and research perspectives. Eur Respir J 2019;53(1):1801887–2018.

[50] Judson MA, Costabel U, Drent M, Wells A, Maier L, Koth L, et al. The WASOG Sarcoidosis Organ Assessment Instrument: an update of a previous clinical tool. Sarcoidosis Vasc Diffuse Lung Dis 2014;31(1):19–27.

[51] Bickett AN, Lower EE, Baughman RP. Sarcoidosis diagnostic score: a systematic evaluation to enhance the diagnosis of sarcoidosis. Chest 2018;154:1052–60.

[52] Prasse A, Kayser G, Warnatz K. Common variable immunodeficiency-associated granulomatous and interstitial lung disease. Curr Opin Pulm Med 2013;19(5):503–9.

[53] Mayer AS, Hamzeh N, Maier LA. Sarcoidosis and chronic beryllium disease: similarities and differences. Semin Respir Crit Care Med 2014;35(3):316–29.

[54] Baughman RP, Valeyre D, Korsten P, Mathioudakis AG, Wuyts WA, Wells A, et al. ERS clinical practice guidelines on treatment of sarcoidosis. Eur Respir J 2021:2004079.

[55] Baughman RP, Judson MA, Wells AU. The indications for the treatment of sarcoidosis: Wells law. Sarcoidosis Vasc Diffuse Lung Dis 2017;34:280–2.

[56] Baughman RP, Wells AU. Advanced sarcoidosis. Curr Opin Pulm Med 2019;25:497–504.

[57] Jeny F, Uzunhan Y, Lacroix M, Gille T, Brillet PY, Nardi A, et al. Predictors of mortality in fibrosing pulmonary sarcoidosis. Respir Med 2020;169:105997. https://doi.org/10.1016/j.rmed.2020.105997. Epub@2020 May 12.

[58] Kirkil G, Lower EE, Baughman RP. Predictors of mortality in pulmonary sarcoidosis. Chest 2018;153(1):105−13.

[59] Walsh SL, Wells AU, Sverzellati N, Keir GJ, Calandriello L, Antoniou KM, et al. An integrated clinicoradiological staging system for pulmonary sarcoidosis: a case-cohort study. Lancet Respir Med 2014;2(2):123−30.

[60] Wells AU, Desai SR, Rubens MB, Goh NS, Cramer D, Nicholson AG, et al. Idiopathic pulmonary fibrosis: a composite physiologic index derived from disease extent observed by computed tomography. Am J Respir Crit Care Med 2003;167(7):962−9.

[61] Nardi A, Brillet PY, Letoumelin P, Girard F, Brauner M, Uzunhan Y, et al. Stage IV sarcoidosis: comparison of survival with the general population and causes of death. Eur Respir J 2011;38(6):1368−73.

[62] Mostard RL, Voo S, van Kroonenburgh MJ, Verschakelen JA, Wijnen PA, Nelemans PJ, et al. Inflammatory activity assessment by F18 FDG-PET/CT in persistent symptomatic sarcoidosis. Respir Med 2011;105(12):1917−24.

[63] Schimmelpennink MC, Vorselaars ADM, van Beek FT, Crommelin HA, Deneer VHM, Keijsers RGM, et al. Efficacy and safety of infliximab biosimilar Inflectra((R)) in severe sarcoidosis. Respir Med 2018;138S:S7−13. https://doi.org/10.1016/j.rmed.2018.02.009.

[64] Baughman RP, Sweiss N, Keijsers R, Birring SS, Shipley R, Saketkoo LA, et al. Repository corticotropin for chronic pulmonary sarcoidosis. Lung 2017;195(3):313−22.

[65] Guleria R, Jyothidasan A, Madan K, Mohan A, Kumar R, Bhalla AS, et al. Utility of FDG-PET-CT scanning in assessing the extent of disease activity and response to treatment in sarcoidosis. Lung India 2014;31(4):323−30.

[66] Vorselaars AD, Verwoerd A, Van Moorsel CH, Keijsers RG, Rijkers GT, Grutters JC. Prediction of relapse after discontinuation of infliximab therapy in severe sarcoidosis. Eur Respir J 2014;43(2):602−9.

[67] Alonso-Coello P, Schunemann HJ, Moberg J, Brignardello-Petersen R, Akl EA, Davoli M, et al. GRADE Evidence to Decision (EtD) frameworks: a systematic and transparent approach to making well informed healthcare choices. 1: Introduction. BMJ 2016;353:i2016. https://doi.org/10.1136/bmj.i2016.

[68] Paramothayan NS, Jones PW. Corticosteroids for pulmonary sarcoidosis. Cochrane Database Syst Rev 2000;4:CD001114.

[69] Gibson GJ, Prescott RJ, Muers MF, Middleton WG, Mitchell DN, Connolly CK, et al. British Thoracic Society Sarcoidosis study: effects of long term corticosteroid treatment. Thorax 1996;51(3):238−47.

[70] Pietinalho A, Tukiainen P, Haahtela T, Persson T, Selroos O, the Finnish Pulmonary Sarcoidosis Study Group. Early treatment of stage II sarcoidosis improves 5-year pulmonary function. Chest 2002;121:24−31.

[71] Sharma OP, Colp C, Williams Jr MH. Course of pulmonary sarcoidosis with and without corticosteroid therapy as determined by pulmonary function studies. Am J Med 1966;41:541−51.

[72] Baughman RP, Winget DB, Lower EE. Methotrexate is steroid sparing in acute sarcoidosis: results of a double blind, randomized trial. Sarcoidosis Vasc Diffuse Lung Dis 2000;17:60−6.

[73] Vorselaars AD, Wuyts WA, Vorselaars VM, Zanen P, Deneer VH, Veltkamp M, et al. Methotrexate versus azathioprine in second line therapy of sarcoidosis. Chest 2013;144:805−12.

[74] Baughman RP, Cremers JP, Harmon M, Lower EE, Drent M. Methotrexate in sarcoidosis: hematologic and hepatic toxicity encountered in a large cohort over a six year period. Sarcoidosis Vasc Diffuse Lung Dis 2020;37(3):c2020001.

[75] Hamzeh N, Voelker A, Forssen A, Gottschall EB, Rose C, Mroz P, et al. Efficacy of mycophenolate mofetil in sarcoidosis. Respir Med 2014;108:1663–9.

[76] Sahoo DH, Bandyopadhyay D, Xu M, Pearson K, Parambil JG, Lazar CA, et al. Effectiveness and safety of leflunomide for pulmonary and extrapulmonary sarcoidosis. Eur Respir J 2011;38:1145–50.

[77] Baughman RP, Lower EE. Leflunomide for chronic sarcoidosis. Sarcoidosis Vasc Diffuse Lung Dis 2004;21:43–8.

[78] Rahaghi FF, Baughman RP, Saketkoo LA, Sweiss NJ, Barney JB, Birring SS, et al. Delphi consensus recommendations for a treatment algorithm in pulmonary sarcoidosis. Eur Respir Rev 2020;29(155):190146–2019.

[79] Baughman RP, Drent M, Kavuru M, Judson MA, Costabel U, Du BR, et al. Infliximab therapy in patients with chronic sarcoidosis and pulmonary involvement. Am J Respir Crit Care Med 2006;174(7):795–802.

[80] Rossman MD, Newman LS, Baughman RP, Teirstein A, Weinberger SE, Miller WJ, et al. A double-blind, randomized, placebo-controlled trial of infliximab in patients with active pulmonary sarcoidosis. Sarcoidosis Vasc Diffuse Lung Dis 2006;23:201–8.

[81] Lower EE, Sturdivant M, Grate L, Baughman RP. Use of third-line therapies in advanced sarcoidosis. Clin Exp Rheumatol 2019;38:834–40.

[82] Crommelin HA, van der Burg LM, Vorselaars AD, Drent M, Van Moorsel CH, Rijkers GT, et al. Efficacy of adalimumab in sarcoidosis patients who developed intolerance to infliximab. Respir Med 2016;115:72–7.

[83] Sweiss NJ, Lower EE, Mirsaeidi M, Dudek S, Garcia JG, Perkins D, et al. Rituximab in the treatment of refractory pulmonary sarcoidosis. Eur Respir J 2014;43(5):1525–8.

[84] Damsky W, Thakral D, Emeagwali N, Galan A, King B. Tofacitinib treatment and molecular analysis of cutaneous sarcoidosis. N Engl J Med 2018;379(26):2540–6.

[85] Rotenberg C, Besnard V, Brillet PY, Giraudier S, Nunes H, Valeyre D. Dramatic response of refractory sarcoidosis under ruxolitinib in a patient with associated JAK2-mutated polycythemia. Eur Respir J 2018;52(6):1801482.

[86] Chopra I, Qin Y, Kranyak J, Gallagher JR, Heap K, Carroll S, et al. Repository corticotropin injection in patients with advanced symptomatic sarcoidosis: retrospective analysis of medical records. Ther Adv Respir Dis 2019;13. https://doi.org/10.1177/1753466619888127.:1753466619888127.

[87] Baughman RP, Barriuso R, Beyer K, Boyd J, Hochreiter J, Knoet C, et al. Sarcoidosis: patient treatment priorities. ERJ Open Res 2018;4(4):00141–2018.

[88] Flaherty KR, Wells AU, Cottin V, Devaraj A, Walsh SLF, Inoue Y, et al. Nintedanib in progressive fibrosing interstitial lung diseases. N Engl J Med 2019;10.

[89] Baughman RP, Shlobin OA, Gupta RG, Engel PJ, Stewart J, Lower EE, et al. Riociguat was effective in increasing time until clinical worsening in sarcoidosis associated pulmonary hypertension: results of a one year double blind, placebo controlled trial. Chest 2021;S0012-3692(21):03613–8. https://doi.org/10.1016/j.chest.2021.07.2162.

[90] Barnett CF, Bonura EJ, Nathan SD, Ahmad S, Shlobin OA, Osei K, et al. Treatment of sarcoidosis-associated pulmonary hypertension: a two-center experience. Chest 2009;135:1455–61.

[91] Boucly A, Cottin V, Nunes H, Jais X, Tazi A, Prevot G, et al. Management and long-term outcomes of sarcoidosis-associated pulmonary hypertension. Eur Respir J 2017;50(4):50–4.

[92] Le Pavec J, Valeyre D, Gazengel P, Holm AM, Schultz HH, Perch M, et al. Lung transplantation for sarcoidosis: outcome and prognostic factors. Eur Respir J 2021:2003358.
[93] Taimeh Z, Hertz MI, Shumway S, Pritzker M. Lung transplantation for pulmonary sarcoidosis. Twenty-five years of experience in the USA. Thorax 2016;71(4):378−9.
[94] Shorr AF, Davies DB, Nathan SD. Predicting mortality in patients with sarcoidosis awaiting lung transplantation. Chest 2003;124(3):922−8.
[95] Gangemi AJ, Myers CN, Zheng M, Brown J, Butler-LeBair M, Cordova F, et al. Mortality for sarcoidosis patients on the transplant wait list in the lung allocation score era: experience from a high volume center. Respir Med 2019;157:69−76. https://doi.org/10.1016/j.rmed.2019.09.001. Epub@2019 Sep 7.:69-76.

Chapter 9

COVID-19 and lung involvement

Jin-Seok You,[1] Rosa Faner,[2] Oriol Sibila[1] and Jacobo Sellarés[1,*]
[1]*Servei de Pneumologia, Institut Clínic Respiratori, Hospital Clínic, Barcelona, Spain;* [2]*Institut d'Investigacions Biomèdiques August Pi i Sunyer (IDIBAPS)-Centro de Investigación Biomedica en Red-Enfermedades Respiratorias (CIBERES), Madrid, Spain*
[*]*Corresponding authors at: sellares@clinic.cat.*

Introduction

Coronaviruses are group of viruses capable of infecting many different animals, including humans, resulting mainly in respiratory diseases that can range from mild to severe [1–4]. Given their high prevalence and wide distribution, large genetic diversity and frequent recombination of their genomes, as well as increasing human–animal interface activities, it is not uncommon for novel coronaviruses to emerge periodically in humans [1].

In 2002 and 2012, respectively, two highly pathogenic coronaviruses with zoonotic origin, severe acute respiratory syndrome coronavirus (SARS-CoV) and Middle East respiratory syndrome coronavirus (MERS-CoV), emerged among humans and caused fatal respiratory illness, making coronaviruses a public health concern [2,5].

In late December 2019, a previously unknown coronavirus was discovered from a cluster of patients with pneumonia of unknown cause in Wuhan, a city in the Hubei province of China [1,4,6]. This virus, initially named 2019-nCoV, was identified as a highly transmissible and pathogenic coronavirus which affected the lung and had a rapid and worldwide spread [1,5,6]. On February 11, 2020, the International Committee on Taxonomy of Viruses (ICTV) named this novel coronavirus as severe acute respiratory syndrome coronavirus 2 (SARS-CoV-2), and on the same day the World Health Organization (WHO) officially designated the disease coronavirus disease 2019 (COVID-19) [1,4,5]. Later, on March 11, 2020, the WHO officially declared the disease a pandemic [6].

The Lung in Autoimmune Diseases. https://doi.org/10.1016/B978-0-323-91083-5.00004-9

COVID-19 can range in severity, depending not only on the viral infection itself and/or secondary infections but is also conditioned by the immune system and the host's response. The disease is often associated with aggressive and uncontrolled inflammation that may lead to acute respiratory distress syndrome (ARDS), multiorgan damage and failure, and death [7,8]. This chapter aims to review the general characteristics of SARS-CoV-2 infection, its interaction with target cells and the resulting immune response, as well as current and potential therapeutic interventions.

Epidemiology

The initial outbreak, on December 2019, only occurred in Wuhan and its surroundings in Hubei Province. By the end of January 2020, COVID-19 had spread to all 31 provinces in mainland China [4]. The first case reported outside of China was on January 13, 2020, from a patient in Thailand that had been in Wuhan [9]. In the following months, the disease spread to all the continents and the WHO officially declared it a pandemic on March 11, 2020 [4,6].

Initial data showed that patients were mainly concentrated at the age of 30–79, accounting for more than 85% of confirmed cases. Prevalence was slightly higher on males and the proportion of infected healthcare workers was around 2% [4,10].

As of July 2021, the cumulative number of cases reported globally was over 187 million and the number of deaths exceeded four million. Cases have been reported from all five continents, most of them announced in America and Europe with 74 and 56 million cases, respectively, with 1.9 and 1.1 million deaths each. Because COVID-19 is an ongoing pandemic, geographic distribution is constantly evolving and situation reports are being released periodically [11,12].

As SARS-CoV-2 continued to circulate and evolve, variants of interest and concern were reported. A variant of interest (VOI) is one with genetic changes affecting virus characteristics such as transmissibility, disease severity, immune escape, diagnostic or therapeutic escape; and with epidemiological impacts suggesting an emerging risk to global public health, like causing significant community transmission or clusters [11].

On the other hand, a variant of concern (VOC) is a SARS-CoV-2 variant that meets the definition of a VOI and has been demonstrated to possess increased transmissibility or detrimental change in COVID-19 epidemiology; or increased virulence or change in clinical disease presentation; or cause decreased effectiveness of public health and social measures or available diagnostics, vaccines and therapeutics. The four VOCs characterized to date are Alpha, Beta, Gamma, and Delta, all of which have demonstrated increased transmissibility. Of those aforementioned variants, Delta has been detected in at least 111 countries and is expected to rise and become the dominant variant globally in the following months [11,12].

Virology

SARS-CoV-2 is a coronavirus that belongs to the betacoronavirus genus in the *Orthocoronavirinae* subfamily. It is an enveloped, positive-sense single-stranded RNA virus with characteristic spikes projecting from its surface [3–5]. These viral particles are generally spherical, its diameter varying from about 60 to 140 nm, and their spikes measure about 9 to 12 nm. On electron micrographs, the negative-stained virions resemble a solar corona, typical of the *Coronaviridae* family [1,4,6].

Through full genome sequencing and phylogenetic analysis, it is known that SARS-CoV-2 is similar to a previously identified SARS-like coronavirus (bat-SL-CoVZC45, MG772933.1) found in bats and pangolins [1,13]. SARS-CoV-2 also shares 79.5% and 50% sequence identity to SARS-CoV and MERS-CoV, respectively [4].

SARS-CoV-2 virions consist of a nucleoprotein (N) which wraps the RNA genome forming a coiled tubular structure, packed by a phospholipid bilayer envelope that is associated with envelop (E) and matrix (M) proteins, and is covered with spike (S) and hemagglutinin-esterase (HE) proteins, the latter being found only in some coronaviruses [4,6].

The genome, 29.9 kb in size, shows the typical betacoronavirus organization consisting of 5′ and 3′ untranslated regions, a replicase complex (ORF1ab) that encodes proteins essential for viral replication/transcription such as RNA dependent RNA polymerase (RdRp), S, E, M, and N genes which are for their respective structural proteins, and several unidentified nonstructural open reading frames [1,6].

Transmission

Human coronaviruses are thought to be of zoonotic origin, and bats are most likely the natural hosts for all presently known CoVs. SARS-CoV-2 shows a high sequence identity to some bat coronaviruses such as RaTG13 previously detected in *Rhinolophus affinis*, a species widespread in China and Southeast Asia. However, bat habitats are generally far from human activity areas, and the virus was probably transmitted to humans by another animal host. Furthermore, bat SARS-like coronaviruses cannot directly infect humans unless they undergo mutation or recombination in animal hosts. For example, animal hosts of SARS-CoV and MERS-CoV are the civet and camel, respectively, before transmission to humans. Regarding the intermediate animal host of SARS-CoV-2, it has been reported that the sequence identity between pangolin origin CoVs and SARS-CoV-2 is very high, suggesting that SARS-CoV-2 may be of pangolin origin [4].

SARS-CoV-2 transmission is mainly person-to-person, through respiratory droplets or secretions which are distributed by coughing or sneezing from infected individuals [4,6,14,15]. Thus, COVID-19 patients are the main source of infection, and those severely ill are more contagious than mild ones. Incubation period is around 3 and 6 days [4,14]. In this period, even without signs or symptoms of respiratory disease, as well as those with asymptomatic infection, are potential sources of transmission [4]. The transmissibility of SARS-CoV-2 is not precisely known, but data show that basic reproduction number (R0) is expected to be around between 2 and 3 [6].

In general, respiratory viruses have the highest transmissibility when the patient is symptomatic, in alignment with the period of peak respiratory viral load. The exact point of transmission for SARS-CoV-2 remains unknown [6]. Moreover, the number of virus RNA copies in some asymptomatic cases can be comparable to those with manifest symptoms, and we can assume that transmission may occur with the illness onset and even with mild or no symptoms [6].

Procedures that induce production of aerosol, such as nebulizer treatment or intubation, are reported to increase the risk of transmission [6]. Transmission by direct and indirect contact may be possible, and recent studies showed that SARS-CoV-2 can remain viable on various surfaces such as stainless steel, plastic, glass, and cardboard at least several hours [6]. SARS-CoV-2 RNA has been detected in stool, whole blood and urine of COVID-19 patients, but whether transmission via such medium is possible is still not precise [4,6].

Pathogenesis

SARS-CoV-2 utilizes the angiotensin-converting enzyme 2 (ACE2) receptor to enter the host cell, similar to SARS-CoV, but with up to 10–20-fold higher affinity [4,15]. ACE2 receptor is a cell membrane protein present in lung, heart, kidney, and intestine tissue. It is highly expressed in the epithelium of the upper respiratory tract, alveolar type II pneumocytes and the enterocytes in the small intestine. SARS-CoV-2 is able to cause respiratory and gastrointestinal symptoms [15]. Naturally, all other organs of the body that express the ACE2 receptor could also be infected and extrapulmonary spread may be observed [4].

However, the presence of the ACE2 receptor is not the sole factor that determines infection of the tissue [15,16]. Cell entry of coronaviruses depends on binding of the viral spike (S) proteins to cellular receptors and subsequent protein priming and fusion [2,4]. The S protein is comprised of two subunits, S1 and S2. The S1 fraction possesses a receptor-binding domain (RBD) which interacts and binds to the ACE2 receptor, and then employs the host's serine protease (TMPRSS2) for S protein priming. The resulting S2 fraction is responsible for the fusion of the virus to the cell membrane and entry [2,4,6].

Once the virus enters the epithelial cells of the upper respiratory tract, it starts to replicate and as the disease progresses, transmits to the lower sections of the airway [4]. Alike SARS-CoV, lung cells once infected show decreased expression of ACE2 receptor [15]. The downregulation of ACE2 expression is associated with acute lung injury and is a pathological mechanism leading to acute lung injury and ARDS [17,18]. Pulmonary inflammation also increases capillary leakage that can cause ARDS [15,19].

In most cases, the immune system can eliminate the virus. However, deficient immunity or hyperinflammation can lead to severe respiratory failure. Thus, the immune response against SARS-CoV-2 and the severity of the inflammation are two major factors that define the outcome in patients with COVID-19 [15,20].

Immune response against COVID-19

SARS-CoV-2 is first recognized by the innate immune system through the identification of pathogen-associated molecular patterns and viral RNA by pathogen-related receptors of the macrophages and epithelial cells. Then, toll-like receptors 3 and 7, cytosolic RNA sensor, RIG-I, and MDA5 contribute to the identification of virus-infected cells and the activation of downstream inflammatory signaling pathways, such as the phosphorylation of nuclear factor-κB (NF-κB), phosphoinositide 3-kinase, mitogen-activated protein kinase, and IFN regulatory factor-3 (IRF-3) [15]. This cascade leads to the induction of innate immune response via production of type 1 interferon (IFN-1) which possesses antiviral function, as well as release of proinflammatory cytokines such as IL-1β, TNF-α, IL-6, and IL-18, and activation of natural killer cells, the latter which exerts a major histocompatibility complex (MHC)-independent immune response that can restrict the pathogenesis of the virus at the early stages of infection [15,21–23].

Through its downstream signaling pathways, IFN-1 activates IFN-induced transmembrane family proteins, which in turn inhibit the entrance of the virus to the host cell. This inhibits the replication of the virus and the infection of the further cells by SARS-CoV-2. It is important to note that although type I IFN-based immune response is initially critical to restrict viral infection, its excessive production leads to severe inflammation and ARDS [15,21].

Dendritic cells that are antigen-presenting cells (APCs) process and present the viral antigen to naïve T cells via the human leukocyte antigens (HLAs), leading to adaptative immune system activation. HLA molecules are very polymorphic with more than 10,000 variants reported so far, these molecules determine the capacity of each individual to recognize and present specific portions of any proteic infectious agent. Accordingly, individual HLA variation has been linked to the efficiency of the immune response to a virus across a population [24]. APCs also produce cytokines that direct the antiviral immune response of the T cells, differentiating them into the different types of effector cells. The cytokines produced by APCs and T cells drive the cellular immune response to SARS-CoV-2 [15].

COVID-19 patients often present with lymphopenia, which demonstrates activation and recruitment to the lung tissue to inhibit the infection by SARS-CoV-2. T cells are the directors of the cellular immunity. Serum levels of Th1-associated cytokines, including IFN-γ, TNF-α, and IL-2, are reported to be increased and activate cytotoxic T cells which destroy virus-infected cells through production of perforin and granzyme. Also, T helper cells may present the viral antigen to the B lymphocytes, which subsequently produce neutralizing antibodies against the spike (S) protein of the virus. The neutralizing antibodies inhibit the replication of the virus and produce humoral immunity, which is one of the main concepts for vaccine design against SARS-CoV-2 [15].

During the cytokine storm, monocytes and Th1 cells produce granulocyte-monocyte colony-stimulating factor (GM-CSF) and IL-6. GM-CSF and IL-6 have a major role in the progression of mild to severe respiratory inflammation and ARDS, and higher serum concentrations of IL-6 are associated with poor clinical outcomes [15,21].

The activation of B cells induces the differentiation of plasma cells and production of neutralizing antibodies that help the eradication of current infection, but also protect the host to further infections. The dynamics of the antibody response are complex, but in most of the patients, these antibodies are present three weeks after infection. First, B cells start their antibody response against the nucleocapsid (N) protein. Then, they produce anti-spike (S) antibodies. These antibodies can be found in patient serum 9 days (IgM) and 14 days (IgG) after infection. Appropriate serum antibody levels prevent the patient from being reinfected.

Immune dysfunction in COVID-19

Dysfunctional immune activity, either as immunodeficiency as well as hyperimmunity with severe or excessive inflammatory response, can result in severe disease and increased mortality. Immunocompromised patients, like those with old age with multiple comorbidities, cancer, immunosuppressive drug therapy, or other immunodeficiencies, are unable to inhibit the replication of the virus and thus susceptible to severe disease. Consequently, SARS-CoV-2 can infect the lower respiratory tract faster and cause pneumonia that can be followed by severe inflammation and ARDS, leading to higher mortality [15].

In addition, SARS-CoV-2 possesses the capability to evade identification by the immune system, which could be the underlying reason for its prolonged incubation period in comparison to other respiratory viruses. Type I IFN, an important antiviral component of the immune system, is decreased in COVID-19 patients as well as in those critically ill, through inhibition of IFN-signal transduction pathways such as IRF-3, resulting in the reduction of the power of the immune system. This mechanism is like the immune evasion acknowledged in SARS and MERS infections, which consists of disturbance in RNA-sensing and type I IFN producing pathways [15,21,23].

The effects of interferons in COVID-19 are time dependent. In the first stages, IFNs hinder disease progression by inhibiting the infection of new host cells. On the contrary, in later stages, IFNs might promote progression by inducing upregulation of ACE-2 in airway epithelial cells, increasing the chance infection of these cells [15].

T lymphocyte cells are a major cellular immunity component and play a key role in the adaptive immune response. T cell exhaustion is associated with severe infection and poor antiviral immune response, and in COVID-19 patients two exhaustion markers, named programmed death-1 (PD-1) and T-cell immunoglobulin and mucin-domain containing-3 (Tim-3), were reported to be highly expressed. This is one of many mechanisms that contribute to severity and understanding the process in order to inhibit or prevent it from happening could lead to improved clinical results. Another plausible immune evasion mechanism is the escaping from the MHC-dependent presentation of its antigens by APCs, thus avoiding the triggering of the adaptive immune response [15,23].

On the other hand, exaggerated immune response, severe inflammation, subsequent ARDS, and further fibrosis lead to lung damage and respiratory failure with bigger impact than the direct cytopathic effects of the virus. Damaged lung cells and macrophages produce chemotactic factors that recall innate immune cells and induce inflammatory response. Then, the inflammatory cells start an uncontrolled production of proinflammatory cytokines and chemokines, which is known as cytokine storm [23,25]. It results in extensive inflammation of the lungs, leakage of fluid to the alveoli and accumulation of inflammatory exudates, and the formation of hyaluronan, which in turn leads to hyaloid membrane formation, ARDS, and even multiple organ failure. CXCL-8, 9, 10, and CCL-2, 3, and 5 are the major produced chemokines in this process, and TGFβ, TNF-α, IFN-γ, IFN-α, IL-1β, 6, 12, 18, and 33, are cytokines that also contribute in its process [15,23,25].

Management of the cytokine storm can reduce lung tissue damage and lead to a better outcome in COVID-19 patient. Multiple strategies, such as using immunomodulatory drugs or targeting inflammatory cytokines can potentially reduce its severity and are discussed in further sections [15,25].

Clinical features

COVID-19 has been considered as a type of self-limiting infectious disease, and most cases with mild symptoms can recover in 1–2 weeks. SARS-CoV-2 infection can cause five different outcomes: asymptomatically infected persons, mild to medium disease which comprises the majority of cases, severe disease, critical disease, and death [4].

Asymptomatic infection

Asymptomatic cases can account to at least one third of SARS-CoV-2 infections [14,26,27]. They can transmit the virus for an extended period, perhaps longer than 14 days, and play a significant role in the COVID-19 pandemic. A small fraction of individuals with positive PCR test but without symptoms may turn out to be presymptomatic and will eventually develop symptoms [26,27]. Both instances are often associated with subclinical lung abnormalities on the CT, which shows that absence of symptoms might not necessarily imply an absence of harm [26].

Clinical manifestations

The incubation period for most cases of COVID-19 is approximately five days, and nearly all infected persons who have symptoms are expected to do so within 12 days of infection [6,14,28,29]. Average duration of hospitalization is around 12 days and severe illness occurs in 15.7% of the patients after admission [29,30]. Duration of viral shedding ranges between 8 and 37 days, the median being at 20 days [30].

The most frequent symptoms are fever, cough, sputum production, and dyspnea. Other less common symptoms include fatigue, myalgia, nausea or vomiting, and diarrhea [6,14,29–32] (Table 9.1). Fever may not always be present [6,29]. Older patients tend to have more systemic symptoms, extensive radiological ground-glass lung changes, lymphopenia, thrombocytopenia, and increased C-reactive protein and lactate dehydrogenase levels [14].

Risk factors for severe disease or death include individuals older in age or with coexisting illness (ages 60 or older), and medical comorbidity such as hypertension, diabetes mellitus, cardiovascular disease, chronic pulmonary disease, or malignancy [29–31]. Other risk factors associated with higher odds of in-hospital death are a higher Sequential Organ Failure Assessment (SOFA) score on admission, elevated D-dimer levels, as well as elevated levels of

TABLE 9.1 Common symptoms and laboratory findings on patients with COVID-19.

Common symptoms	Common laboratory findings	
Fever	Lymphocytes	Decreased
Cough	Neutrophils	Elevated
Sputum production	C-reactive protein	Elevated
Dyspnea	Serum ferritin	Elevated
Fatigue or myalgia	Lactate dehydrogenase	Elevated
Nausea or vomiting	D-dimer	Elevated
Diarrhea	Erythrocyte sedimentation rate	Elevated
Headache	Lnterleukin-6	Elevated
	Aspartate aminotransferase	Elevated
	Alanine aminotransferase	Elevated

blood IL-6, high-sensitivity cardiac troponin I, lactate dehydrogenase, and lymphopenia. These findings could help clinicians to identify at an early stage patients with worse prognosis [30].

Approximately 15% of individuals affected by COVID-19 develop severe disease, and 5% to 6% are critically ill with respiratory failure and/or multiple organ dysfunction or failure [31]. Disease progression is usually seen in the form of pneumonia. Further worsening, over the course of 7 to 10 days after initiating symptoms, may translate into ARDS and respiratory failure, thromboembolic complications such as deep vein thrombosis or pulmonary embolism, acute kidney injury and sepsis, either attributed to secondary infection or directly caused by SARS-CoV-2 infection [29,30]. In some cases, marked inflammatory or autoimmune responses such as Guillain-Barré syndrome may appear [33,34].

Patients may need invasive mechanical ventilation, renal replacement therapy, vasopressor infusion, or other critical care measures. They also have elevations in leukocytes, neutrophils, and creatinine kinase, and in computed tomography extended ground-glass opacities, interstitial infiltration, and/or multiple patchy consolidations in both lung fields [31].

Complications

Several complications of COVID-19 have been described. ARDS is a major complication that arises in a median of eight days after symptom onset [32]. ARDS is a life-threatening lung condition that prevents enough oxygen from getting to the lungs and into the circulation, accounting for mortality of most respiratory disorders and acute lung injury [4].

Inflammatory complications may arise during SARS-CoV-2 infection. Clinical findings showed exuberant inflammatory responses, further resulting in uncontrolled pulmonary inflammation, likely a leading cause of case fatality. Rapid viral replication and cellular damage, virus-induced ACE2 downregulation and shedding, and antibody-dependent enhancement are responsible for aggressive inflammation caused by SARS-CoV-2. The initial onset of rapid viral replication may cause massive epithelial and endothelial cell death and vascular leakage, triggering the production of proinflammatory cytokines and chemokines. Loss of pulmonary ACE2 function has been proposed to be related to acute lung injury because ACE2 downregulation and shedding can lead to dysfunction of the renin-angiotensin system, and further enhance inflammation and cause vascular permeability [4].

Thromboembolic disease is another common complication among COVID-19 patients. In patients receiving at least standard doses of thromboprophylaxis, the incidence of the composite events venous and arterial thromboembolism, including deep vein thrombosis and pulmonary embolism, is around 31% [35]; most patients have elevated D-dimer and fibrinogen levels [36]. It is more frequent in severely ill patients and particularly in those in the intensive care unit (ICU). Pulmonary embolism is the most frequent thrombotic complication [35,36], and age and coagulopathy are independent predictors of thrombotic complications [35]. Unless contraindicated, pharmacological thrombosis prophylaxis should be started in all hospitalized patients, and physicians should be vigilant for signs of thrombotic complications and order appropriate diagnostic tests at a low threshold in order to promptly switch to high-prophylactic or therapeutic doses [35,36].

Laboratory findings

The most frequent laboratory abnormalities found on patients with COVID-19 are lymphocytopenia, neutrophilia, and thrombocytopenia [10,15,37–39]. The pulmonary infiltration of the lymphocytes, apoptosis/pyroptosis of the lymphocytes, lateral margination, and infection of the lymphocytes by SARS-CoV-2 are the most common reasons leading to lymphopenia [7,15] and has been proposed as a prognostic marker for COVID-19 [39]. Other findings include elevated inflammatory markers, like C-reactive protein ($\geq$10 mg/L), lactate dehydrogenase ($\geq$250 U/L), serum ferritin (>300 μg/L), and D-dimer ($\geq$0.5 mg/L); liver and kidney dysfunction; and coagulopathies (Table 9.1), with patients with severe disease having more prominent laboratory abnormalities [14,29,30,38].

Imaging findings

The most frequent radiographic and CT patterns are ground-glass opacities (GGOs) and local or bilateral patchy shadowing. Interstitial abnormalities may also be present. In some cases, no abnormal images may be found; paired with the fact that not all patients develop fever, diagnosis in mild cases may be complicated [14,29]. Lung abnormalities are predominantly found in peripheral middle and lower regions, and often show a multiple or bilateral onset and an asynchronous process [40].

The imaging findings of COVID-19 can be classified broadly in three stages: an early rapid progressive stage ($\leq$7 days), an advanced stage (8–14 days), and an absorption stage (>14 days) [40]. In the early rapid progressive stage, GGOs plus a reticular pattern, GGO plus consolidation, and GGO alone were all common signs. In the advanced stage, GGO plus reticular pattern or consolidation were the dominant findings. Finally, in the absorptive stage, repairing signs like subpleural lines, bronchus distortion, and fibrotic strips can be found [40] (Fig. 9.1).

Pathology findings

Histological examination of lung tissue shows involvement of alveoli and bronchioles with diffuse alveolar damage as the main finding, along with

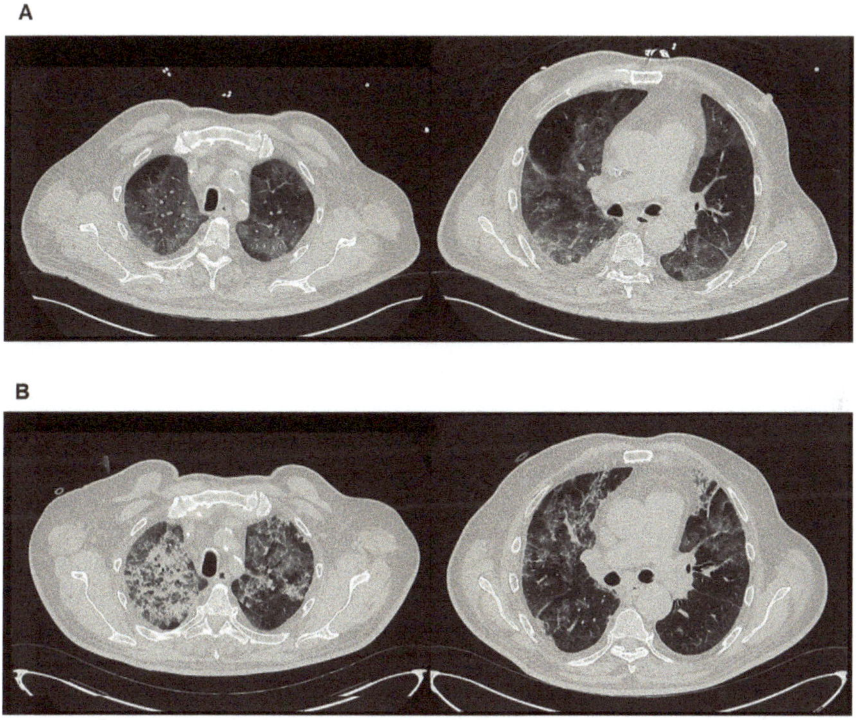

FIGURE 9.1 **Chest CT images from a patient with COVID-19.** (A) Early progressive stage with bilateral ground-glass. (B) Advanced stage with ground-glass opacities and consolidation.

cellular fibromyxoid exudates filling its lumina, consisting in protein-rich edema fluid, fibrin, cellular debris, macrophages, neutrophils, and lymphocytes. Epithelial necrosis with desquamation of pneumocytes, hyaline membrane formation, and pulmonary edema can be observed and is suggestive of ARDS [4,19,31,41].

Multinucleated syncytial cells with atypical enlarged pneumocytes characterized by large nuclei, amphophilic granular cytoplasm, and prominent nucleoli can be identified in the intra-alveolar spaces, indicating viral cytopathic-like changes. In addition, interstitial involvement with mononuclear inflammatory infiltrates, dominated by lymphocytes, can be found in the lungs [4,31,41].

In areas with more advanced lesions, organizing-stage diffuse alveolar damage with pronounced fibroblastic proliferation, partial fibrosis, and pneumocyte hyperplasia result in interstitial thickening. Alveoli are collapsed and its walls are thickened and lined by cuboidal epithelial cells characteristic of type II pneumocyte hyperplasia. These pulmonary pathological findings resemble those seen in SARS and MERS [4,19,31,41].

Diagnosis

Diagnostic approach

COVID-19 is a viral respiratory disease and as such, it should be suspected in all febrile and/or respiratory symptomatic patients, especially if the person has had close contact (within six feet during more than a few minutes while not wearing a face mask or other personal protective equipment) or has recently been to a high SARS-CoV-2 infection prevalence location. There are no specific clinical features, and in the pandemic context, clinicians should have a low threshold for suspicion. In the absence of fever or pulmonary complications, COVID-19 should also be considered if the patient has disease-related symptoms like, for example, diarrhea, taste or olfactory loss, and thromboembolic events.

Ideally, all suspected cases should be tested as soon as possible after symptom onset. This is in order to control transmission, to monitor SARS-CoV-2 transmission rates and severity, to mitigate the impact of COVID-19 in healthcare and social care settings, to detect clusters or outbreaks in specific settings, and to maintain COVID-19 elimination status once achieved. If this is not possible, testing strategies or priorities should be established. When testing is limited or unavailable, patients with history of exposure, compatible clinical course, and no other evident explanation of symptoms, may be presumptively diagnosed as probable COVID-19. If hospitalization is not necessary, self-isolation at home and monitoring is an option.

Soon after initial outbreak, diagnosis based on the detection of the viral sequence by nucleic acid amplification testing (NAAT) via reverse-transcription polymerase chain reaction (RT-PCR) became available and is the main method of diagnosis [4,13]. It is used for qualitative and quantitative SARS-CoV-2 detection in samples collected from the upper respiratory tract, including nasal or nasopharyngeal swabs [42]. Another frequently used test is the detection of SARS-CoV-2 antigens. A positive RT-PCR for SARS-CoV-2 generally confirms the diagnosis of COVID-19. However, patients can have detectable SARS-CoV-2 RNA for weeks after the onset of symptoms, and furthermore this test does not determine time of infection [43]. Also, RNA detection does not necessarily indicate infectiousness, which is determined by viral load. For example, patients who are beyond day 10 of symptoms and have less than 100,000 viral RNA copies per ml of sputum are considered to have little residual risk of infectivity [44]. A negative RT-PCR for SARS-CoV-2 generally excludes the diagnosis of COVID-19. However, false-negative results may happen and if clinical suspicion is high, the test should be repeated. Many biotechnology companies have successfully developed nasopharyngeal swabs and nucleic acid detection kits [4]. It has been shown that patients with SARS-CoV-2 infection possess acute serological responses. Combined with immunochromatography, colloidal gold, and other technologies, relevant detection reagents have been developed rapidly [4].

Compatible laboratory or imaging findings can further support the diagnosis. With the rapid spread of COVID-19, CT is an especially important tool for establishing diagnosis and severity [40]. The majority of COVID-19 cases have similar features on CT images including bilateral distribution of patchy shadows and GGOs predominantly in middle and lower lung fields, as mentioned previously [4,31]. To note, there is a small proportion of COVID-19 patients with negative RT-PCR tests and lung abnormalities on CT imaging, suggesting that CT could detect lesions earlier in the disease [40]. However, clinical picture and thoracic imaging alone are not specific enough to make a definite diagnosis [42].

In some patients, a second-line investigation like bronchoalveolar lavage (BAL) is often required to diagnose or exclude SARS-CoV-2 infection [42]. In a study, BAL was performed on patients after at least one negative or indeterminate upper respiratory swab due to clinical or radiological suspicion for COVID-19 [42]. High concordance between swabs and BAL were observed, the latter being the gold standard to detect pathogens in the presence of pulmonary infiltrates [42]. It seems that BAL has a limited role in the diagnosis of COVID-19 if thoracic imaging and upper respiratory tract swabs are concordantly negative, but it might be necessary in patients with a negative swab to establish a different diagnosis [42].

Management

General management

Management of patients with COVID-19 is based mainly on symptomatic control and supportive therapy, including supplemental oxygen, mechanical ventilator support when needed, antibiotics for prevention of secondary bacterial infection, and body fluid management. In most cases, outpatient management is appropriate, since approximately 80% of patients develop a mild disease which does not warrant medical intervention or hospitalization [45].

Bacterial superinfection and pneumonia are not a prominent feature and empiric therapy is not routinely administered, but its clinical features may overlap with those of COVID-19, and treatment is reasonable when the diagnosis is uncertain or there is clinical suspicion. Because of higher risk of thromboembolic complications, all hospitalized patients should receive pharmacological thrombosis prophylaxis, unless contraindicated [35,36,46].

Based on the pathogenesis of COVID-19, many drugs—new and existing, those that target the virus itself or modulate the immune response—are being researched and clinical trials are being launched.

Dexamethasone and other glucocorticoids

In patients hospitalized with COVID-19, the use of dexamethasone, oral or intravenous, at a dose of 6 mg daily for up to 10 days or until discharge, has shown to lower 28-day mortality in patients who were receiving respiratory support [47]. When compared to usual care alone, there was an absolute reduction in mortality of 2.8% (22.9% vs. 25.7%; age-adjusted rate ratio, 0.83; 95% CI, 0.75 to 0.93) [47]. Incidence of death was lower among patients receiving invasive mechanical ventilation (29.3% vs. 41.4%; rate ratio, 0.64; 95% CI, 0.51 to 0.81) and among those receiving oxygen without invasive mechanical ventilation (23.3% vs. 26.2%; rate ratio, 0.82; 95% CI, 0.72 to 0.94) [47].

The use of dexamethasone in patients who are receiving oxygen was also associated with a lower risk of invasive mechanical ventilation or, for those already receiving invasive mechanical ventilation, a greater chance of successful cessation [47]. The benefit was also clear in patients who were being treated more than seven days after symptom onset, when inflammatory lung damage is more likely [47]. However, there was no found benefit among patients who did not require oxygen, and results were consistent with possible harm in this subgroup [47].

A prospective meta-analysis of clinical trials of critically ill patients with COVID-19 showed that administration of systemic corticosteroids was associated with lower 28-day all-cause mortality, when compared with usual care or placebo [48]. Other treatment strategies analyzed were dexamethasone intravenous 20 mg daily for five days followed up by 10 mg daily for five days; hydrocortisone intravenous 200 mg daily for seven days, continuous or in bolus dosing every 6 h; and methylprednisolone intravenous 40 mg every 12 h for seven days [48]. Therefore, when dexamethasone is not available, it is reasonable to use other glucocorticoids at equivalent doses.

The ORs for the association between corticosteroids and mortality were similar and the optimal dose and duration of treatment could not be assessed [48]. There was no suggestion of an increased risk of serious adverse events [48]. However, patients receiving glucocorticoids should be monitored due to risk of hyperglycemia and increased risk of infections, and prophylaxis treatment for *Strongyloides* is reasonable for patients from endemic areas. In the absence of compelling contraindications, a corticosteroid regimen should be a component of standard care for critically ill patients with COVID-19 [48].

Finally, inhaled corticosteroids [49] has been tested in a recent trial in patients with mild COVID-19 symptoms, showing that early administration of inhaled budesonide reduced the likelihood of needing urgent medical care and reduced time to recovery after early COVID-19. Further studies are necessary to confirm the routine use of inhaled corticosteroids in COVID-19.

Remdesivir

Remdesivir, recently recognized as a promising antiviral drug against a wide array of RNA viruses in-vitro, is an adenosine analog which incorporates into nascent viral RNA chains resulting in premature termination [50]. It is approved by the Food and Drug Administration (FDA) for the treatment of COVID-19 in hospitalized adult and pediatric patients and can be administered in a five-day course (200 mg day one, 100 mg daily days 2−5) or extended to a 10-day course (100 mg daily days 6−10) if there is no clinical improvement. Remdesivir is not recommended in patients with renal impairment with an estimated glomerular filtration rate (eGFR) < 30 mL/min per 1.73 m2 unless the potential benefit outweighs the potential risk [51].

In patients with nonsevere COVID-19 disease, hospitalized with peripheral capillary oxygen saturation (SpO_2) >94% on room air, remdesivir appeared to yield better clinical status and higher discharge rates, although not statistically significant. Treatment with remdesivir also failed to show or to exclude a statistically significant reduction in mortality or time to recovery when compared with no remdesivir [52−54].

In hospitalized patients with $SpO_2 \leq 94\%$ on room air, including patients on supplemental oxygen, on mechanical ventilation, and extracorporeal membrane oxygenation (ECMO), initial data showed treatment with remdesivir trended toward greater clinical improvement at 28 days, a shorter median time to recovery and decreased need for mechanical ventilation [52,53,55,56]. According to the WHO-sponsored SOLIDARITY trial, there was no difference in overall 28-day mortality between patients randomly assigned to open-label remdesivir and those assigned to standard care [52]. In another study, ACTT-1, remdesivir resulted in a faster time to recovery, defined as discharge from the hospital or continued hospitalization without need for supplemental oxygen or ongoing medical care. Further analysis showed that recovery was only statistically significant among patients who were on low-flow oxygen at baseline [53]. A double-blind RCT in China involving patients with severe COVID-19, stopped early for poor enrollment, stated that time to clinical improvement was not statistically different with remdesivir compared with placebo for 10 days [55].

In a meta-analysis of four trials that included the trials mentioned above, remdesivir did not reduce mortality (OR 0.9, 95% CI 0.7−1.12) or need for mechanical ventilation (OR 0.90, 95% CI 0.76−1.03) compared with standard of care or placebo [57,58]. Among those who were not on mechanical ventilation at baseline, there appeared to be a trend toward lower mortality with remdesivir but without statistical significance. In this population, remdesivir is suggested over no antiviral treatment, prioritizing those requiring low-flow supplemental oxygen [51,59].

Baricitinib and JAK inhibitors

Janus kinase (JAK) is a family of intracellular tyrosine kinases that mediates intracellular transcription factors. It is involved in the phosphorylation of the signal transducer and activator of transcription (STAT) protein family in the JAK-STAT pathway, which results in the production of several proinflammatory cytokines, including IL-6. Inhibition of JAK could reduce the production of proinflammatory cytokines and restrict cytokine storm in severe COVID-19 patients [15,60].

Baricitinib is a selective inhibitor of JAK 1 and 2 and blocks the intracellular signaling pathway of inflammatory cytokines, including interleukin-2, interleukin-6, interleukin-10, interferon-γ, and granulocyte-macrophage colony-stimulating factor. In addition, it limits SARS-CoV-2 entry and infectivity by inhibiting adaptor-associated protein kinase 1 receptor [61,62] and improves lymphocyte counts in patients with COVID-19 [62].

The US FDA has issued an emergency use authorization (EUA) to permit the emergency use of baricitinib, in combination with remdesivir, for treatment of suspected or laboratory confirmed COVID-19 in hospitalized adults and pediatric patients two years of age or older requiring supplemental oxygen, invasive mechanical ventilation, or ECMO. It is administered as a 4 mg daily dose, either orally or through a nasogastric tube, for 14 days or until hospital discharge. Patients with an eGFR of less than 60 mL per minute are recommended a dose of 2 mg once daily [62,63].

Baricitinib plus remdesivir was superior to remdesivir alone for the treatment of hospitalized patients with COVID-19, with a shorter time to recovery and a greater improvement in clinical status. However, it did not detect a difference in mortality. Because of this reason, added to the fact that dexamethasone showed a significant benefit in survival, and because baricitinib and dexamethasone have not been compared directly, it is not the first drug to be considered. The safety and efficacy of using both baricitinib and a glucocorticoid are uncertain, and there is no evidence supporting the use of baricitinib alone [62].

Tocilizumab and IL-6 pathway inhibitors

In response to cytokines, inflammatory cells are recruited, and an immune response is exerted. In some cases, these inflammatory immune cells lead to an uncontrolled production and cytokine storm, of which IL-6 is one of the most important contributors [64].

Tocilizumab is a humanized monoclonal antibody against the interleukin-6 receptor (IL-6R) that can inhibit the inflammatory pathway induced by IL-6. It was granted an EUA for the treatment of COVID-19 in the United States in June 2021 [15,65,66] and can be administered in hospitalized adults and pediatric patients (two years of age and older) who are receiving systemic corticosteroids and require supplemental oxygen, noninvasive or invasive mechanical ventilation, or ECMO. It is given 8 mg/kg up to 800 mg as a single dose and is recommended in individuals with severe or rapidly progressing disease, those who require high-flow oxygen or greater respiratory support and have either been admitted to the ICU within the prior 24 h or have significantly increased inflammatory markers [59,67].

Overall, it is an effective treatment for hospitalized COVID-19 patients who have hypoxia and evidence of inflammation (CRP $\geq$75 mg/L), and studies have shown that treatment reduces mortality at day 28, increases the chances of successful hospital discharge, and reduces the chances of requiring invasive mechanical ventilation, compared to standard care alone or placebo [67–69]. These benefits are consistent across all patient groups, including those receiving invasive mechanical ventilation, noninvasive respiratory support, or no respiratory support other than simple oxygen [67].

Although tocilizumab inhibits the destructive effects of the SARS-CoV-2 on lung tissue, like other immunosuppressive drugs, uncontrolled or unnecessary application could be associated with adverse effects, including an increase in hepatic enzymes and opportunistic infections [15,25].

Convalescent plasma and antibody-based therapies

Antibody-based treatments are a form of passive immunotherapy that can improve the immune response and inhibit SARS-CoV-2 infection and progression. This can be achieved by the infusion of the SARS-CoV-2 convalescent plasma from recovered patients, as demonstrated previously for the treatment of multiple diseases, including SARS [70] and MERS [71].

Convalescent plasma can restrict viral infection and modulate the immune response. It contains neutralizing IgM and IgG antibodies, which inhibit viral entry to the host cell activating the complement system, inducing phagocytosis of the virus, and activating antibody-dependent cellular toxicity [72]. Convalescent plasma also contains immune-modulatory cytokines and autoantibodies that control the hyperinflammatory process and the cytokine storm [15,73].

In the United States, EUA has been granted for high-titer convalescent plasma among hospitalized patients with COVID-19 who are early in the course of disease or have impaired humoral immunity [74].

Use of convalescent plasma in patients with COVID-19 has also been reported in numerous clinical trials [75–77], and data suggest that plasma with higher antibody titers administered earlier in the disease are associated with better outcomes, with lower 30-day mortality rates [76]. However, many studies, including a meta-analysis of four published RCTs, have not demonstrated a clear clinical benefit of convalescent plasma, and neither a difference in mortality, duration of hospitalization or use of mechanical ventilation were detected with convalescent plasma compared with placebo or standard of care [78,79].

It is uncertain whether convalescent plasma is beneficial in COVID-19, but it is safe and well tolerated and an early administration within the clinical course of the disease can potentially improve patient outcomes with relatively low risk [79,80]. Low antibody levels in some of the recovered patients, limited access to large doses of convalescent plasma, and the possibility of adverse reactions are the main limitations and challenges of convalescent plasma therapy [15].

Conclusion

COVID-19 is caused by SARS-CoV-2 infection and mainly affects the lung. Depending on the host's immune and inflammatory response, it may develop a disease that can range from asymptomatic or mild to severe and life-threatening. A competent immune system is crucial in eliminating the virus and controlling the disease, and either deficient immunity or hyper-inflammation can lead to uncontrolled disease and progression, respiratory failure, and death. Since being declared a pandemic by the WHO on March 2020, a global effort is being made to research and develop potential treatment. By understanding the virus and its pathogenesis, including its structure, mechanism of entry, host's response, and immune and inflammatory mediators involved, targeted therapies can be designed and developed.

Take-home messages

SARS-CoV-2 emerged in late December 2019 and since then it has spread across the globe, resulting in an ongoing pandemic. The virus continues to circulate and evolve, with variants of interests and concern emerging periodically.

Entry to the host cell involves binding between the host's ACE2 receptor and the viral S protein. The S1 fraction possesses a RBD and the S2 fraction mediates fusion and entry.

The cytotoxic effects of the virus stimulate the release of proinflammatory cytokines in an attempt to control the infection. Deficient immunity or hyperinflammation can lead to severe and uncontrolled disease.

Several therapeutic interventions have been proposed and numerous clinical trials are being conducted. Remdesivir incorporates into nascent viral RNA and mediates premature termination. Dexamethasone, baricitinib, and tocilizumab aim to control the host's excessive inflammatory response by acting on different pathways. Finally, convalescent plasma, with its neutralizing IgM and IgG antibodies, restricts viral infection and modulates immune response.

References

[1] Zhu N, Zhang D, Wang W, et al. A novel coronavirus from patients with pneumonia in China, 2019. N Engl J Med 2020;382(8):727–33. https://doi.org/10.1056/nejmoa2001017.

[2] Hoffmann M, Kleine-Weber H, Schroeder S, et al. SARS-CoV-2 cell entry depends on ACE2 and TMPRSS2 and is blocked by a clinically proven protease inhibitor. Cell 2020;181(2):271–280.e8. https://doi.org/10.1016/j.cell.2020.02.052.

[3] V'kovski P, Kratzel A, Steiner S, Stalder H, Thiel V. Coronavirus biology and replication: implications for SARS-CoV-2. Nat Rev Microbiol 2021;19(3):155–70. https://doi.org/10.1038/s41579-020-00468-6.

[4] Jin Y, Yang H, Ji W, et al. Virology, epidemiology, pathogenesis, and control of COVID-19. Viruses 2020;12(4):372. https://doi.org/10.3390/v12040372.

[5] Hu B, Guo H, Zhou P, Shi ZL. Characteristics of SARS-CoV-2 and COVID-19. Nat Rev Microbiol 2021;19(3):141–54. https://doi.org/10.1038/s41579-020-00459-7.

[6] Park SE. Epidemiology, virology, and clinical features of severe acute respiratory syndrome-coronavirus-2 (SARS-COV-2; Coronavirus Disease-19). Kor J Pediatr 2020;63(4):119–24. https://doi.org/10.3345/cep.2020.00493.

[7] Zirui Tay M, Meng Poh C, Rénia L, MacAry PA, Ng LFP. The trinity of COVID-19: immunity, inflammation and intervention. Nat Rev Immunol 2019. https://doi.org/10.1038/s41577-020-0311-8.

[8] Cao W, Li T. COVID-19: towards understanding of pathogenesis. Cell Res 2020;(April):1–3. https://doi.org/10.1038/s41422-020-0327-4.

[9] WHO statement on novel coronavirus in Thailand. 2020. https://www.who.int/news/item/13-01-2020-who-statement-on-novel-coronavirus-in-thailand. [Accessed 24 July 2021].

[10] Goyal P, Choi JJ, Pinheiro LC, et al. Clinical characteristics of Covid-19 in New York city. N Engl J Med 2020;382(24):2372–4. https://doi.org/10.1056/NEJMC2010419.

[11] Coronavirus disease (COVID-19) situation reports. https://www.who.int/emergencies/diseases/novel-coronavirus-2019/situation-reports. [Accessed 24 July 2021].

[12] COVID-19 situation update worldwide, as of week 28. July 22, 2021. https://www.ecdc.europa.eu/en/geographical-distribution-2019-ncov-cases. [Accessed 24 July 2021].

[13] Baay M, Lina B, Fontanet A, et al. SARS-CoV-2: virology, epidemiology, immunology and vaccine development. Biologicals 2020;66:35–40. https://doi.org/10.1016/j.biologicals.2020.06.005.

[14] Chan JFW, Yuan S, Kok KH, et al. A familial cluster of pneumonia associated with the 2019 novel coronavirus indicating person-to-person transmission: a study of a family cluster. Lancet 2020;395(10223):514–23. https://doi.org/10.1016/S0140-6736(20)30154-9.

[15] Esmaeilzadeh A, Elahi R. Immunobiology and immunotherapy of COVID-19: a clinically updated overview. J Cell Physiol 2021;236(4):2519–43. https://doi.org/10.1002/jcp.30076.

[16] Li W, Moore MJ, Vasllieva N, et al. Angiotensin-converting enzyme 2 is a functional receptor for the SARS coronavirus. Nature 2003;426(6965):450–4. https://doi.org/10.1038/nature02145.

[17] Imai Y, Kuba K, Rao S, et al. Angiotensin-converting enzyme 2 protects from severe acute lung failure. Nature 2005;436(7047):112. https://doi.org/10.1038/NATURE03712.

[18] Kuba K, Imai Y, Penninger JM. Angiotensin-converting enzyme 2 in lung diseases. Curr Opin Pharmacol 2006;6(3):271–6. https://doi.org/10.1016/J.COPH.2006.03.001.

[19] Rockx B, Kuiken T, Herfst S, et al. Comparative pathogenesis of COVID-19, MERS, and SARS in a nonhuman primate model. Science 2020;368.

[20] Zhang F, Gan R, Zhen Z, et al. Adaptive immune responses to SARS-CoV-2 infection in severe versus mild individuals. Signal Transduction Targeted Ther 2020;5(1):1−11. https://doi.org/10.1038/s41392-020-00263-y.
[21] Li X, Geng M, Peng Y, Meng L, Lu S. Molecular immune pathogenesis and diagnosis of COVID-19. J Pharm Anal 2020;10(2):102−8. https://doi.org/10.1016/J.JPHA.2020.03.001.
[22] Florindo HF, Kleiner R, Vaskovich-Koubi D, et al. Immune-mediated approaches against COVID-19. Nat Nanotechnol 2020;15(8):630−45. https://doi.org/10.1038/s41565-020-0732-3.
[23] Vabret N, Britton GJ, Gruber C, et al. Immunology of COVID-19: current state of the science. Immunity 2020;52(6):910−41. https://doi.org/10.1016/J.IMMUNI.2020.05.002.
[24] Iturrieta-Zuazo I, Rita CG, García-Soidán A, et al. Possible role of HLA class-I genotype in SARS-CoV-2 infection and progression: a pilot study in a cohort of Covid-19 Spanish patients. Clin Immunol 2020:219. https://doi.org/10.1016/J.CLIM.2020.108572.
[25] Mehta P, Mcauley DF, Brown M, et al. Correspondence COVID-19: consider cytokine storm syndromes and. Lancet 2020;6736(20):19−20. https://doi.org/10.1016/S0140-6736(20)30628-0.
[26] Oran DP, Topol EJ. Prevalence of asymptomatic SARS-CoV-2 infection: a narrative review. Ann Intern Med 2020;173(5):362−7. https://doi.org/10.7326/M20-3012.
[27] Oran DP, Topol EJ. The proportion of SARS-CoV-2 infections that are asymptomatic A systematic review background: asymptomatic infection seems to be a nota. Ann Intern Med 2021. https://doi.org/10.7326/M20-6976.
[28] Lauer SA, Grantz KH, Bi Q, et al. The incubation period of coronavirus disease 2019 (COVID-19) from publicly reported confirmed cases: estimation and application. Ann Intern Med 2020. https://doi.org/10.7326/M20-0504.
[29] Guan W, Ni Z, Hu Y, et al. Clinical characteristics of coronavirus disease 2019 in China. N Engl J Med 2020;382(18):1708−20. https://doi.org/10.1056/nejmoa2002032.
[30] Zhou F, Yu T, Du R, et al. Clinical course and risk factors for mortality of adult inpatients with COVID-19 in Wuhan, China: a retrospective cohort study. Lancet 2020;395(10229):1054−62. https://doi.org/10.1016/S0140-6736(20)30566-3.
[31] Schaller T, Hirschbühl K, Burkhardt K, et al. Postmortem examination of patients with COVID-19. J Am Med Assoc 2020;323(24):2518−20. https://doi.org/10.1001/jama.2020.8907.
[32] Wang D, Hu B, Hu C, et al. Clinical characteristics of 138 hospitalized patients with 2019 novel coronavirus-infected pneumonia in Wuhan, China. J Am Med Assoc 2020;323(11):1061−9. https://doi.org/10.1001/jama.2020.1585.
[33] Leisman DE, Ronner L, Pinotti R, et al. Cytokine elevation in severe and critical COVID-19: a rapid systematic review, meta-analysis, and comparison with other inflammatory syndromes. Lancet Respir Med 2020;8(12):1233−44. https://doi.org/10.1016/S2213-2600(20)30404-5.
[34] Toscano G, Palmerini F, Ravaglia S, et al. Guillain−barré syndrome associated with SARS-CoV-2. N Engl J Med 2020;382(26):2574−6. https://doi.org/10.1056/nejmc2009191.
[35] Klok FA, Kruip MJHA, van der Meer NJM, et al. Incidence of thrombotic complications in critically ill ICU patients with COVID-19. Thromb Res 2020;191:145−7. https://doi.org/10.1016/j.thromres.2020.04.013.
[36] Helms J, Tacquard C, Severac F, et al. High risk of thrombosis in patients with severe SARS-CoV-2 infection: a multicenter prospective cohort study. Intensive Care Med 2020;46(6):1089−98. https://doi.org/10.1007/s00134-020-06062-x.

[37] Huang C, Wang Y, Li X, et al. Clinical features of patients infected with 2019 novel coronavirus in Wuhan, China. Lancet 2020;395(10223):497–506. https://doi.org/10.1016/S0140-6736(20)30183-5.

[38] Rokni M, Ahmadikia K, Asghari S, Mashaei S, Hassanali F. Comparison of clinical, para-clinical and laboratory findings in survived and deceased patients with COVID-19: diagnostic role of inflammatory indications in determining the severity of illness. BMC Infect Dis 2020;20(1). https://doi.org/10.1186/S12879-020-05540-3.

[39] GM B, A G, L K, et al. Predictors of COVID-19 severity: a literature review. Rev Med Virol 2021;31(1):1–10. https://doi.org/10.1002/RMV.2146.

[40] Zhou S, Zhu T, Wang Y, Xia L. Imaging features and evolution on CT in 100 COVID-19 pneumonia patients in Wuhan, China. Eur Radiol 2020. https://doi.org/10.1007/s00330-020-06879-6.

[41] Xu Z, Shi L, Wang Y, et al. Pathological findings of COVID-19 associated with acute respiratory distress syndrome. Lancet Respir Med 2020. https://doi.org/10.1016/S2213-2600(20)30076-X.

[42] Geri P, Salton F, Zuccatosta L, et al. Limited role for bronchoalveolar lavage to exclude COVID-19 after negative upper respiratory tract swabs: a multicentre study. Eur Respir J 2020;56(4). https://doi.org/10.1183/13993003.01733-2020.

[43] He X, Lau EHY, Wu P, et al. Temporal dynamics in viral shedding and transmissibility of COVID-19. Nat Med 2020;26(5):672–5. https://doi.org/10.1038/s41591-020-0869-5.

[44] Wölfel R, Corman VM, Guggemos W, et al. Virological assessment of hospitalized patients with COVID-2019. Nature 2020;581(7809):465–9. https://doi.org/10.1038/s41586-020-2196-x.

[45] Xu K, Cai H, Shen Y, et al. Management of corona virus disease-19 (COVID-19): the Zhejiang experience. Zhejiang da Xue Xue Bao Yi Xue Ban 2020;49(1):147–57. https://doi.org/10.3785/J.ISSN.1008-9292.2020.02.02.

[46] Thachil J, Tang N, Gando S, et al. ISTH interim guidance on recognition and management of coagulopathy in COVID-19. J Thromb Haemostasis 2020;18(5):1023–6. https://doi.org/10.1111/JTH.14810.

[47] Recovery Collaborative Group, Horby P, Lim WS, et al. Dexamethasone in hospitalized patients with Covid-19. N Engl J Med 2021;384(8):693–704. https://doi.org/10.1056/nejmoa2021436.

[48] WHO Rapid Evidence Appraisal for COVID-19 Therapies (REACT) Working Group, Sterne JAC, Murthy S, et al. Association between administration of systemic corticosteroids and mortality among critically ill patients with COVID-19: a meta-analysis. J Am Med Assoc 2020:1–12. https://doi.org/10.1001/jama.2020.17023.

[49] Ramakrishnan S, Nicolau D v, Langford B, et al. Inhaled budesonide in the treatment of early COVID-19 (STOIC): a phase 2, open-label, randomised controlled trial. Lancet Respir Med 2021. https://doi.org/10.1016/S2213-2600(21)00160-0.

[50] Wang M, Cao R, Zhang L, et al. Remdesivir and chloroquine effectively inhibit the recently emerged novel coronavirus (2019-nCoV) in vitro. Cell Res 2020. https://doi.org/10.1038/s41422-020-0282-0.

[51] Bhimraj A, Morgan RL, Hirsch Shumaker A, et al. Infectious diseases Society of America Guidelines on the treatment and management of patients with COVID-19. Clin Infect Dis 2020. https://doi.org/10.1093/cid/ciaa478.

[52] WHO Solidarity Trial Consortium, Pan H, Peto R, et al. Repurposed antiviral drugs for Covid-19 — interim WHO solidarity trial results. N Engl J Med 2021;384(6):497–511. https://doi.org/10.1056/nejmoa2023184.

[53] Beigel JH, Tomashek KM, Dodd LE, et al. Remdesivir for the treatment of Covid-19 — final report. N Engl J Med 2020;383(19):1813–26. https://doi.org/10.1056/nejmoa2007764.
[54] Spinner CD, Gottlieb RL, Criner GJ, et al. Effect of remdesivir vs standard care on clinical status at 11 Days in patients with moderate COVID-19: a randomized clinical trial. J Am Med Assoc 2020;324(11):1048–57. https://doi.org/10.1001/jama.2020.16349.
[55] Wang Y, Zhang D, Du G, et al. Remdesivir in adults with severe COVID-19: a randomised, double-blind, placebo-controlled, multicentre trial. Lancet 2020;395(10236):1569–78. https://doi.org/10.1016/S0140-6736(20)31022-9.
[56] Goldman JD, Lye DCB, Hui DS, et al. Remdesivir for 5 or 10 Days in patients with severe Covid-19. N Engl J Med 2020;383(19):1827–37. https://doi.org/10.1056/nejmoa2015301.
[57] Wilt TJ, Kaka AS, MacDonald R, Greer N, Obley A, Duan-Porter W. Remdesivir for adults with COVID-19: a living systematic review for American College of physicians practice points. Ann Intern Med 2021;174(2):209–20. https://doi.org/10.7326/M20-5752.
[58] Kaka AS, MacDonald R, Greer N, et al. Major update: remdesivir for adults with COVID-19 : a living systematic review and meta-analysis for the American College of physicians practice points. Ann Intern Med 2021;174(5):663–72. https://doi.org/10.7326/M20-8148.
[59] COVID-19 Treatment Guidelines Panel. Coronavirus Disease 2019 (COVID-19) Treatment Guidelines. National Institutes of Health; 2021. https://www.covid19treatmentguidelines.nih.gov/. [Accessed 24 July 2021].
[60] Favalli EG, Biggioggero M, Maioli G, Caporali R. Baricitinib for COVID-19: a suitable treatment? Lancet Infect Dis 2020;20(9):1012–3. https://doi.org/10.1016/S1473-3099(20)30262-0.
[61] Richardson P, Griffin I, Tucker C, et al. Baricitinib as potential treatment for 2019-nCoV acute respiratory disease. Lancet 2020;395(10223):e30–1. https://doi.org/10.1016/S0140-6736(20)30304-4.
[62] Kalil AC, Patterson TF, Mehta AK, et al. Baricitinib plus remdesivir for hospitalized adults with Covid-19. N Engl J Med 2021;384(9):795–807. https://doi.org/10.1056/nejmoa2031994.
[63] Fact sheet for healthcare providers emergency use authorization (EUA) of baricitinib. https://www.fda.gov/media/143823/download. [Accessed 24 July 2021].
[64] Tanaka T, Narazaki M, Kishimoto T. Immunotherapeutic implications of IL-6 blockade for cytokine storm. Immunotherapy 2016;8(8):959–70. https://doi.org/10.2217/IMT-2016-0020.
[65] Liu B, Li M, Zhou Z, Guan X, Xiang Y. Can we use interleukin-6 (IL-6) blockade for coronavirus disease 2019 (COVID-19)-induced cytokine release syndrome (CRS)? J Autoimmun 2020;111. https://doi.org/10.1016/J.JAUT.2020.102452.
[66] Coronavirus (COVID-19) update: FDA authorizes drug for treatment of COVID-19. FDA; 2021. https://www.fda.gov/news-events/press-announcements/coronavirus-covid-19-update-fda-authorizes-drug-treatment-covid-19. [Accessed 24 July 2021].
[67] Ghosn L, Chaimani A, Evrenoglou T, et al. Interleukin-6 blocking agents for treating COVID-19: a living systematic review. Cochrane Database Syst Rev 2021;2021(3). https://doi.org/10.1002/14651858.CD013881.
[68] Investigators TR-C. Interleukin-6 receptor antagonists in critically ill patients with Covid-19. N Engl J Med 2021;384(16):1491–502. https://doi.org/10.1056/NEJMOA2100433.
[69] Abani O, Abbas A, Abbas F, et al. Tocilizumab in patients admitted to hospital with COVID-19 (recovery): a randomised, controlled, open-label, platform trial. Lancet 2021;397(10285):1637–45. https://doi.org/10.1016/S0140-6736(21)00676-0.

[70] Cheng Y, Wong R, Soo YO, et al. Use of convalescent plasma therapy in SARS patients in Hong Kong. Eur J Clin Microbiol Infect Di 2005;24(1):44–6. https://doi.org/10.1007/S10096-004-1271-9.

[71] Ko JH, Müller MA, Seok H, et al. Suggested new breakpoints of anti-MERS-CoV antibody ELISA titers: performance analysis of serologic tests. Eur J Clin Microbiol Infect Di 2017;36(11):2179–86. https://doi.org/10.1007/S10096-017-3043-3.

[72] Rojas M, Rodríguez Y, Monsalve DM, et al. Convalescent plasma in Covid-19: possible mechanisms of action. Autoimmun Rev 2020;19(7). https://doi.org/10.1016/J.AUTREV.2020.102554.

[73] Bloch EM, Shoham S, Casadevall A, et al. Deployment of convalescent plasma for the prevention and treatment of COVID-19. J Clin Invest 2020;130(6):2757–65. https://doi.org/10.1172/JCI138745.

[74] FDA In Brief: FDA Updates Emergency Use Authorization for COVID-19 Convalescent Plasma to Reflect New Data. FDA; 2021. https://www.fda.gov/news-events/fda-brief/fda-brief-fda-updates-emergency-use-authorization-covid-19-convalescent-plasma-reflect-new-data. [Accessed 24 July 2021].

[75] Salazar E, Christensen PA, Graviss EA, et al. Treatment of coronavirus disease 2019 patients with convalescent plasma reveals a signal of significantly decreased mortality. Am J Pathol 2020;190(11):2290–303. https://doi.org/10.1016/J.AJPATH.2020.08.001.

[76] Joyner MJ, Carter RE, Senefeld JW, et al. Convalescent plasma antibody levels and the risk of death from Covid-19. N Engl J Med 2021;384(11):1015–27. https://doi.org/10.1056/NEJMOA2031893.

[77] Liu STH, Lin HM, Baine I, et al. Convalescent plasma treatment of severe COVID-19: a propensity score-matched control study. Nat Med 2020;26(11):1708–13. https://doi.org/10.1038/S41591-020-1088-9.

[78] Janiaud P, Axfors C, Schmitt AM, et al. Association of convalescent plasma treatment with clinical outcomes in patients with COVID-19: a systematic review and meta-analysis. J Am Med Assoc 2021;325(12):1185–95. https://doi.org/10.1001/JAMA.2021.2747.

[79] Piechotta V, Chai KL, Valk SJ, et al. Convalescent plasma or hyperimmune immunoglobulin for people with COVID-19: a living systematic review. Cochrane Database Syst Rev 2020;7(7). https://doi.org/10.1002/14651858.CD013600.PUB2.

[80] Joyner MJ, Bruno KA, Klassen SA, et al. Safety update: COVID-19 convalescent plasma in 20,000 hospitalized patients. Mayo Clin Proc 2020;95(9):1888–97. https://doi.org/10.1016/J.MAYOCP.2020.06.028.

Index

'*Note*: Page numbers followed by "f" indicate figures, "t" indicate tables, and "b" indicate boxes.'

A

Abatacept, 31
Acute lupus pneumonitis (ALP), 46–48
ANCA-associated vasculitis (AAV)
  bronchoalveolar lavage (BAL), 154
  C-reactive protein (CRP) levels, 155
  chest X-rays, 153–154
  computed tomography (CT), 153–154
  eosinophilic granulomatosis with polyangiitis (EGPA). *See* Eosinophilic granulomatosis with polyangiitis (EGPA)
  granulomatosis with polyangiitis (GPA). *See* Granulomatosis with polyangiitis (GPA)
  lung involvement, 160–162
  pulmonary manifestations, 153–157
    diffuse alveolar hemorrhage (DAH), 153–155, 154f
    interstitial lung disease (ILD), 155–156, 156f
    nonspecific pulmonary opacities, 157
    pleural effusion, 157
    pulmonary embolism, 157
Anti-MDA5 syndrome
  clinical spectrum, 118–119
  clinical vignette, 122b
  diagnosis of, 118–119
  ILD, 119–120
  prognostic biomarkers, 120–121
  scleromyositis, 121–122
Antibody-based therapies, 205–206
Antifibrotic drugs, 32
Antifibrotic therapy, 44–45, 93–94
Antisynthetase syndrome, 111–118
  anti-ARS detection, 114–115
  clinical spectrum, 112–113
  clinical vignette, 117b–118b
  comment, 117b–118b
  definition, 111–112
  diagnosis, 113–114
  immunosuppressive therapy, 126–127
  prognostic factors, 116–118
  rapidly progressive ILD management, 127–129
  recognition, 113–114
Asthma, 159–160
Asymptomatic infection, 195–196

B

Baricitinib, 204
Bone morphogenetic protein receptor type 2 (BMPR2), 77
Bronchoalveolar lavage (BAL), 62–63, 83–85

C

C-reactive protein (CRP) levels, 155
CC-chemokine ligand 2 (CCL2), 75–76
Chest X-rays, 153–154
Computed tomography (CT), 153–154
Connective tissue disease (CTD), 1
Connective tissue growth factor (CTGF), 75
Convalescent plasma, 205–206
Conventional disease-modifying antirheumatic drugs, 28–30
Coronaviruses 2019 (COVID-19)
  antibody-based therapies, 205–206
  asymptomatic infection, 195–196
  Baricitinib, 204
  clinical features, 195–198
  clinical manifestations, 196–197, 196t
  complications, 197–198
  convalescent plasma, 205–206
  dexamethasone, 202
  diagnosis, 200–201
  diagnostic approach, 200–201
  epidemiology, 190
  general management, 201
  IL-6 pathway inhibitors, 204–205
  imaging findings, 198
  immune dysfunction, 194–195
  immune response, 193–194

Coronaviruses 2019 (COVID-19) (*Continued*)
Janus kinase (JAK), 204
laboratory findings, 198
management, 201–206
other glucocorticoids, 202
pathogenesis, 192–195
pathology findings, 198–199
Remdesivir, 203
Sequential Organ Failure Assessment (SOFA), 196–197
Tocilizumab, 204–205
transmission, 191–192
virology, 191
Cyclophosphamide (CYC), 29, 80, 90

D

Dexamethasone, 202
Diffuse alveolar hemorrhage (DAH), 46

E

Eosinophilic granulomatosis with polyangiitis (EGPA)
pulmonary manifestations
asthma, 159–160
pulmonary nodules, 157, 158f
European Respiratory Society (ERS), 180

F

Forced vital capacity (FVC), 44–45

G

Gastro-oesophageal reflux disease (GORD), 75–76
Genetic susceptibility, 75
Glucocorticoids (GCs), 27–32
Granulomatosis with polyangiitis (GPA)
pulmonary manifestations
large-airway involvement, 159
pulmonary nodules, 157, 158f

H

Haematopoietic stem cell transplantation (HSCT), 94
High-resolution computed tomography (HRCT), 80–85, 82f–83f

I

Idiopathic interstitial pneumonia (IIP), 1
IL-6 pathway inhibitors, 204–205
Immune dysfunction, 194–195
Immune response, 193–194
Inflammatory myopathies (IM)
diagnosis, 108
disease severity assessment, 108–109
interstitial lung disease (ILD), 107–135
antifibrotic treatment, 129–130
arthritis, 131–134
clinical spectrum of, 111–122
clinical vignette, 132b–133b
comment, 133b–134b, 138b
lung transplantation, 130–131
management strategy, 124–135
mixed connective tissue disease (MCTD), 135–138
monitoring of, 109
myositis-related autoantibodies, 109–110
pathogenesis of, 123–124
pulmonary hypertension, 134–135
treatment approach, 124–135
lung in, 105–106
myositis-related autoantibodies, 109–110
obstructive sleep apnea syndrome (OSAS), 106–107
ventilatory failure, 107
Interstitial lung disease (ILD), 1, 42–45, 43f
azathioprine, 29–30
biological disease-modifying antirheumatic drugs, 30–32
abatacept, 31
antifibrotic drugs, 32
Janus kinase inhibitors (JAKi), 31–32
lung transplantation, 32
rituximab, 31
tocilizumab, 30
tumor necrosis factor inhibitors (TNFi), 30
clinical manifestations, 23
conventional disease-modifying antirheumatic drugs, 28–30
cyclophosphamide, 29
cystic lung disease, 61
diagnostic imaging, 23–25, 24f–25f
different diagnostic methods, 25–26
glucocorticoids (GCs), 27–32
histology, 59–61
imaging studies, 59–61
inflammatory myopathies (IM), 107–135
anti-MDA5 syndrome. *See* Anti-MDA5 syndrome
antifibrotic treatment, 129–130

antisynthetase syndrome. *See* Antisynthetase syndrome
arthritis, 131–134
clinical spectrum of, 111–122
clinical vignette, 132b–133b, 136b–138b
comment, 133b–134b, 138b
lung transplantation, 130–131
management strategy, 124–135
mixed connective tissue disease (MCTD), 135–138
monitoring of, 109
myositis-related autoantibodies, 109–110
pathogenesis of, 123–124
pulmonary hypertension, 134–135
treatment approach, 124–135
leflunomide, 29
lymphocytic interstitial pneumonia, 61
methotrexate, 28–29
mycophenolate mofetil (MMF), 29
nonspecific interstitial pneumonia, 59
organizing pneumonia, 60–61
overview, 58–59
pathogenesis, 21–22, 22f
pulmonary function tests in, 61–62, 62f
rheumatoid arthritis (RA), 21
risk factors, 21–22, 22f
systemic sclerosis (SSc)
antifibrotic therapies, 93–94
bronchoalveolar lavage (BAL), 83–85
clincal presentation, 77–78
cyclophosphamide, 90
diagnosis of, 78–86
epidemiology, 73–74
haematopoietic stem cell transplantation (HSCT), 94
high-resolution computed tomography (HRCT), 80–85, 82f–83f
lung biopsy, 85–86
monitoring, 88–89
mycophenolate mofetil, 90
prognosis, 89
progression, 88–89
screening for, 86–88
targeted therapies, 91–93
therapy, 26–32, 27t
usual interstitial pneumonia, 60
Interstitial pneumonia with autoimmune features (IPAF)
classification, 6–10
clinical domain, 6–8
connective tissue disease (CTD), 1
criticisms, 14–15
epidemiology, 5–6
idiopathic interstitial pneumonia (IIP), 1
interstitial lung disease (ILD), 1
mechanisms of disease, 10–12
genetics, 11–12
immune system, 10–11
morphologic domain, 8–10
potential shortcomings, 14–15
prognosis, 12–13
serologic domain, 8
treatment, 13–14

J

Janus kinase inhibitors (JAKi), 31–32, 180, 204

L

Large-airway involvement, 159
Leflunomide, 29
Lung biopsy, 63
Lung magnetic resonance imaging (LMRI), 82
Lung transplantation, 32, 182
Lung ultrasound (LUS), 81–82
Lymphoma, 65

M

Methotrexate, 28–29
Morphologic domain, 8–10
Mycophenolate mofetil (MMF), 29, 44, 80

N

Nintenanib, 180
Nonspecific interstitial pneumonia (NSIP), 77

O

Obstructive sleep apnea syndrome (OSAS), 106–107

P

Pirfenidone, 180
Platelet-derived growth factor (PDGF), 77
Pleural disease, 65–66
Pleural involvement, 41–42
Positron emission tomography (PET), 82–83
Prognosis, 12–13
Pulmonary amyloidosis, 66

Pulmonary arterial hypertension, 45–46, 66
Pulmonary artery pressure, 180
Pulmonary function tests (PFTs), 57–58, 78
Pulmonary manifestations
asthma, 159–160
large-airway involvement, 159
pulmonary nodules, 157, 158f
Pulmonary nodules, 157, 158f
Pulmonary vasculitis, 46

R

Remdesivir, 203
Repository corticotropin injection (RCI), 180
Rheumatoid arthritis (RA), 21
Rituximab, 31

S

Sarcoidosis
anti-inflammatory therapy, 179
computer tomography (CT), 169
diagnosis of, 176–178, 176f, 177t
European Respiratory Society (ERS), 180
lung transplantation, 182
lymphatic involvement, 169–171, 171f
parenchymal lung involvement, 172–174, 172f–173f
pulmonary fibrosis, 180
pulmonary sarcoidosis, 169
pulmonary vascular involvement, 174–176, 175t
repository corticotropin injection (RCI), 180
treatment, 178–182, 178t, 179f
Sequential Organ Failure Assessment (SOFA), 196–197
Serologic domain, 8
Shrinking lung syndrome (SLS), 48–50, 49f
Sjogren's syndrome (SS)
airway disease
histology, 56–57
imaging studies, 56–57
overview, 56
pulmonary function tests (PFTs), 57–58
treatment, 58
bronchoalveolar lavage (BAL) cell, 62–63
interstitial lung disease
cystic lung disease, 61
histology, 59–61
imaging studies, 59–61
lymphocytic interstitial pneumonia, 61
nonspecific interstitial pneumonia, 59
organizing pneumonia, 60–61
overview, 58–59
pulmonary function tests in, 61–62, 62f
usual interstitial pneumonia, 60
lung biopsy, 63
lymphoma, 65
pleural disease, 65–66
pulmonary amyloidosis, 66
pulmonary arterial hypertension, 66
treatment, 63–64, 65f
Systemic lupus erythematosus (SLE)
acute lupus pneumonitis (ALP), 46–48
antifibrotic therapy, 44–45
diffuse alveolar hemorrhage (DAH), 46
forced vital capacity (FVC), 44–45
glucocorticoids (GCs), 44
interstitial lung disease, 42–45, 43f
mycophenolate mofetil (MMF), 44
pleural involvement, 41–42
pulmonary arterial hypertension, 45–46
pulmonary vasculitis, 46
shrinking lung syndrome (SLS), 48–50, 49f
Systemic sclerosis (SSc), lung involvement in
clincal presentation
interstitial lung disease, 77–78
pulmonary arterial hypertension, 78
COVID-19, 94–95
epidemiology, 73–74
interstitial lung disease (ILD). *See* Interstitial lung disease (ILD); systemic sclerosis (SSc)
pathogenesis, 74–77
lung fibrosis, 75–76
pulmonary arterial hypertension, 77
pulmonary arterial hypertension, 74

T

Tocilizumab, 30, 204–205
Transforming growth factor-β (TGFβ), 75–76
Tumor necrosis factor inhibitors (TNFi), 30

U

Ultra-short time (UTE), 82

V

Ventilatory failure, 107

FSC
www.fsc.org
MIX
Papier | Fördert gute Waldnutzung
FSC® C083411

Kolibri 360 GmbH
Ferdinand-Jühlke-Straße 7
99095 Erfurt, Deutschland
produktsicherheit@kolibri360.de

Natural Disaster Research, Prediction and Mitigation

Volcanic Eruptions

Triggers, Role of Climate Change and Environmental Effects

NATURAL DISASTER RESEARCH, PREDICTION AND MITIGATION

Additional books in this series can be found on Nova's website under the Series tab.

Additional e-books in this series can be found on Nova's website under the e-book tab.

NATURAL DISASTER RESEARCH, PREDICTION AND MITIGATION

VOLCANIC ERUPTIONS

TRIGGERS, ROLE OF CLIMATE CHANGE AND ENVIRONMENTAL EFFECTS

TRENT MILBURN
EDITOR

nova publishers
New York

Additional color graphics may be available in the e-book version of this book.

Library of Congress Cataloging-in-Publication Data

Volcanic eruptions : triggers, role of climate change, and environmental effects / Trent Milburn, editor.
pages cm. -- (Natural disaster research, prediction and mitigation)
Includes index.
ISBN 978-1-63463-308-6 (hardcover)
1. Volcanic eruptions. 2. Volcanic activity prediction. 3. Volcanoes--Environmental aspects. 4. Volcanic ash, tuff, etc. I. Milburn, Trent, editor.
QE522.V63 2014
551.21--dc23
2014039720

Published by Nova Science Publishers, Inc. † New York

CONTENTS

Preface **vii**

Chapter 1 The Impact of Volcanic Ash Fallout on Industrial Facilities: Natural-Technological Hazards in Wastewater Treatments (Screening Processes) **1**
M. F. Milazzo, G. Ancione, P. Primerano, E. Salzano and G. Maschio

Chapter 2 A Possible Link between Sun's Variability and Volcanic Activity **23**
Paolo Madonia, Francesco Parello and Dalila Pitarresi

Chapter 3 Extreme Pointer Years in Tree-Ring Records of Central Spain As Evidence of the Eruption of the Huaynaputina Volcano (Peru, 1600 AD) **39**
Mar Génova Fuster

Chapter 4 The Seismic Signatures of the Volcanic Crises: A Review **53**
Mauro Palo

Chapter 5 Effect of Volcanic Eruptions on Stratospheric Ozone and Irradiance **117**
Susana B. Diaz and Alejandro A. Paladini

Chapter 6 Volcanic Complex Puyehue-Cordón Caulle: Impact of Volcanic Ash on Insects in Patagonia, Argentina **141**
V. Fernández-Arhex, A. L. Pietrantuono M. E. Amadio and O. Bruzzone

Index **159**

PREFACE

Natural catastrophic events such as volcano eruptions have greatly affected environments in wide regions around the world. Ash and gases impelled by these eruptions into the atmosphere carry large volumes of particles of different sizes (nanometer and ultrafine) that are scattered around the earth. However, the greater accumulation of different grain size was observed in the range of 10 kilometers from the center of the volcano, causing devastating effect. The most important consequences of this type of event are loss of habitats for flora and fauna. This book discusses the triggers of volcanic eruptions, as well as environmental effects and the role they play in climate change.

Chapter 1 – In recent years, worldwide attention focused on the hazards derived from the interaction between an extreme natural phenomena and critical infrastructures and/or chemical and process industry (Natural-Technological hazards or Na-Techs). Amongst different Na-Techs, this chapter focuses on the study of those triggered by volcanic ash emissions. Ash fallouts can directly endanger human health due to the inhalation of solid particles or indirectly compromise the safety of people due to the damage of critical structures, infrastructures, transport systems, chemical plants and lifelines. The effects of the impact on chemical plants and lifelines could also be significant on ecosystems. In this framework, this work focuses on volcanic Na-Techs in wastewater treatments (WWTs); the main aim is the definition of the conditions leading to failures *in primary treatments* due to volcanic ash fallouts. The estimation of the threshold amounts of ash causing damages will be shown for a case study (Mt. Etna, Italy).

Chapter 2 – Sun inconstancy has the ability to control global climate, that in turn acts as a trigger for volcanic activity. Looking for possible Sun-Earth connections the authors analysed the time distribution of eruptions of volcanoes located on the northern hemisphere, from the Caribbean Sea to the East Mediterranean Sea, with a particular detail on the most active Italian volcanoes. The compared analysis between sunspot and volcanic cycles suggested that volcanic eruptions are more frequent during minima of Sun activity, with about 3 eruptions out of 4 occurring at relative minima of the quasi-11 year Sun cycle. Not so evident are the long term (centennial time scale) relationships between Sun and volcanic system variability: since the former is controlled by much more complex mechanisms the analysis of correlations between eruptions and Sun activity cannot prescind from geodynamical discriminants, which play a fundamental role in driving magma migration toward the Earth's surface.

Chapter 3 – The interpretation of the pointer years in tree-ring records depends on their position in the dendrochronological sequences and on their significance. It has been demonstrated that the pointer years, which present themselves over wide geographical areas, tend to be associated with determinate macro-climatic events. Several studies have related negative pointer years to macro-climatic events on a global scale, such as those derived from major volcanic eruptions. Here are presented the results matching the negative pointer year's record of *Pinus sylvestris* tree-ring chronologies with those determined in certain historical timber in the central Iberian Peninsula (Spain). Today there is an extensive *Pinus sylvestris* dendrochronological database in central Spain that has enabled the development of a regional chronology extended from 1513 to 2005. Finding that the probable time span of the studied wood coming from the Royal Old Mint of Segovia, which was built using these nearby pine forest, these historical woods have been crossdated with the oldest tree-ring series of this dendrochronological database assembled in a master chronology. The Mint chronologies and the master chronology have been matched in the period 1558-1723, with 1600 and 1601 being recognized as common negative pointer years in all tree ring series reaching that period, coinciding with many growth anomalies dated in the tree rings of the Northern Hemisphere at high latitudes. Just like these dendrochronological studies it has been inferred that these anomalies were the effect of the eruption of Huaynaputina, which occurred in Peru at the beginning of 1600 AD. It should be noted that this is the first time that have been determined the effects of this eruption in the tree-ring records of Southern Europe.

Chapter 4 – Volcano seismology is considered a good proxy of the internal conditions of the volcanic systems. In particular, the volcanic crises are anticipated by a loading process triggered by an overall upward magma migration inducing gas exsolution and stress build up within the feeding system and the hosting rocks. This process activates brittle failures within the volcanic edifice and pressurized magmatic fluids flowing through magma-filled cavities, generating the two end-members of the volcano seismicity: Volcano-Tectonic and Long-Period events, respectively. Volcano seismicity follows the disequilibrium conditions within the plumbing system preceding and accompanying the volcanic crises, exhibiting modifications of the source process in respect to the inter-eruptive phase in terms of wavefield properties and statistics of the earthquake occurrence. Although some common correlations between seismic activity and magma dynamics during the eruptive crises have been identified, a wide variability of behaviors appears as well, with a sharp dependence on the volcano and on the eruptive episode. Here I critically review the characteristics of the volcano seismicity before and during the volcanic crises, describing the source process of the volcanic earthquakes in terms of both the seismologic parameters and the statistical properties of the point process ruling their occurrence times and magnitude.

Chapter 5 – Major volcanic eruptions can inject large amounts of sulfur into the stratosphere, increasing the stratospheric aerosol layer for several years. In the last decades, this effect was observed after the eruptions of El Chichón, in 1982, and Mt. Pinatubo, in 1991, which had a considerable contribution to ozone depletion. The natural variability of atmospheric ozone occurs in time scales ranging from day to day, to decadal. Atmospheric circulation, chemistry, and radiative processes play important roles in the variability of ozone. Large volcanic eruptions reaching the stratosphere could cause significant temporary changes. The effect of a volcanic eruption on stratospheric ozone is largest when large chlorine and bromine levels are present in the atmosphere. How past volcanic eruptions have changed stratospheric ozone was studied using models. It was concluded that eruptions of El Chichon and Pinatubo resulted in globally total ozone losses and severe ozone depletion in the lower stratosphere. Earlier eruptions (Krakatau, Santa Maria and Agung) resulted in globally total ozone increases and almost no ozone changes in the stratosphere. This difference in ozone response was caused by the amount of ozone depleting substances present in the atmosphere, which increased the availability of chlorine and caused a change in the chemistry, during the last decades. In the mid-1990s, a maximum in stratospheric ozone depletion was observed, as consequence of ozone response to volcanic aerosols from Mt. Pinatubo, superimposed to the depletion produced by halocarbons.

One of the reasons that make stratospheric ozone important is the attenuation of solar ultraviolet (UV) radiation while it trespasses the atmosphere. Radiation reaching the Earth's surface is influenced by scattering and absorption processes in the atmosphere and the ground. Sun-Earth distance, atmospheric gases and aerosols, solar zenith angle (SZA), clouds and surface albedo are the main factors that determine radiation at ground-level. The effect of volcanic eruptions on UV radiation is complex. On one side, depletion of stratospheric ozone results in an increase in UV radiation. In addition, volcanic eruptions increase the aerosol amount and change aerosol size composition, producing important variation in optical properties of the atmosphere. As a result, a decrease is usually observed in direct UV radiation, due to absorption produced by the emitted particles. At the same time, an increase in the diffuse radiation may be experienced, resulting from scattering increase. As consequence of these two processes the effect on global UV radiation is difficult to anticipate.

In this chapter, the authors present a review of the effect of major volcanic eruptions on the ozone layer and UV radiation. The authors also introduce their own results on the effect of Puyehue-Cordon Caulle volcanic complex eruption, in 2011, which did not affect globally the ozone layer but produced a large regional impact on aerosols and UV radiation.

Chapter 6 – In June 4th 2011, there was a major volcanic eruption of the Puyehue-Caulle complex (PCC) in southern Andean range near the Argentina-Chile border. This event covered with ashes over 7.5 million hectares in Argentinean Patagonia during for a year and affecting the flora and fauna, including the insect. In this chapter the authors present different case studies which evaluated the effect of volcanic ash on survival, motivation and use of habitat in different species of insects. Laboratory bioassays results have shown that the ash does not affect the species studied in the same way, and also there are differences between guilds of phytophagous insects. Phloem-sucking insects are not strongly affected, actively choose their habitats for living and are capable of discriminate unfavorable habitats (i.e., presence of volcanic ash). On the other hand on orthopteran species, the volcanic ash has a strong aversive and insecticidal effect similar to that of inert dust. In this case the volcanic ash could potentially have a protective effect against insect pests, reducing the damage they can cause to grasslands and pastures. The impact of the ashes from PCC on the insect community may be radical in the acute deposition phase, with substantial qualitative effects in the chronic phase of exposure. The recovery of populations affected by ash in desert areas where dry ash persists will be slower, and this will have tangible and long-term consequences for insect host plants, and on the development of populations of vertebrate insectivores. By contrast, the presence of ash in humid regions will impact the ecosystem by the addition of nutrients, which in combination with water retention by the ash will lead to a qualitative and quantitative recovery of the populations under favorable conditions. Therefore the authors propose that the ash can generate two types of responses on insects: direct (on individuals) or indirect (on individual-environment interactions).

Chapter 7 – This study objectively investigates the potential for rainfall that can trigger earthquakes with a Richter magnitude (local magnitude) of ML ≥ 6.0 using rainfall information for the period from January 1995 to August 2012. Lin (2013) determined that typhoons triggered small earthquakes, especially after the occurrence of the Chi-Chi earthquake from January 1995 to July 2012. The results of a chi-square test performed after the Chi-Chi earthquake indicate that earthquakes are likely to have a significant positive relationship with rainfall. The results revealed a significant difference between the correlations of daily-accumulated rainfall values and earthquake activities before and after the Chi-Chi earthquake. The significant difference has been discussed in terms of changes in crustal conditions after the Chi-Chi earthquake.

In: Volcanic Eruptions
Editor: Trent Milburn

ISBN: 978-1-63463-308-6

Chapter 1

THE IMPACT OF VOLCANIC ASH FALLOUT ON INDUSTRIAL FACILITIES: NATURAL-TECHNOLOGICAL HAZARDS IN WASTEWATER TREATMENTS (SCREENING PROCESSES)

M. F. Milazzo[1,*], G. Ancione[1], P. Primerano[1], E. Salzano[2] and G. Maschio[3]

[1]Dipartimento di Ingegneria Elettronica, Chimica e Ingegneria Industriale, University of Messina, Messina, Italy

[2]Istituto Ricerche sulla Combustione, Consiglio Nazionale delle Ricerche, Napoli, Italy

[3]Dipartimento di Ingegneria Industriale, University of Padova, Padova, Italy

ABSTRACT

In recent years, worldwide attention focused on the hazards derived from the interaction between an extreme natural phenomena and critical infrastructures and/or chemical and process industry (Natural-

[*] Corresponding author: mfmilazzo@unime.it.

Technological hazards or Na-Techs). Amongst different Na-Techs, this chapter focuses on the study of those triggered by volcanic ash emissions. Ash fallouts can directly endanger human health due to the inhalation of solid particles or indirectly compromise the safety of people due to the damage of critical structures, infrastructures, transport systems, chemical plants and lifelines. The effects of the impact on chemical plants and lifelines could also be significant on ecosystems. In this framework, this work focuses on volcanic Na-Techs in wastewater treatments (WWTs); the main aim is the definition of the conditions leading to failures *in primary treatments* due to volcanic ash fallouts. The estimation of the threshold amounts of ash causing damages will be shown for a case study (Mt. Etna, Italy).

1. INTRODUCTION

Natural events may cause several damages to lifelines, such as electrical power grids, water distribution systems, gas and oil pipelines, etc. The lifelines' disruption affects whole cities and even entire countries [1]; the literature gives several examples, some of them are: the electrical power outages occurred during the Kocaeli (1999) and Kobe (1995) earthquakes [2, 3], the blackouts due to the floods occurred in France [1] and the catastrophic impact on the wastewater treatment plants due to the eruption of St. Helen in 1980 [4].

Technological risks triggered by natural events are commonly named Na-Tech events [1]; De Rademaeker et al. [5] indicated, amongst several prioritised research topics related to the process safety, the category "*Natural hazard triggering technological disasters*" as emerging issues. The literature shows some approaches addressing the quantification of Na-Tech risks caused by many types of natural events (such as lightning, earthquakes, floods, volcanic eruptions, etc.) in the chemical and process industry [6-8]. Even prior to 2010 few works were published, the research dealing with study of the potential impact of volcanic ash fallouts has grown after the recent eruption of the Eyjafjallajökull volcano (Iceland). The most significant contributions are due to the following authors: Spence et al. [9] used a deterministic approach to evaluate the vulnerability of buildings; Rasà et al. [10] qualitatively described the effects of volcanic ash fallout from Etna on building, electric motors and other systems; Baxter et al. [11] analysed the reduction of functionality of water treatment systems (either industrial or civil installation) and the hazards related to the transportation of hazardous materials; other authors analysed the fragilities of atmospheric storage tanks [12] and filtering systems [13], then they developed procedures for the vulnerability mapping [14].

The aim of this work is to focus on volcanic Na-Techs in wastewater treatments (WWTs). Ancione and co-workers recently identified the most vulnerable equipment of a typical wastewater treatment and defined the causes of damage and their potential effects [15]. Compared to the previous literature, the present work gives a further contribution to the definition of the conditions leading to damages in *primary treatments* (or *mechanical treatments*) and, in particular, it focuses on screening processes. This chapter is structured as follows: Section 2 provides an overview on wastewater treatments, then points at the main equipment of *primary treatments* and their failure modes; Section 3 gives a description of the approach for the estimation of the ash thickness on screens leading to their functionality reduction; Section 4 describes the case-study which will be used to apply the approach proposed in Section 3; and, finally Section 5 shows the results and gives some discussion about them.

2. Wastewater Treatments

Wastewater treatments are designed to achieve improvements in the wastewater quality. The general principle is to remove/reduce the following pollutants from the sewage:

- *Suspended solids*: physical particles that can clog channels as they settle under gravity;
- *Biodegradable organics*: materials that can serve as food for microorganisms;
- *Pathogenic bacteria and other disease*: these are most relevant if water is used for drinking or people would be in close contact with it;
- *Nutrients, including nitrates and phosphates*: these can lead to high concentrations of unwanted algae, which can themselves become heavy loads of biodegradable organic material.

In the context of WWTs, a widely used terminology refers to three levels of wastewater treatment, as shown in Figure 1, these are primary, secondary and tertiary (or advanced).

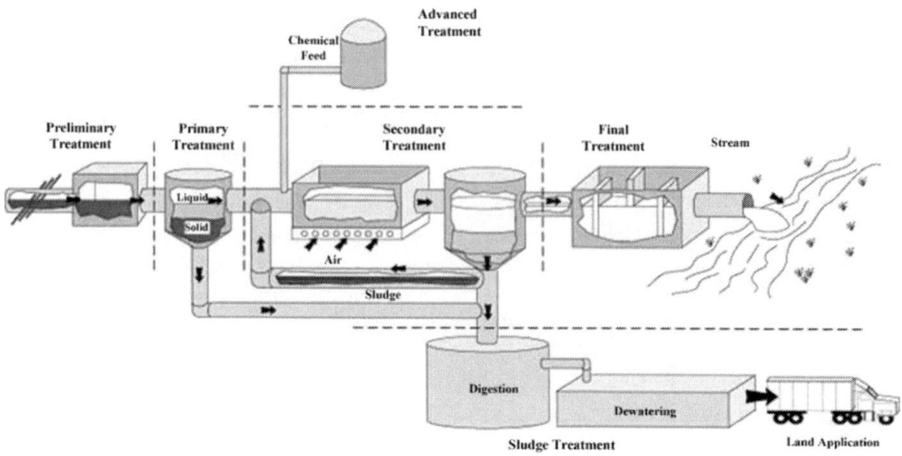

Figure 1. Wastewater Treatment plant (adapted from [16]).

Each levels of treatment is described below:

- *Primary (mechanical) treatment* deals with the removal of gross, suspended and floating solids from raw sewage. It includes screening to trap solid objects and sedimentation by gravity to remove suspended solids. This level is also referred to as *mechanical treatment*, although chemicals are often used to accelerate the sedimentation process.
- *Secondary (biological) treatment* removes the dissolved organic matter that escapes primary treatment, by means of microbes consuming the organic matter as food, and converting it to carbon dioxide, water and energy for their own growth and reproduction. The biological treatment is followed by additional settling tanks (*secondary sedimentation*) to remove more of the suspended solids.
- *Tertiary treatment* is simply an additional treatment, which can remove more than 99% of all the impurities from sewage, producing an effluent of almost drinking-water quality. The related technology is very expensive, requiring a high level of technical know-how and well trained plant operators, a steady energy supply, chemicals and specific equipment.

This contribution aims at the identification of the conditions leading to failures in *primary treatments*. The main equipment in a typical *primary treatment* includes screens, comminutors/grinders and grit removal; their characteristics are not reported here, but are described in [17]. Solids in the wastewater can interfere with the downstream processes (biological and chemical treatments) or may also cause mechanical wear and increase maintenance on the equipment. The main failure modes, associated with the presence of volcanic ash in the raw sewage, were identified by Ancione et al. [15] by an extensive literature analysis; with reference to the *primary treatments* the most relevant identified failure modes are the following:

- *Screens' clogging*: Screens could clog due to a deposit formation, this may occur when the particles' size in raw stream is greater than their openings. The malfunction is underlined by a variability (reduction) of flow-rate [18];
- *Incomplete grit removal*: Grit removals cannot give a complete deposition of ash, during the stream's passing in the channels. This causes abrasion and wear of mechanical equipment, grit deposition in pipelines and accumulation in anaerobic digesters and aeration basins [18].

3. METHODOLOGY

Modern plants for the wastewater treatment sometimes use both coarse screens and fine screens. Coarse screens remove large solids, rags and debris and typically have openings of 6 mm or larger. Fine screens are typically used to remove material that may create operating and maintenance problems in downstream processes, their typical opening sizes are 1.5 to 6 mm; very fine screens with openings of 0.2 to 1.5 mm placed after coarse or fine screens can reduce suspended solids to levels near those achieved by primary clarification.

The variability of flow-rate due to the ash accumulation is correlated to the screen's pressure drop (ΔP); thus the ΔP is the main indicator to underline the malfunctions. Given the dimension of ash particles, the effects of accumulation should be study for fine and very fine screens, anyway it is worth noting that this type of equipment is not included in all plants. The ΔP in fine screens can be calculated as suggested by the literature [19], then the length of deposit causing the critical pressure drop can be quantified by means of the methodology given in next Section.

3.1. Condition for the Screen Clogging

The pressure drop in fine screen can be calculated by using the following equation [19]:

$$\Delta P = \frac{\rho}{2 \cdot C} \cdot \left(\frac{Q}{A_s} \right)^2 \tag{1}$$

where: ΔP = pressure drop [Pa]; C = coefficient of discharge for the fine screen (typically this value for clean screens is 0.60, for dirty screens is 0.4 and for very dirty screens is 0.25); A_s = effective open area of submerged screen [m^2]; ρ = fluid (wastewater) density [kg/m^3].

The methodology for the estimation of the ash deposit threshold on a fine screen causing malfunctions is based on the assumption that the accumulation is a granular bed and the sewage represents the fluid passing through it. The literature [20] suggests estimating the bed dimension by means of the Darcy's equation in case of streamline flows and the Carman's equation for transition and turbulent flows. In the fluid dynamic, the parameter, which permits to determine the flow's regime is the Reynolds number (Re):

$$\text{Re} = \frac{D_{eq} \cdot \rho \cdot u_l}{\mu} \tag{2}$$

where: D_{eq} = equivalent diameter of the pore space [m]; μ = fluid viscosity [kg/m·s]; ρ = fluid density [kg/m^3]; u_l = average velocity through the pore channels [m/s].

The equivalent diameter and the average velocity through the pore channels depend on the characteristics of granular bed, i.e., the specific surface area S and the voidage e:

$$D_{eq} = \frac{e}{S \cdot (1 - e)} \tag{3}$$

$$u_l = \frac{u}{e} \tag{4}$$

Hence:

$$\mathrm{Re} = \frac{u \cdot \rho}{S \cdot \mu \cdot (1 - e)} \tag{5}$$

where: e = voidage or porosity, it represents the fraction of the volume of the bed which is not occupied by solid material [dimensionless]; S = specific surface area of the particles, it is the surface area of the particles divided by their volume [m^{-1}]; u = average velocity of the flow [m/s].

The following rules are given in the fluid dynamic to define the regime of a fluid flow in granular beds:

Re < 10 laminar (or streamline) flow

Re > 2000 turbulent flow

According to the Darcy law, the average velocity is directly proportional to the driving pressure and inversely proportional to the thickness of the bed:

$$Q = \frac{K}{\rho \cdot g} \cdot A_{tot} \cdot \frac{\Delta P}{l} \tag{6}$$

where: Q = volumetric flow rate [m^3/s]; A_{tot} = cross-sectional area [m^2], in this case it is effective open area of submerged screen (A_s); l = thickness of the porous medium [m]; g = gravity acceleration [m/s^2]; K = constant, it depends on the characteristics of the porous medium (intrinsic permeability, B) and the fluid characteristics (viscosity μ and density ρ) [m/s].

If the flow regime is transition or turbulent, the Carman's equation has to be used:

$$\frac{R'}{\rho u_l^2} = \frac{e^3}{S \cdot (1 - e)} \cdot \frac{(-\Delta P)}{l} \cdot \frac{1}{\rho \cdot u^2} \tag{7}$$

where: R' = component of the drag force per unit area of particle surface in the direction of motion.

The $(R'/\rho \cdot u_l^2)$ of the Carman's equation represents the friction coefficient, which is dimensionless and is correlated to the Reynolds number as follows:

$$\frac{R'}{\rho u_l^2} = 5\,\mathrm{Re}^{-1} + 0.4\,\mathrm{Re}^{-0,1} \tag{8}$$

3.2. Ash Characterisation

Some experimental tests were made to characterise the volcanic ash and obtain size distribution, density, specific surface area, voidage and permeability. The results of ash characterisation are needed in order to apply the methodology described above. The following experimental tests were performed:

- Analysis of the size distribution;
- Density determination;
- Specific surface area measurement (BET method) and voidage determination;
- Determination of the permeability.

3.2.1. Analysis of the Size Distribution

The sieving is the method used to determine the size distribution of the volcanic particles. The analysis makes use of special sieves arranged in a column; each of them retains the fraction of granules having larger dimensions compared with those of the holes of the sieve. The sieves must be stacked in such a way that the top has the larger mesh and the others have a gradually smaller mesh going down to the bottom. At the base of the column, there is a plate which is used to collect the granules with smaller diameters than the holes of the sieve with the lower mesh. The column is placed on a mechanical shaker for 20 min and, after the shaking, the solid fractions retained by each sieve is weighted. The weight of each solid fraction is then compared to the weight of the total solid to obtain the percentage of solid retained by each sieve.

3.2.2. Density Determination

The density determination was performed according to the EN 1097-3 standard [22]. The density is the *loose bulk density*, which is defined as the mass of the dried particles (not compressed), contained in a container, divided by the volume they occupy (tank volume). The total volume includes particles volume, inter-particles void volume and internal pore volume. According to this definition, the density determination was executed by using a container, whose volume and weight are known. It was filled with the volcanic ash and, subsequently, weighed. The weight and the volume of the ash allowed determining the density.

3.2.3. Specific Surface Area Measurement and Voidage

The determination of the specific surface area (*S*) have been executed by nitrogen adsorption, measurements were made using a Micromeritics ASAP 2020 sorption apparatus. The samples (~ 1 mg) were outgased in vacuum at 250°C for at least 16 h. The *S* values were calculated by applying the BET model (S_{BET}).

Assuming that the samples are composed by spherical particles (ideal sample), the *e* data from Coulson et al. [20] were plotted against *d* (particle's diameter) and then the voidage of the volcanic ash samples was extrapolated from the derived graph.

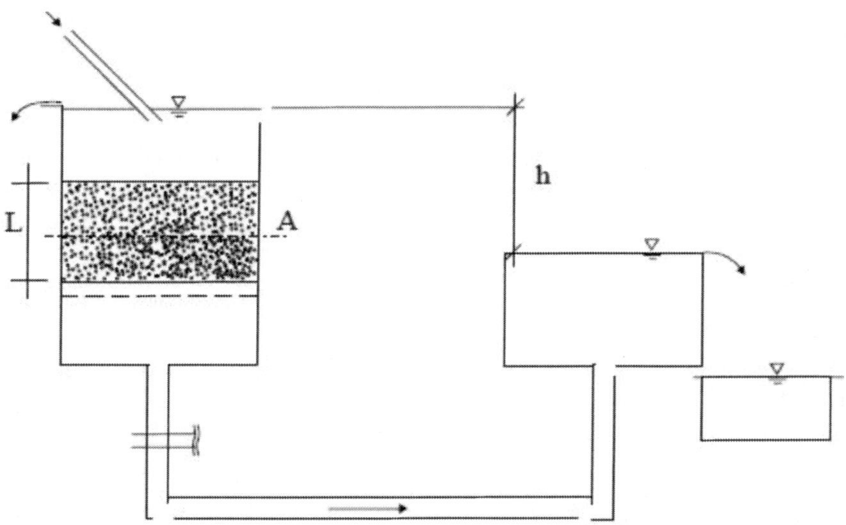

Figure 2. Permeameter at constant head.

3.2.4. Determination of the Permeability

Permeability (or hydraulic conductivity, *K*) refers to the ease with which water can flow through a granular solid. It is determined by using the constant head (load) test method (according to the standard ASTM D 2434 [23], which is used only for permeable materials ($K > 10^{-4}$ cm/s). A homemade permeameter at constant head was made for our experiments (see scheme in

Figure 2). The sample was subjected to a fixed piezometric load (Δh); then, the volume of water, passing through it during a certain time (t), was measured. The value of K is given by the equation:

$$K = \frac{L}{\Delta h \cdot A} \cdot \frac{V}{t} \tag{9}$$

where: L = length of the porous medium (sample) [m]; A = cross section of the porous medium (sample) [m^2]; V = volume of water collected during the time t [m^3]; Δh = piezometric load [m].

4. Case-Study

The case study is a WWT located in the surrounding Mt. Etna (South Italy). This volcano is 3300 m high and is characterised by both basaltic explosive behaviour and effusive activity. Mt. Etna has five main craters (Figure 3): North-East Crater (NEC), Voragine (VOR), Bocca Nuova (BN), South-East Crater (SEC) and New South-East Crater (NSEC). This last crater emerged very recent, i.e., during an eruption occurred in 2014.

The volcanic activity in particular during 2001, 2002–2003 and 2013 was characterised by an explosive style and for many weeks produced stable tephra and gas columns in the atmosphere [24, 25]. Two reasons oriented towards the choice of this case-study [13]: (*i*) an increased trend to give explosive eruptions with ash emission has recently been observed [26]; (*ii*) the expected damage due to ash fallout is expected to be larger because of the increased urbanization and number of industrial infrastructures installed in the recent years. The area close to the volcano is characterized by the presence of the city of Catania (300 thousand inhabitants), by many small urban centres and agricultural and industrial areas. In the Southern area there is one of the most complex industrial sites of Europe (Priolo-Augusta-Melilli), which could be involved during specific weather conditions. The whole *primary treatment* of a typical WWT is schematised in Figure 4, but the scope of this study is to focus on a fine screen.

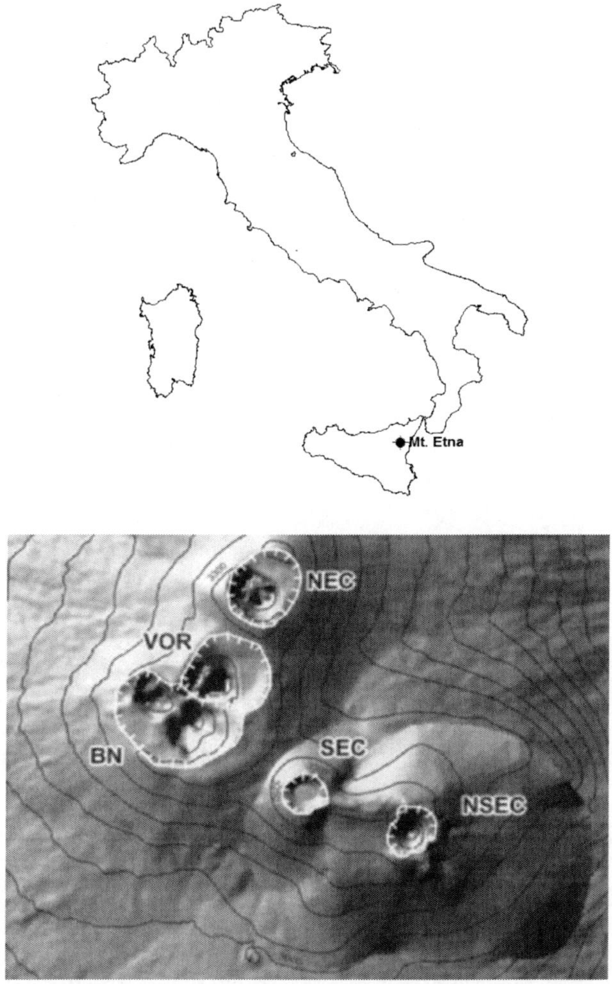

Figure 3. Location of Mt. Etna (Italy) five main craters.

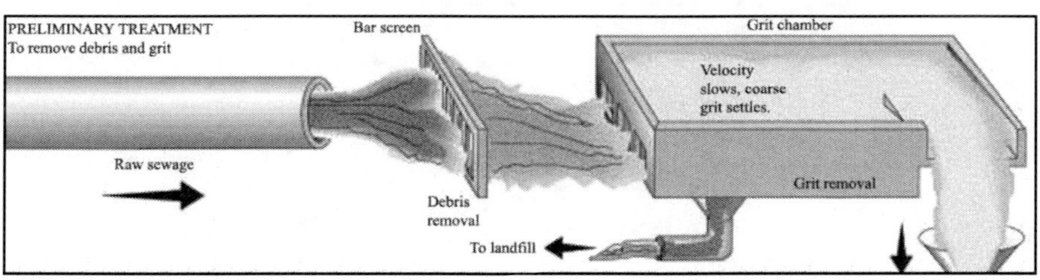

Figure 4. Primary treatment.

Two samples of ash produced by eruptions of Mt. Etna were used for the investigations needed for this study. The first sample (ID=1) was collected close to the Cratere Silvestri (coordinates: lat. 37°41'55.73"N , long. 15°0'16.94"E; distance 5.5 km from the main crater) and the second one (ID=2) was taken in urban area of Messina during the eruption of the 23rd February 2013 (coordinates: lat. 38°10'16.66"N, long: 15°31'25.56"E; distance 65 km from the main crater). To apply the methodology given in Section 3.1, the ash must be characterised to determine its main parameters as indicated in Section 3.2 (ϕ, ρ, S, e and K). Then, the Reynolds number for the wastewater stream, flowing in the granular bed (ash deposit), was calculated to make possible the choice of the approach for the computation of the thicknesses of the deposit (Darcy or Carman approach). The characteristics of the square opening fine screen, chosen in this study, are given in Table 1; some parameters of the screen are shown in Figure 5.

Table 1. Fine screen characteristics

Parameter	Symbol	Unit	Value
Wastewater flow rate	Q	m^3/s	0.8
Wastewater velocity	u	m/s	0.7
Area of submerged screen	A	m^2	1.14
Effective open area of submerged screen	A_s	m^2	0.285
Opening size	c	m	$0.5 \cdot 10^{-4}$
Vertical opening distance	U_1	m	10^{-3}
Horizontal opening distance	U_2	m	10^{-3}
Bar spacing	b_1	m	$0.5 \cdot 10^{-3}$
Bar thickness	b_2	m	$0.5 \cdot 10^{-3}$

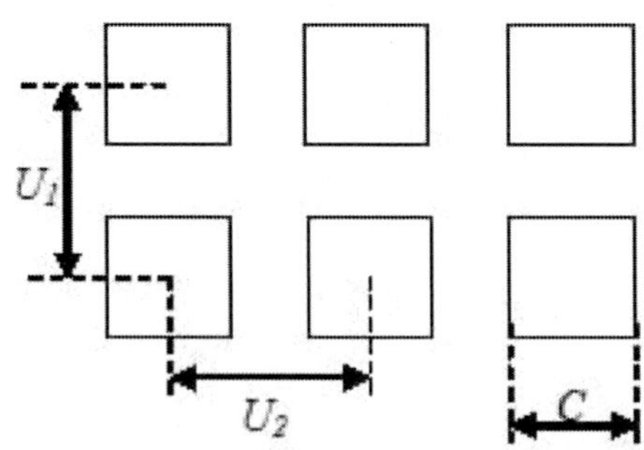

Figure 5. Square opening fine screen.

5. Results and Discussion

In this Section, the results derived by the application of the proposed methodology are presented; some comments are also given on the resulting critical ash thicknesses.

5.1. Size Distribution

The size distribution of the ash samples was calculated by Milazzo et al. [27] and presented using the Krumbein parameter $\phi = -\log_2(d/d_o)$, where: d = diameter of the particle [mm]; d_o = reference diameter, which is equal to 1 mm to make the equation dimensionally consistent [28].

By analysing the results of Milazzo and coworkers (Figure 6), the prevailing diameters for the ash particles are:

- 0.1 ÷ 2 mm (ϕ = 3.3 ÷ -1) for the sample 1;
- 0.15 ÷ 2 mm (ϕ = 2.7 ÷ -1) for the sample 2.

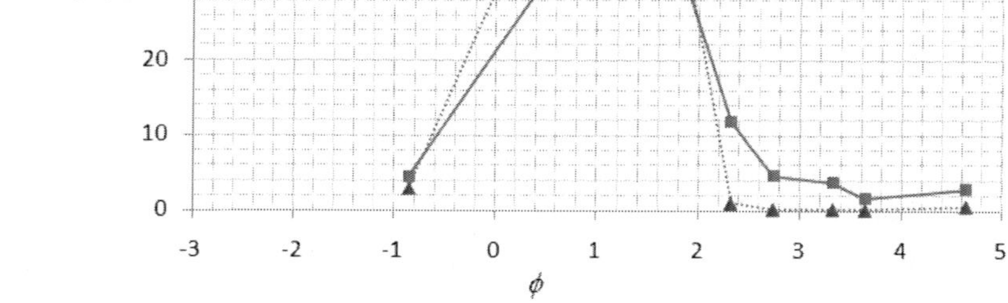

Figure 6. Size distribution for the samples of volcanic ash.

Form the size distribution analysis other data were obtained, these are given in Table 2.

Table 2. Diameter of particles

Sample ID	Average weighted diameter (m)	Maximum diameter (m)	Minimum diameter (m)
1	$4.3 \cdot 10^{-4}$	$2 \cdot 10^{-3}$	$1 \cdot 10^{-4}$
2	$5 \cdot 10^{-4}$	$2 \cdot 10^{-3}$	$1.5 \cdot 10^{-4}$

5.2. Density

The ash density of both the samples was also calculated by Milazzo et al. [27], their results are given in Table 3.

Table 3. Ash densities

Sample ID	Density (kg/m^3)
1	1,594
2	832

5.3. Specific Surface Area and Voidage

The measurements of the specific surface area provided a very low S value, which was close to the sensitivity limit of the sorption apparatus; therefore further investigation would be required. However, the specific surface area can be actually considered with certainty lower than 2 m^2/g. The measured value is higher than that indicated for the sands by Jury and Horton [29], even if the size distribution analysis shows some analogies amongst the particles' size, reflecting probably a higher porosity for our samples. Further elaborations were performed, as indicated by Coulson et al. [20], to achieve the specific surface area; the calculation makes use of the following formula and is based on the assumption that the samples are composed of spherical and smooth particles (with the same dimensions):

$$S = \frac{6}{d \cdot \rho \cdot 1000} \qquad (10)$$

In equation (11) the diameter of the particle (*d*) is expressed in m, thus the calculated specific surface area (*S*) has the unit m^2/g.

The specific surface area was calculated using the average weighted diameter of the particles and, then, also their maximum and minimum values. The results are given in Table 4 and allowed verifying the influence of the particles' diameter and the specific surface area on the pressure drop.

Table 4. Specific surface area

Sample ID	S (m^2/g) BET method	S (m^2/g) Coulson et al. [20]		
		d = average weighted diameter	d = maximum diameter	d = minimum diameter
	S_{BET}	S_{av}	S_{min}	S_{max}
1	< 0.17	$9 \cdot 10^{-3}$	$1.9 \cdot 10^{-3}$	$3.8 \cdot 10^{-2}$
2	< 0.17	$1.3 \cdot 10^{-2}$	$3.3 \cdot 10^{-3}$	$4.5 \cdot 10^{-2}$

The results given in Section 5.1, related to the prevailing diameters for the particles, allowed estimating the voidage by using the plot *e* vs. *d* (Figure 7). The calculated average value of *e* (average weighted voidage) is ~ 0.392 for both the samples.

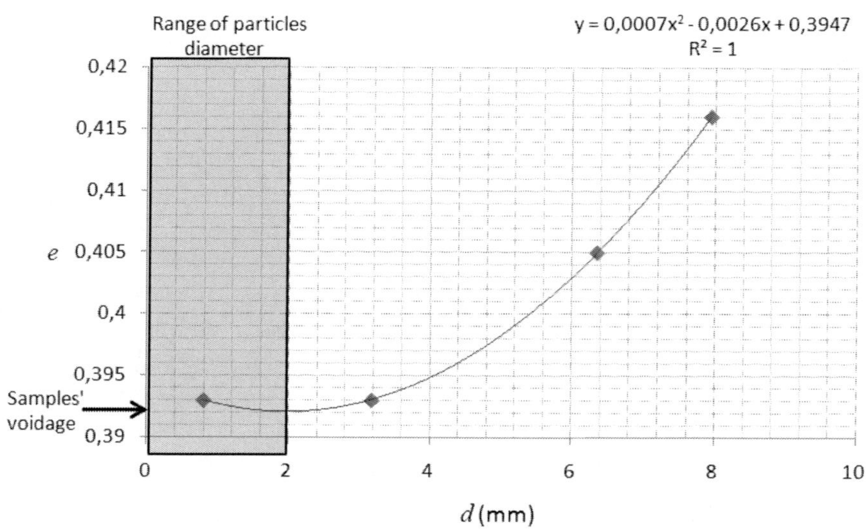

Figure 7. Voidage vs. diameter for spherical particles (data source: Coulson et al. [20]).

5.4. Permeability

The measurements made possible the calculation of *K*, which resulted close to $2.5 \cdot 10^{-5}$ m/s. It can be stated that the ash samples from Etna have an average permeability according to the International classification of soils, because *K* is comprised in the range $10^{-3} \div 10^{-5}$ m/s. The intrinsic permeability (*B*) was close to $2.4 \cdot 10^{-12}$ m^2.

5.5. Flow Regime for the Wastewater

By using some results from the ash characterisation and equations (2-4), the regime flow for the wastewater inside the pore channels was identified. The results are shown in Table 5, each case gave a transition regime flow.

Table 5. Flow characteristics

Sample ID	u_l (m/s)	S (m^{-1})	Re	Regime
1	1.79	S_{av}	82	Transition
2	1.79	S_{av}	95	Transition
1	1.79	S_{min}	384	Transition
2	1.79	S_{min}	384	Transition
1	1.79	S_{max}	19	Transition
2	1.79	S_{max}	29	Transition

5.6. Critical Ash Deposit on Fine Screens

Malfunctions and reductions of the stream flow-rate are defined by means of the screen's pressure drop (see also: Metcalf et al. [19]; Milazzo et al. [30]). The ΔP was calculated with the equation (1), by choosing the proper *C* value (typically 0.60 for clean screens, 0.40 for dirty screens and 0.25 for very dirty screens), thus results were:

- $\Delta P_o \sim 6570$ Pa (initial screen's pressure drop)
- $\Delta P_1 \sim 9850$ Pa (dirty screen pressure drop)
- $\Delta P_2 = 15760$ Pa (very dirty screen pressure drop)

It is worth noting that the extreme event, which is the total screen clogging, was not considered in this work, since cleaning operations were assumed to be executed before the occurrence of a total blockage.

As proposed in Section 5.3 and given the regime flows identified in Table 5, the thicknesses of the ash deposit on the screen were calculated by using the Carman equation. Results are shown in Table 6, where l_1 and l_2 are, respectively, the thicknesses of the ash deposit causing a pressure drop equal to ΔP_1 and ΔP_2. It can be evidenced that a very small quantity of ash is enough to clog this type of screen.

Table 6. Thickness of ash deposit

Sample ID	S (m^{-1})	$R'/(\rho \cdot u^2)$ (dimensionless)	l_1 (mm)	l_2 (mm)
1	S_{av}	0.32	< 1	< 1
2	S_{av}	0.30	< 1	< 1
1	S_{min}	0.23	~ 2	~ 4
2	S_{min}	0.23	~ 2	~ 4
1	S_{max}	0.56	< 1	< 1
2	S_{max}	0.46	< 1	< 1

5.7. Discussion

The deposit thicknesses causing the critical pressure drops are very small, in some cases these do not reach the value of 1 mm. This observation allows stating that the presence of few quantities of volcanic ash, with the characteristics similar to those emitted by Mt. Etna, causes instantly the system clogging. It should be underlined that the study was focused on fine screens because the size distribution analysis of the volcanic samples showed that these are the only typology able to retain such particles, even if fine screens are not always installed in wastewater treatments. If such screens are not included within the plant, the particles' removal is provided by grit chambers, these are also affected by the presence of ash but the study of such equipment is currently in progress [31].

Some comments can be made on the ash characteristics. The specific surface areas, identified through the BET method are very small, i.e., < 2 m^2/g. The BET measures, being very close to the sensitivity limit of the sorption apparatus, need of further investigations, thus a numerical calculation of S was also made by assuming a smooth and spherical shape and the same dimension for the particles. The calculation was carried out assuming that the diameter of the spheres is equal to the average weighted diameter and, subsequently, equal to the maximum and minimum diameter of the particles. It was found that S clearly increases as d decreases and, by assuming a constant diameter (as in the case of the maximum diameter, which is the same for both the samples), S is greater for the sample having a lower density (ID = 2), reflecting a higher porosity. It must evidenced that the sample 2 was collected at about 65 km away from the main crater, thus it is supposed that it is composed by light particles, which were transported at greater distances during the ash cloud dispersion. As regards the voidage, it was calculated by an extrapolation procedure from data of Coulson et al. [20]; but it must be recalled that in the range of prevailing diameters, identified by the size distribution analysis, the plot unfortunately does not provide a detail estimate. As shown in Figure 6, both the samples have approximately the same value of e.

By applying the approach for the calculation of the critical thicknesses, it was observed that the flow had always a transition regime; the increase of S (related to the decrease of the diameter of the particles) causes the decrease of the Reynolds number up to bring the flow close to the laminar regime. It must be recalled that S rises also as the porosity increases. Consequently, the critical thickness increases with the decrease of S and, thus, with the increase of d. Finally the increase of the voidage of the particles increases also the accumulation of ash, further details on this investigations are given [30].

CONCLUSION

In this chapter the conditions leading to failures or malfunctions of screens, with the respect to the phenomenon of volcanic ash emission, were determined. The estimation of the threshold amounts of ash causing the reduction of functionality of fine screens was made for a case-study in the surrounding of Mt. Etna, by using literature data and experimental results from the ash characterisation.

The study is based on two main assumptions: (*i*) the sewage characteristics were assumed to be equal to those of water, and (*ii*) the particles were assumed having a smooth and spherical shape and the same size. Even if these approximations were necessary to simplify the application of the proposed approach, the results gave a valid support in addressing alternative solutions for the ash removal and more efficient management (frequent cleaning operations).

Finally the work provided the base for the construction of the vulnerability maps related to these facilities located in the area affected by the fallout of volcanic ash, according to the methodology presented by Milazzo et al. [8].

REFERENCES

[1] Cruz, A. M.; Steinberg, L. J.; Arellano, A. L. V.; Nordvik, J. P.; Pisano, F. State of the art in Natech risk management. Report no. 21292, *European Commission Directorate General Joint Research Centre*, EUR, 2004.

[2] Tang, A. Izmit (Kocaeli), Turkey, earthquake of August 17, 1999 including Duzce earthquake of November 12, 1999: lifeline performance; *American Society of Civil Engineers: Reston, US*, 2000.

[3] Erdik M. Seismic design practice into the next century: research and application; Proceedings of the Sixth SECED Conference on seismic design practice into the next century: Oxford, UK, 1998.

[4] Zais, D. May 18, 1980: The Day the Sky Fell Managing the Mt. St. Helens Volcanic Ashfall on Yakima, Washington, U.S.A. [available online: www.volcanoes.usgs.gov; accessed 06.08.2014].

[5] De Rademaeker, E.; Suter, G.; Pasman, H.; Fabiano, B. Process Saf Environ 2014, in press, doi: 10.1016/j.psep.2014.03.007.

[6] Antonioni, G.; Bonvicini, S.; Spadoni, G.; Cozzani, V. *Reliab. Eng. Syst. Safe* 2009, 94, 1442-1450.

[7] Girgin, S.; Krausmann, E. *J. Loss Prevent. Proc.* 2013, 26, 949-960.

[8] Milazzo, M. F.; Ancione, G.; Salzano, E.; Maschio, G. J Risk Res 2014, in press, doi: 10.1080/13669877.2014.961515.

[9] Spence, R. J. S.; Baxter, P. J.; Zuccaro, G. *J. Volcanol Geoth. Res.* 2004, 133, 321-343.

[10] Rasà R.; Tripodo A.; Casella S.; Szilagyi M. L. Contributi alla valutazione della pericolosità e rischio vulcanico nell'area etnea ed alla mitigazione dei danni attesi. Carta Tematica di Rischio Vulcanico della Regione Sicilia Ed. C.R.P.R. - Regione Sicilia Palermo, 2007, (in Italian).

[11] Baxter, P. J.; Bernstein, R. S.; Falk, H.; French, J.; Ing, R. Disasters, 1982, 6, 268-276.
[12] Milazzo, M. F.; Ancione, G.; Basco, A.; Lister, D.; Salzano, E.; Maschio, G. Nat Hazards 2013, 66, 939-953, doi: 10.1007/s11069-012-0518-5.
[13] Milazzo, M. F.; Ancione, G.; Salzano, E.; Maschio, G. Reliab Eng Syst Safe 2013, 120, 106-110, doi: 10.1016/j.ress.2013.05.008.
[14] Milazzo, M. F.; Ancione, G.; Salzano, E.; Maschio, G. Chem Eng Trans 2013, 31, 901-906, doi: 10.3303/CET1331151.
[15] Ancione, G.; Salzano, E.; Maschio, G.; Milazzo, M. F. Chem Eng Trans 2014, 36, 433-438, doi: 10.3303/CET1436073.
[16] Rensselaer Polytechnic Institute web-site: [http://www.rpi.edu/; accessed 08.08.2014].
[17] USEPA 2003. Wastewater Technology Fact Sheet. Screening and Grit Removal. Document no. EPA832-F-03-011 [available online: http://www.epa.gov/ owm/mtb/ mtbfact.htm; accessed 06.08.2014]
[18] Blong, R. J. Volcanic hazards: a sourcebook on the effects of eruptions; Academic Press: Sydney, AU, 1984.
[19] Metcalf, L.; Eddy, H. P.; Tchobanoglous, G. Wastewater engineering: treatment, disposal, and reuse; McGraw-Hill: New York, US, 2004.
[20] Coulson, J. M.; Richardson, J. F.; Backhurst, J. R.; Harker, J. H. Chemical engineering: Particle technology and separation processes, (5th ed.); Butterworth-Heinemann: Oxford, UK 2002; Vol. 2, pp 191-203.
[21] Coulson, J. M.; Richardson, J. F.; Backhurst, J. R. Chemical Engineering: Fluid flow, heat transfer, and mass transfer (6th ed.); Butterworth-Heinemann: Oxford, UK, 1999; Vol. 1, pp 195-212.
[22] EN 1097-3. Tests for mechanical and physical properties of aggregates - Part 3: Determination of loose bulk density and voids.
[23] ASTM D 2434. Standard Test Method for Permeability of Granular Soils (Constant Head).
[24] Palumbo A. *J. Volcanol. Geoth. Res.* 1998, 83, 167-171.
[25] Global Volcanism Program web-site [http://www.volcano.si.edu/; accessed 07.08. 2014].
[26] Branca S.; Del Carlo P. Eruptions of Mt. Etna during the past 3,200 years: a revised compilation integrating the historical and stratigraphic records. "Mt. Etna: Volcano Laboratory" *Geophys. Monogr.* 2004, 143, 1-27.

[27] Milazzo, M. F.; Primerano, P.; Ancione, G.; Salzano, E.; Maschio, G. Chem Eng Trans 2014, 36, 487-492; doi: 10.3303/CET1436082.

[28] Krumbein, W. C. Size frequency distributions of sediments. *J. Sediment Petrol.* 1934, 4, 65–77.

[29] Jury, W. A.; Horton, R. *Soil. Physics.* Wiley & Sons, 2004.

[30] Milazzo M. F.; Ancione G.; Salzano E.; Maschio G. Study of volcanic Na-Tech risks in primary wastewater treatments. *Proceeding European Safety & Reliability Conference*, ESREL 2014, Wroclaw, PL, 2014.

[31] Ancione G.; Milazzo M. F.; Salzano E.; Maschio G. The impact of volcanic ash fallout on industrial facilities: Natural-Technological hazards in wastewater treatments (Grit removal). Volcanic Ash: *Chemical Composition, Environmental Impact and Health Risks; Nova Publication, in preparation.*

In: Volcanic Eruptions
Editor: Trent Milburn
ISBN: 978-1-63463-308-6

Chapter 2

A Possible Link between Sun's Variability and Volcanic Activity

Paolo Madonia[1*], Francesco Parello[2†] and Dalila Pitarresi[2]

[1]Istituto Nazionale di Geofisica e Vulcanologia, Sez. di Palermo, Palermo, Italia

[2]Università degli Studi di Palermo, Dipartimento di Scienze della Terra e del Mare (DiSTeM), Palermo, Italia

Abstract

Sun inconstancy has the ability to control global climate, that in turn acts as a trigger for volcanic activity. Looking for possible Sun-Earth connections we analysed the time distribution of eruptions of volcanoes located on the northern hemisphere, from the Caribbean Sea to the East Mediterranean Sea, with a particular detail on the most active Italian volcanoes. The compared analysis between sunspot and volcanic cycles suggested that volcanic eruptions are more frequent during minima of Sun activity, with about 3 eruptions out of 4 occurring at relative minima of the quasi-11 year Sun cycle. Not so evident are the long term (centennial time scale) relationships between Sun and volcanic system variability: since the former is controlled by much more complex mechanisms the analysis of correlations between eruptions and Sun

* Email: paolo.madonia@ingv.it; Via Ugo La Malfa 153, 90146 Palermo, Italia.
† Email: parello@unipa.it; Via Archirafi 36, 90123 Palermo, Italia.

activity cannot prescind from geodynamical discriminants, which play a fundamental role in driving magma migration toward the Earth's surface.

INTRODUCTION

One of the most evident influences of Sun inconstancy on Earth's natural systems and cycles is its ability to control global climate. This happens through three main processes (Krivova and Solanki, 2004): (i) variations in total irradiance, (ii) changes in stratospheric chemistry due to changes in UV irradiance and (iii) changes in cloud cover caused by sun-induced variations in cosmic ray flux.

The combination of these processes has been the main responsible for the global warming/cooling cycles of the planet Earth until the XIX century at least, when anthropogenic emissions of greenhouse gases started to play a relevant role as modulators of the global climatic system. Anthropogenic disturbances apart, maxima of solar activity correspond to warm periods and vice-versa; the most evident sign of increased solar activity is the increased number of sunspots, whose main cycle has a period of quasi-11 years.

Global climate and/or local weather at minor scale may influence volcanic activity, triggering eruptions and/or unrest episodes. Mason et al. (2004) analysed global volcanic activity during the last three hundred years, highlighting its seasonality at a statistically significant degree. This pattern was observed mainly along the Pacific "Ring of Fire" and more locally at some other volcanoes. In the author's opinion, the pattern of seasonality is caused by the annual Earth surface deformation that accompanies the movement of surface water mass during the hydrological cycle. Neuberg (2000) studied records of seismovolcanic activity from different volcanoes, including Stromboli. The comparison of these signals with theoretical body tides in the spectral domain revealed strong evidence against a correlation between seismovolcanic activity and tidal stress. By contrast, other parameters such as air temperature and barometric pressure showed the same diurnal and semi-diurnal time patterns of seismicity and may be then considered as possible external modulators of volcanic activity. Mc Guire et al. (1997) analysed the frequency of explosive activity of Mediterranean volcanoes, based on dated tephra layers in deep-sea sediment cores, and its relationship with the rate of late Quaternary sea-level changes. They found a nonlinear correlation between the two parameters, tentatively explained in terms of dynamic responses of the volcanoes to stress changes at various spatial scales.

The ultimate mechanism was identified on climate-driven growth and decay of large ice sheets, which can influence the eruptive chronologies of distant volcanic edifices via changes in global sea level. In particular, the authors highlighted a marked low of explosive eruptions from Mt. Etna during a sea-level stand occurred between 22 and 15 ky B.P. Rampino et al. (1979) found a major volcanic eruption frequency coinciding with cooling trends of decadal or longer duration. The driving mechanism was identified in variations in climate leading to stress changes on the earth's crust, for instance by loading and unloading of ice and water masses and by axial and spin-rate changes that might augment volcanic potential.

Similar findings were retrieved by Kutterolf et al. (2013), which detected Milankovitch periodicities in ash plume deposits recorded in marine sediments along the Pacific Ring of Fire. They identified variability in volcanic activity, driven by crustal stress changes associated with ice age mass redistribution, supporting the idea of a causal link between climatic variations, continental stress field, and volcanism.

The common conclusion of the above mentioned studies is that volcanic processes can be influenced by climatic changes. Since these are controlled by solar cycles, theoretically Sun's activity might influence volcanic activity via the Earth's climate. The exploration of this theoretical link entails giant problems, due to the extreme complexity of climate and geodynamic systems. What we propose in this paper is a basic "black box" approach, aimed to highlight preliminary clues of a possible link between solar and volcanic activities.

Methods

We considered onset dates of eruptions and unrests of volcanoes from 6 different areas, located along a West-East transect, extended in latitude between 10°N and 40°N: Caribbean Sea, Cape Verde Islands, Azores Islands, Canary Islands, Italy and Greece (Figure 1): volcanoes of the South Italian volcanic district (Vesuvio, Etna, Stromboli and Vulcano islands) have been particularly detailed. The structure of the analyzed volcanic database has been determined accounting for: i) limited extension in latitude for avoiding too huge differences in the coupled Sun-Earth system; ii) their location in islands or in close proximity of sea coast, i.e., in areas strongly influenced by sea level changes, invoked by McGuire et al. (1997) as the main climate-driven parameter potentially able to trigger volcanic activity; iii) the availability of a reliable and well documented historical record of their eruptions (especially Etna, with a little less than 150 eruptions occurred.

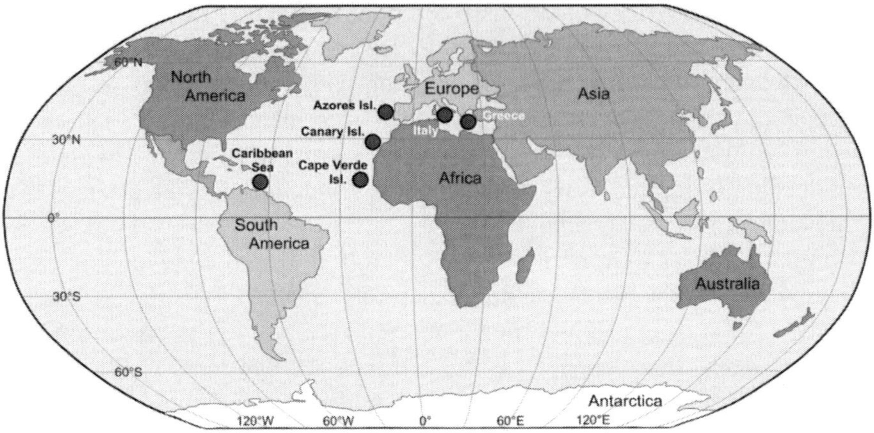

Figure 1. Location of the studied volcanic areas.

Onset dates of volcanic eruptions reported in this study derive from the Smithsonian Institution Global Volcanic Program on-line catalogue, available at the URL http://www.volcano.si.edu/, integrated with the data published by Arrighi et al. (2001) for Vesuvio, Capaldi et al. (1978) and Giacomelli and Scandone (2007) for Stromboli.

The sources for the number of sunspots are the graphs published by Lanzerotti (2001) and Vaquero (2007), integrated for the most recent period (2000-2010) with the data published online by the Australian Space Weather Agency at the URL: www.ips.gov.au/Solar/1/6.

VOLCANOLOGICAL SETTING OF THE STUDIED AREAS

In order to achieve if the geodynamic context in which a volcanic edifice is located has a relevance or not in its possible response to Sun variability, the main characteristics of each studied area are briefly outlined hereafter, moving from the Caribbean Sea to Greece.

Volcanism of Caribbean Sea is linked to the Lesser Antilles island arc, about 850 km long with a curvature radius of about 450 km. The Lesser Antilles arc results from the subduction of the Atlantic beneath the Caribbean plate, with relatively slow current convergence rates (2–4 cm/y) as reported by

Feuillet et al. (2002), and magma productivity between 3 and 5 km^3/m.y./km (MacDonald et al., 2000). Volcanism along the arc started ~40 m.y. ago (Bouysse et al., 1990).

The volcanic Cape Verde Archipelago is located in the East Central Atlantic, 600 to 900 km from the western African coast. Composed of 10 principal islands and some islets, Cape Verde Rise represents a hotspot swell, associated with an underlying mantle plume, by dynamic uplift (Pim et al., 2008) and characterized by low magma production rates with some 0.026 km^3 y^{-1} of magma added to the crust, corresponding to a volume flux of ≈28 m^3 s^{-1} , which is only ≈9% of the one calculated for Hawaii (Holm et al., 2008).

The Canary archipelago comprises seven main volcanic islands and several islets that form a chain extending for ~500 km across the eastern Atlantic, with its eastern edge only 100 km from the NW African coast. The Canary Islands developed in a geodynamic setting characterized by oceanic lithosphere formed during the first stage of opening of the Atlantic at 180-150 Ma and lying close to the passive continental margin of the African plate. Magmatic activity in the Canary Islands started during the Cretaceous and subaerial volcanism during the Miocene (Carracedo et al., 2002). It is generally assumed that the archipelago originated from residual old plume material in the upper mantle. On the other hand, the long period of eruptive activity in this archipelago (> 20 Ma in some islands), their morphological and structural features, seismic signature and geochemical evolution present problems for that model (Hoernle and Schmincke, 1993). A comprehensive model is proposed by Viñuela (http://www.mantleplumes.org/WebpagePDFs/Canary.pdf), suggesting that magmatic systems are feed by a mantle anomaly, but tensional stages generate fractures that work as preferential pathways for magma liberation, whereas tectonic compressive phases produce island uplifts.

The Azores archipelago is located in the North Atlantic Ocean at about 1500 km from the European continent and 3900 km from the North America east coast. It is formed by nine volcanic islands and a few islets, dispersed along a 600 km NW-SE direction axis. The islands rise from the so called Azores Plateau, a thick and irregular area of the oceanic crust roughly limited by the 2000 meters bathymetric curve (Gente et al., 2003). The islands are associated with a region of positive gravity and residual depth anomaly, which has been interpreted as the surface expression of a mantle plume in the zone where the American, Eurasian and Nubian lithospheric plates meet, forming the Azores Triple Junction (Searle, 1980; Luís *et al.*, 1994, McKenzie and O'Nions, 1995). The genesis of the magmas building the Azores has been attributed to an enriched mantle source (Yang et al., 2006). However, the geological evolution of the islands appears to have been greatly influenced by regional deformation, in particular by sea-floor spreading along the Mid-Atlantic ridge, and distension/transtension along the diffuse boundary between the Nubian and the Eurasian plates (Haase and Beier, 2003).

The Italian peninsula is one of the most complex geodynamic settings on Earth (Doglioni et al., 1999; Wezel, 1985). One expression of this complexity is the wide variety of Plio-Quaternary magmatism in Italy, that ranges from ultrabasic to acid and from sub-alkaline to ultra-alkaline, covering almost entirely the compositional field of igneous rocks occurring worldwide. In the present study we considered the most active volcanoes during the last centuries: Vesuvio, Etna, Stromboli and Vulcano.

Vesuvio is a composite volcanic system comprising the Vesuvio cone, the main present elevation of the volcanic edifice (1281 m a.s.1.) formed after the famous 79 A.D. plinian eruption that destroyed the roman cities of Ercolano and Pompei, and the pre-existing Mt. Somma caldera. Vesuvio eruptive activity has been characterized by the alternation between quiescent and active phases, lasting up to several centuries. During the active phases, both effusive and explosive eruptions occurred. In the period 79-1631 A.D. only two major explosive eruptions took place, in 472 and 1631 A.D. After the 1631 eruption, numerous effusive episodes occurred until the last one in 1944, often accompanied by explosive phases with production of tephra deposits volumetrically smaller than those of the Middle Age (Arrighi et al., 2001).

Etna is the largest subaerial active volcano in Europe, with an elliptical base of 38x47 km and a maximum elevation of about 3300 m. Throughout its eruptive history, started about 200 ky B.P. and accredited for more than 230 eruptions since historical sources are available, Etna has been characterized by a dominant effusive activity, even if pyroclastic deposits are common in the Holocene sequence.

Stromboli is a strato-volcano that rises 3000 m from the floor of the southern Tyrrhenian Sea up to a maximum elevation of 924 m a.s.l.. It is considered one of the most active volcanoes in the world because of its persistent mild explosive activity, known as strombolian activity, that is going on almost for the last 2000 years. This normal activity is episodically interrupted by lava effusions and more violent explosions, which are referred to as major explosions and paroxysms (Barberi et al., 1993).

Vulcano island is located along a NW-SE–trending strike-slip fault system and owes its present behaviour to multiple collapse and cone-growth phases that succeeded along its eruptive history (Peccerillo et al., 2006). The most recent volcanic cycle began 6 ky B.P. and built up the “La Fossa” cone (about

450 m a.s.l.), whose last eruption lasted from 1888 to 1890 A.D. At present, Vulcano is characterized by shallow seismicity and intense fumarolic activity.

Volcanism of Greece is linked to the Aegean region, where the African plate subducts beneath the Eurasian plate forming the Aegean volcanic arc, (Fytikas et al.,1985; Keller, 1982). The Aegean volcanic arc comprises the smaller volcanic centers of Sousaki, Aegina, Poros and Methana, and the larger accumulations of Milos, Santorini, Nisyros, Yali and Kos. Erupted lavas of these volcanoes are late-Miocene to Quaternary in age. Methana, Nisyros and Santorini have records of eruptions during historical times (Fytikas et al., 1985).

The geodynamic characterization of the volcanic areas delineated by the above discussed references is summarized in Table 1.

Table 1. Summary of geodynamic characterization of the studied volcanic areas (see main text for references)

Volcanic area	Geodynamic context
Caribbean Sea	Subduction
Cape Verde islands	Hot spot (mantle source)
Canary islands	Complex (mantle source modified by regional tectonic)
Azores islands	Complex (mantle plume, seafloor spreading, plate motion)
Vesuvio	Subduction
Etna	Intraplate (mantle source unmodified by subduction
Stromboli	Subduction
Vulcano	Subduction
Aegean Sea	Subduction

TIME DISTRIBUTION OF VOLCANIC ACTIVITY COMPARED TO SUN CYCLES

In the evaluation of the possible coupling between Sun cycles and volcanic activity the approach we followed was the "black.-box" model: we simply compared the time patterns of eruptions and sunspot number (hereafter referred as Ss), looking for any possible link between these two. In doing this we focused a particular attention on volcanic cycles (hereafter referred as VCs), i.e., any group of at least three consecutive eruptions whose time occurrence rate was clearly higher with respect to adjacent periods, in these

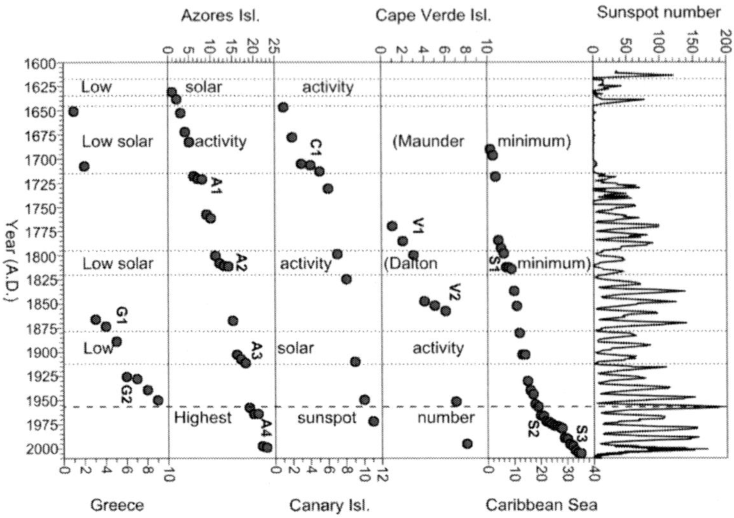

Figure 2a. From the right to the left: sunspot number, cumulative number of eruptions in the Caribbean Sea, Cape Verde Islands, Canary Islands, Azores Islands and Greece. Volcanic cycles for each area (three consecutive eruptions at least) were identified by progressively numbered abbreviations.

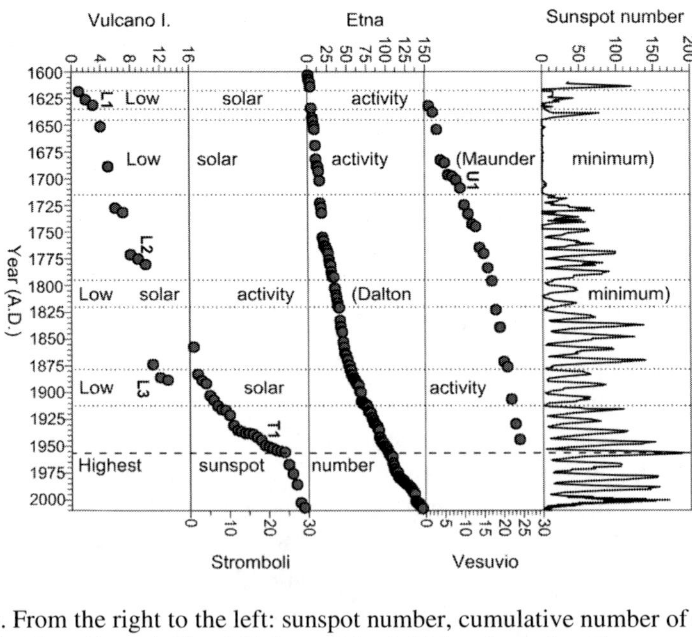

Figure 2b. From the right to the left: sunspot number, cumulative number of eruptions of Vesuvio, Etna, Stromboli and Vulcano Island. Volcanic cycles (three consecutive eruptions at least) were identified by progressively numbered abbreviations.

including prolonged absence of volcanic activity. For a better evidence of VCs we plotted eruptions using a cumulative curve. Data from volcanoes located in the same area were grouped together and presented in Figure 2a, with the exception of Italy where, due to the highest detail, we considered each volcano separately (Figure 2b).

Based on the two above mentioned figures a total of 17 VCs were recognized, 3 in the Caribbean Sea, 2 in Cape Verde Isl., 1 in Canary Isl., 4 in Azores Isl. and a total of 5 in Italy: 1 at Vesuvio, 1 at Stromboli and 3 at Vulcano Isl.; the Etna record is so continuous that no differentiation in VCs can be done. Comparing VCs frequencies with centennial Ss variations, 8 VCs out of the total of 17 occurred during periods of reduced solar activity, 7 at maxima and the remaining 2 during variable periods. If VCs are grouped for each of the 6 volcanic areas, Canary Isl., Azores Isl. and Italy show higher frequencies during solar minima (1 out of 1, 3 out of 4 and 3 out of 5, respectively), the Caribbean during maxima (2 out of 3), Cape Verde Isl. and Greece both during minima and maxima. Accordingly to the above considerations, no systematic relationships between volcanic activity and centennial Sun cycles can be assessed.

The next step consisted in subdividing the eruptions for different classes of Ss, i.e., associating to each eruption onset date the corresponding Ss observed on the Sun. Results are plotted on the bar chart of Figure 3. As shown in the figure, the distribution of eruptions upsets that one of Ss, with the 73% of eruptions occurred when sunspot number was lower than 60, condition under which the Sun spent the 76% of its time. The strong similarity of the two frequency distributions suggests the absence of any cause-effect relationship between the two parameters, since the probability that an eruption occurs during low Ss phases is higher just because the Sun spends the most of its time under this condition.

Conversely, the clue of a possible link between VCs and Sun cycles is more evident if intra- quasi-11 year cycle variations of Ss are considered. Due to the huge variability of the quasi-11 year cycles, whose range between minima and maxima varies between 0 and 200 ca, the absolute sunspot number could be not indicative. As illustrated in the sketch at the upper left corner of Figure 4, the same absolute value of Ss may correspond to the upper or the lower half of two different cycles, characterized by different Ss ranges.

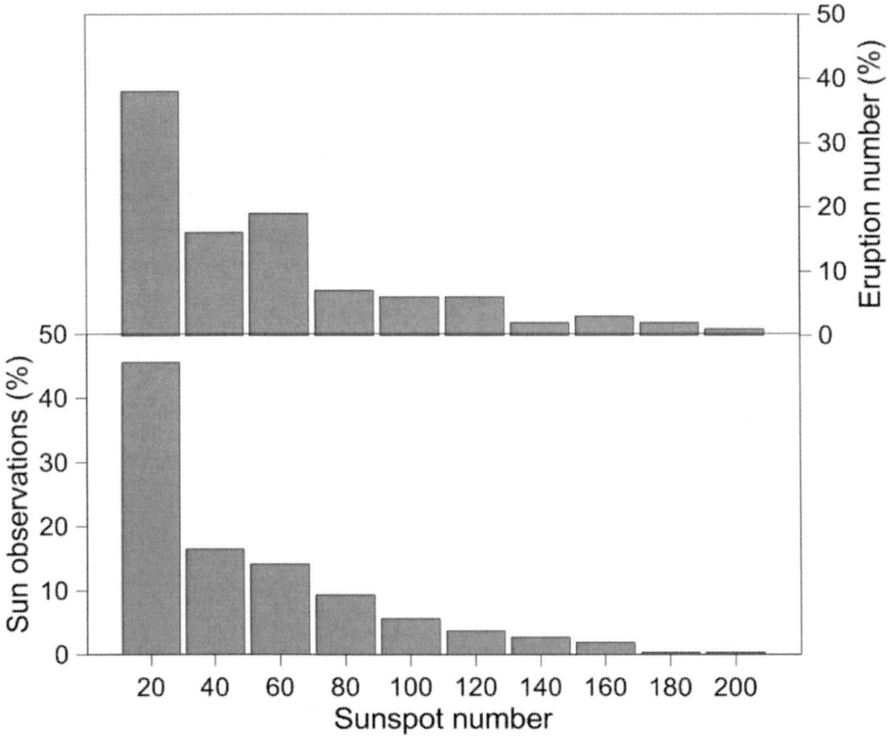

Figure 3. From the top to the bottom, numbers of eruptions and sun observations grouped for rising classes of sunspot number (values are expressed in %).

Thus, each quasi-11 year cycle was subdivided in two halves, using the median peak amplitude as a divide between the low and high part of the cycle; eruptions were then classified on the basis of their position within the peak. As evidenced in Figure 4, the highest frequencies of eruptions are observed during relative minima of quasi-11 year Sun cycles in all the considered areas. Canary Isl. showed the wider differences, with 90.9 % of the eruptions occurred during lower half peaks against 9.1 % during the higher ones, whereas Stromboli has the lowest differences, with 55.2% and 44.8 respectively. In total, 71.9% of the eruptions took place during quasi-11 year cycle minima and only 28.1% during maxima.

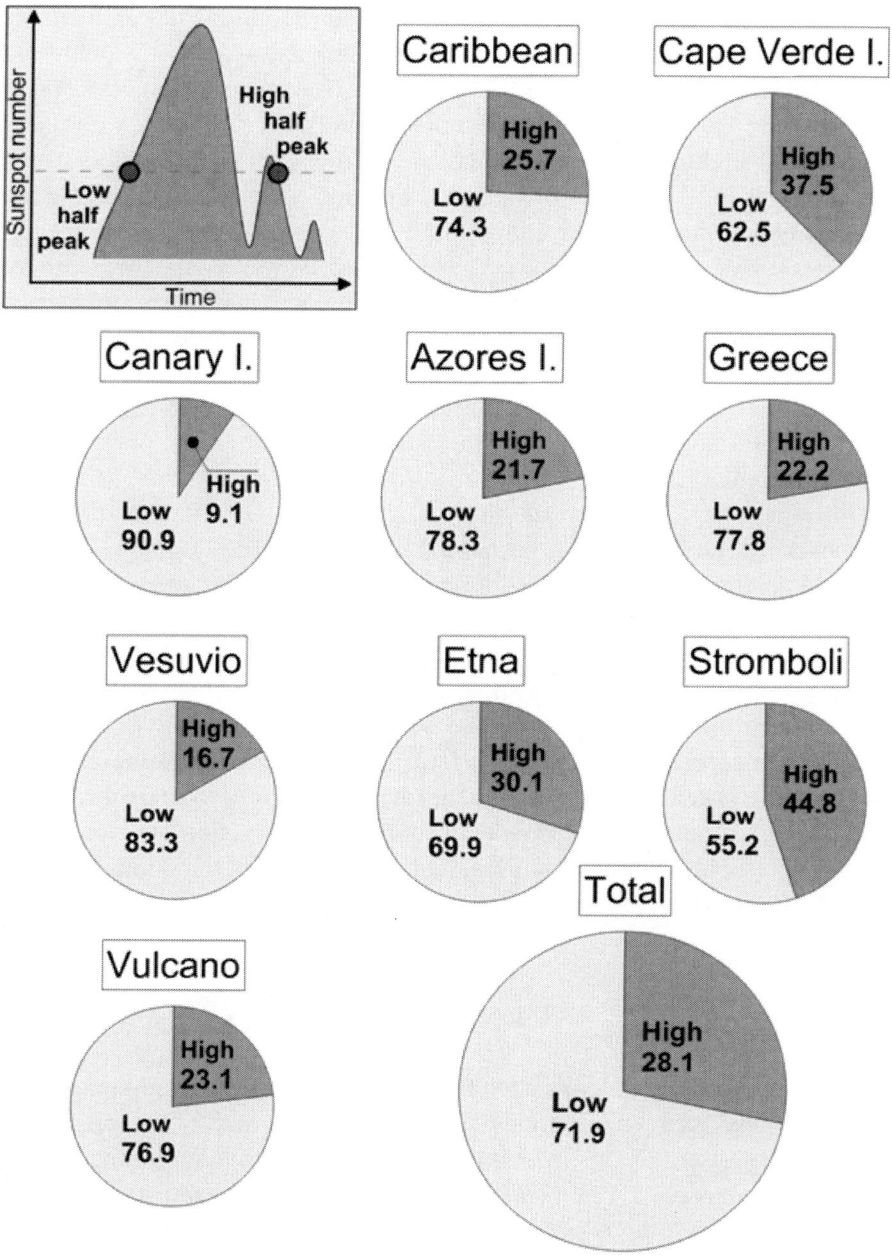

Figure 4. Pie charts showing the classification of eruptions according to their position on the corresponding quasi-11 year solar cycle (upper or lower halves of the cycle, as illustrated in the sketch in the upper left corner).

This finding could suggest that Earth's climate variability, driven by Sun's cycle, could affect at a certain extent volcanic activity. Most of the published papers on the relationship between climate and volcanic eruptions (Mason et al., 2004; Mc Guire et al., 1997; Rampino et al., 1979) point to a common opinion: global climate and related sea level changes act as modulators of the stress field acting on the Earth's crust, triggering volcanic eruptions by the variation of confining pressures, promoting the ascent of fresh magma batches and destabilizing already weakened volcanoes. However, the response of volcanoes to Sun cycles is not unambiguous. Sun activity is only an external force able to lower the eruptive energetic threshold of a volcano while it is following its own evolution, in its turn driven by lithospheric parameters like plate motion rate and rheology, regional seismic activity and so on. These latter are fully independent of the Sun's state, so eruptions can occur also in absence of Sun anomalies.

In other words, volcanoes are characterized by different energetic thresholds whose overcoming can lead to unrests and eruptions. If the threshold is low, they can be significantly influenced by solar activity: a volcano that is following its own evolution, completely independent of the Sun, will overcome the unrest threshold and erupt in close time relation with Ss cycles. Conversely, if the threshold is high, Sun activity will affect it only at a very little extent and a volcano will erupt at a certain time that is completely independent of Sun state. Last, if a volcano is pulsating at a very low background activity, far from the threshold, an impulsive energetic trigger like a strong earthquake could suddenly enhance its energetic state close to the eruptive threshold, whose overcoming can now occur via the combination of Sun and volcanic activity oscillations.

CONCLUSION

Volcanic systems are controlled by complex mechanisms and the analysis of correlations between eruptions and Sun activity cannot prescind from geodynamical discriminants, which play a fundamental role in driving magma migration toward the Earth's surface. Despite the complications induced by geodynamic factors, the compared analysis between Ss cycles and frequency of eruptions suggests that volcanic eruptions are more frequent during minima of Sun's quasi-11 year cycle, when about 3 eruptions out of 4 occurred in the studied area. This finding can be interpreted as a preliminary clue that Earth's climate variability, driven by Sun's cycle, could act as a possible trigger for volcanic activity. However, since this effect is a mere external forcing of the eruptive energetic threshold of a volcano, a direct link between eruptions and Sun's cycles must be excluded. Sun's activity cannot awaken a dormant volcano, but it could trigger the onset of an eruption in a volcano that is independently undergoing pre-eruptive conditions.

REFERENCES

Arrighi S, Principe C, Rosi M (2001) Violent strombolian and subplinian eruptions at Vesuvius during post-1631 activity. *B Volcanol* 63:126-150 doi: 10.1007ls004450100130.

Barberi F, Rosi M, Sodi A (1993) Volcanic hazard assessment at Stromboli based on review of historical data. *Acta Vulcanol* 3:173-187

Bouysse P, Westercamp D (1990) Subduction of Atlantic aseismic ridges and late Cenozoic evolution of the Lesser Antilles island arc. Tectonophysics 175:349–380 doi:10.1016/0040-1951(90)90180-G

Capaldi G, Del Pezzo E, Ghiara MR, Guerra I, La Volpe L, Lirer L, Lo Bascio A, Luongo G, Martini M, Munno R, Pece R, Rapolla A, Scarpa R (1978) Stromboli and its 1975 eruption. *B Volcanol* 41(3):259-285

Carracedo JC, Pérez FJ, Ancochea E, Meco J, Hernán F, Cubas CR, Casillas R, Rodriguez E, Ahijado A (2002) Cenozoic volcanism II: The Canary Islands, in Gibbons W, Moreno T (eds) The Geology of Spain. The Geological Society of London, UK, pp. 439-472

Doglioni C, Harabaglia P, Merlini S, Mongelli F, Peccerillo A, Piromallo C (1999). Orogens and slabs vs their direction of subduction. *Earth-Sci Rev* 45:167-208.

Feuillet N, Manighetti I, Tapponnier P, Jacques E (2002) Arc parallel extension and localization of volcanic complexes in Guadeloupe, Lesser Antilles. J Geophys Res 107:1-29 doi:10.1029/2001JB000308

Fytikas M, Innocenti F, Manetti P, Mazzuoli R, Peccerillo A, Villari L (1985) Tertiary to Quaternary evolution of the volcanism in the Aegean region, in Dixon JE, Robertson AHF (eds) The Geological Evolution of the Eastern Mediterranean. Blackwell Publ., Oxford, UK

Gente P, Dyment J, Maia M, Goslin J (2003). Interactions between the MAR and the Azores hot spot during the last 85 Myr: emplacement and rifting of the hot spot-derived plateaus. *Geochem Geophy Geosy* 4:1-23 doi: 10.1029/2003GC000527

Giacomelli L, Scandone R (2007) *Vulcani d'Italia.* Liguori, Napoli, Italy.

Haase KM, Beier C (2003) Tectonic control of ocean island basalt sources on São Miguel, Azores. Geophy Res Lett 30(16) doi: 10.1029 /2003GL017500.

Hoernle KAJ, Schmincke HU (1993) The role of partial melting in the 15-Ma geochemical evolution of Gran Canaria: A blob model for the Canary hotspot. *J Petrol* 34:599-626.

Holm PM, Grandvuinet T, Friis J, Wilson JR, Barker AK, Plesner S (2008) An 40Ar-39Ar study of the Cape Verde hot spot: Temporal evolution in a semistationary plate environment. *J Geophys Res* 113:B08201.

Keller J (1982) Mediterranean island arcs, in Thorpe RS, Wiley J (eds) Andesites. Chichester, UK, pp. 307-325

Krivova NA, Solanki SK (2004) Solar variability and global warming: a statistical comparison since 1850. *Adv Space Res* 34:361-364.

Kutterolf S, Jegen M, Mitrovica JX, Kwasnitschka T, Freundt A, Huybers PJ (2013) A detection of Milankovitch frequencies in global volcanic activity. Geology 41(2):227-230

Lanzerotti LJ (2001) Space weather effects on technologies, in Song P, Singer HJ, Siscoe GL (eds) *Space Weather. Geoph Monog Series*, vol. 125, AGU, Washington D.C., USA, pp. 11-22.

Luis JF, Miranda JM, Galdeano A, Patriat P, Rossignol J, Mendes C, Victor LA (1994) The Azores triple junction evolution since 10 Ma from aeromagnetic survey of the Mid-Atlantic Ridge. *Earth Planet Sc Lett* 125:439-459.

Mason BG, Pyle DM, Dade WB, Jupp T (2004) Seasonality of volcanic eruptions. J Geophys Res 109:B04206 doi: 10.1029/2002JB002293

Macdonald R, Hawkesworth CJ, Heath E (2000) The Lesser Antilles volcanic chain: a study in arc magmatism. *Earth-Sci Rev* 49:1-76.

McGuire WJ, Howarth RJ, Firth CR, Solow AR, Pulle AD, Saunders SJ, Stewart IS, Vita-Finzi C (1997) Correlation between rate of sea-level change and frequency of explosive volcanism in the Mediterranean. *Nature* 389:473-476 doi: 10.1038/38998

McKenzie D, O'Nions RK (1995) The source regions of ocean island basalts. *J Petrol* 36:133-159.

Neuberg J (2000) External modulation of volcanic activity. *Geophys J Int* 142:232-240.

Peccerillo A, Frezzotti ML, De Astis G, Ventura G (2006) Modeling the magma plumbing system of Vulcano (Aeolian Islands, Italy) by integrated fluid-inclusion geobarometry, petrology, and geophysics. *Geology* 34:17-20 doi: 10.1130/g22117.1

Pim J, Peirce C, Watts AB, Grevemeyer I, Krabbenhoft A (2008) Crustal structure and the origin of the Cape Verdes Rise. *Earth Planet Sc Lett* 272:422-428.

Rampino MR, Self S, Fairbridge RW (1979) Can Rapid Climatic Change Cause Volcanic Eruptions?. *Science* 206(4420):826-829 doi: 10.1126/science.206.4420.826.

Searle RC (1980) Tectonic pattern of the Azores spreading center and triple junction. *Earth Planet Sc Lett* 51:415-434.

Vaquero JM (2007) Historical sunspot observations: A review. *Adv Space Res* 40(7):929-941 doi: 10.1016/j.asr.2007.01.087.

Wezel FC (1985) Structural Features and Basin Tectonics of the Tyrrhenian Sea, in Stanley DJ, Wezel FC (eds) *Geological Evolution of the Mediterranean Basin*. Springer-Verlag, New York, USA, pp. 153-194.

Yang T, Shen Y, Van der Lee S, Solomon SC, Hung SH (2006) Upper mantle structure beneath the Azores hotspot from finite-frequency seismic tomography. *Earth Planet Sc Lett* 250:11-26.

In: Volcanic Eruptions
Editor: Trent Milburn

ISBN: 978-1-63463-308-6

Chapter 3

EXTREME POINTER YEARS IN TREE-RING RECORDS OF CENTRAL SPAIN AS EVIDENCE OF THE ERUPTION OF THE HUAYNAPUTINA VOLCANO (PERU, 1600 AD)

Mar Génova Fuster*
Universidad Politécnica de Madrid, Spain

ABSTRACT

The interpretation of the pointer years in tree-ring records depends on their position in the dendrochronological sequences and on their significance. It has been demonstrated that the pointer years, which present themselves over wide geographical areas, tend to be associated with determinate macro-climatic events. Several studies have related negative pointer years to macro-climatic events on a global scale, such as those derived from major volcanic eruptions. Here are presented the results matching the negative pointer year's record of *Pinus sylvestris* tree-ring chronologies with those determined in certain historical timber in the central Iberian Peninsula (Spain). Today there is an extensive *Pinus sylvestris* dendrochronological database in central Spain that has enabled the development of a regional chronology extended from 1513 to 2005. Finding that the probable time span of the studied wood coming from the Royal Old Mint of Segovia, which was built using these nearby pine

* mar.genova@upm.es

forest, these historical woods have been crossdated with the oldest tree-ring series of this dendrochronological database assembled in a master chronology. The Mint chronologies and the master chronology have been matched in the period 1558-1723, with 1600 and 1601 being recognized as common negative pointer years in all tree ring series reaching that period, coinciding with many growth anomalies dated in the tree rings of the Northern Hemisphere at high latitudes. Just like these dendrochronological studies it has been inferred that these anomalies were the effect of the eruption of Huaynaputina, which occurred in Peru at the beginning of 1600 AD. It should be noted that this is the first time that have been determined the effects of this eruption in the tree-ring records of Southern Europe.

1. Introduction

Dendroclimatic studies are valuable for examining the time distribution of climate events, because the length of tree-ring series provides an extended context to assess such changes. One of the features to assess these changes is pointer years: years with markedly wider or narrower tree-ring width compared to neighbouring tree rings. The interpretation of the pointer years depends on their position in the dendrochronological sequences and on their significance, whether individual, local or regional [1], although at the regional level only the climatic interpretation is possible. Furthermore, pointer years are also used to support the correct dating in historical or archaeological material [1, 2, 3, 4].

In general, the study of the relationship between pointer years and climatic factors has represented only a marginal interest in dendrochronology, especially with the growing application of information technology, because this relationship is not easy to define. Nevertheless, in certain cases and using qualitative techniques, it has indeed been demonstrated that the pointer years, which present themselves over wide geographical areas, tend to be associated with determinate macro-climatic events [5, 6, 7, 8, 9, 10, 11]. Evident climatic interpretations such as severe winter frosts, unusual summer droughts, or excessive cold springs can explain most of the negative pointer years. Other authors have related negative pointer years to macro-climatic events on a global scale, such as those derived from the major volcanic eruptions [5, 6, 12, 7, 9, 11].

In this context, the results presented here matching the record of pointer years of regional significance in the central Iberian Peninsula with the pointer years recorded in certain historical timber. A *Pinus sylvestris* dendrochronological database of the central Iberian Peninsula (Sierra de Guadarrama) has been developed in which extreme growth values and pointer years have been already identified [11]. Furthermore, a set of pieces from a wooden deck of *Pinus sylvestris*, exposed during archaeological work in the Royal Old Mint of Segovia (Spain) has also been studied [4]. This paper updates and reviews the results of these two earlier studies about the significant effects on tree rings of an extreme event happened in the early 17th century and related to a volcanic eruption.

2. Study Area

The Sierra de Guadarrama forms part of the eastern half of the Central System Range in the Iberian Peninsula. It extends in a southwest–northeast direction in the Spanish provinces of Madrid, Segovia and Ávila. It is one of the most important forested areas of continental Spain, with a clear-predominance, especially above 1000 m altitude, of one of the best Spanish representations of *Pinus sylvestris* forest.

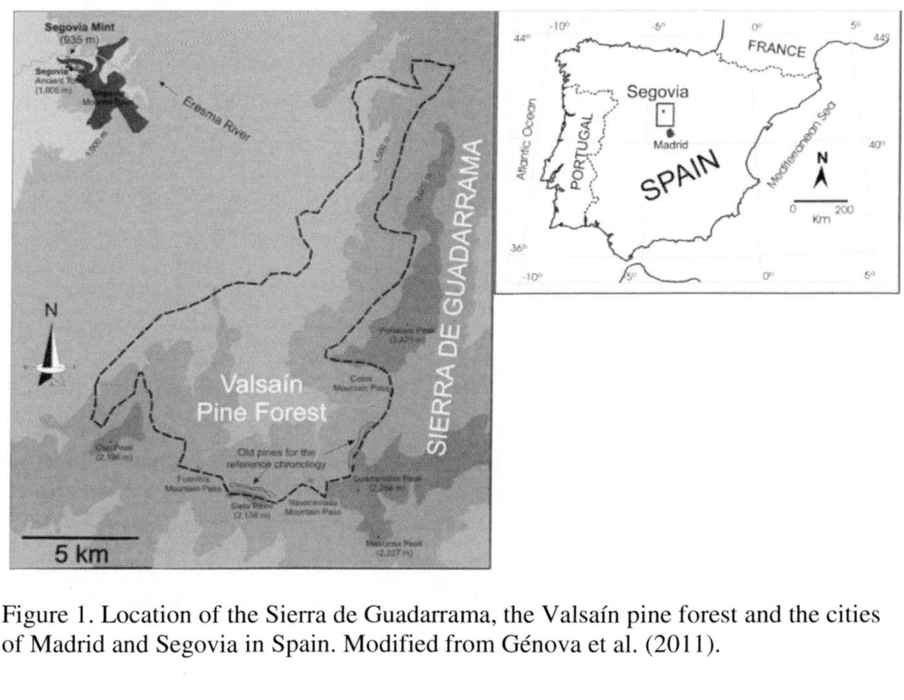

Figure 1. Location of the Sierra de Guadarrama, the Valsaín pine forest and the cities of Madrid and Segovia in Spain. Modified from Génova et al. (2011).

By the end of the 19th and beginning of the 20th centuries the area was practically deforested, especially on its southerly slopes, due to repeated fires, war and grazing and the large-scale extraction of wood which had been taking place since the Middle Ages. Consequently, the greater part of the pine woods derives from successive afforestation from that time on [13, 14, 15]. Nevertheless, the northern slopes still preserve some of finest natural Scots pine forests that exist in Spain: the Valsaín Forest (Figure 1). This is one of the few state-owned forests in Spain and has been precisely managed since the 18th century. Thus, although it has been drawn upon as a source of timber without interruption until the present day, it has been kept in an excellent state of conservation.

3. MATERIAL

3.1. Living Tree-Ring Chronologies

Over a period of several decades different sites in the Sierra de Guadarrama had been extensively sampled, and currently there is a *Pinus sylvestris* dendrochronological database of 394 individual growth sequences from 201 trees compiled in 13 local chronologies, and the regional chronology extends from 1513 to 2005 [11]. The dendrochronological samples of living Scots pines had been extracted principally from the highest areas and the northern slopes of the Sierra de Guadarrama, availing of what remains of the original forest that still preserves some aged trees (Figures 1 and 2).

3.2. Timber samples of the Royal Old Mint of Segovia

The Royal Old Mint of Segovia is a complex of historic buildings on the outskirts of this city in central Spain, 90 km north of Madrid, and which was declared a UNESCO World Heritage Site in 1985 (Figure 3). This Royal Mint has a long and fascinating history originating in the collaborative effort on the part of governments and technicians to implement a better system for producing coinage in Spain [16].

The building was designed by the famous architect Juan de Herrera, who also oversaw the completion of the El Escorial Monastery, with the

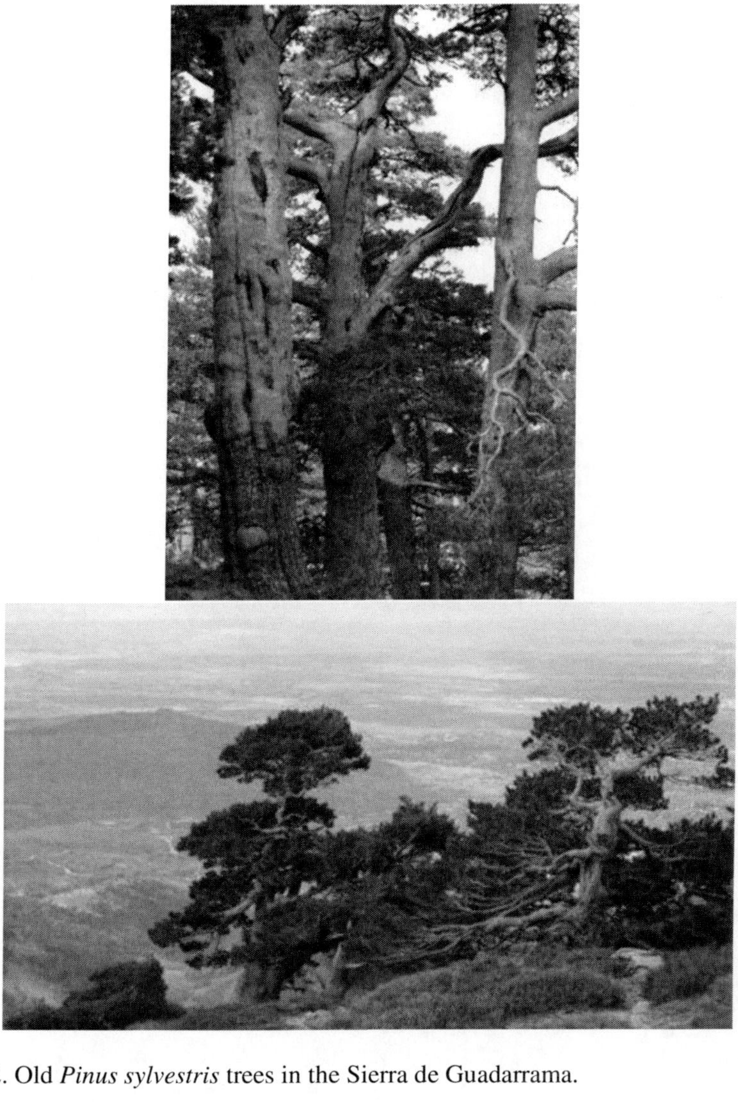

Figure 2. Old *Pinus sylvestris* trees in the Sierra de Guadarrama.

collaboration of German and Austrian engineers [16]. For many years the Segovia Mint was the most prestigious coin factory in Europe. After nearly three centuries of producing some of the world's largest gold and silver coins, the Mint was finally closed in 1869, when Spanish coin production was centralized in Madrid. Today the Segovia Mint is considered one of the oldest, most advanced, and most complete industrial monuments still standing in the world [17], and in recent years it has been undergoing restoration to house a living and working museum of minting technology and the history of coinage in Europe. During archaeological research work in the complex of the Mint for its restoration as a museum, various wood elements appeared in the bed of the old hydraulic canal or mill race; among them was an outstanding wooden deck covered by layers of clay, loam deposits, and debris. Wood was covering the ancient rock canal, originally built in the late 16th century (Juan de Herrera, ca. 1583–1590). This old canal was overlaid with a masonry structure: the canal "Sabatini," named after the famous-Italian architect who built this upper canal in the late 18th century (ca. 1771). The wood used in its construction, according to [18], came from the nearby Valsaín forests of *Pinus sylvestris* (Sierra de Guadarrama).

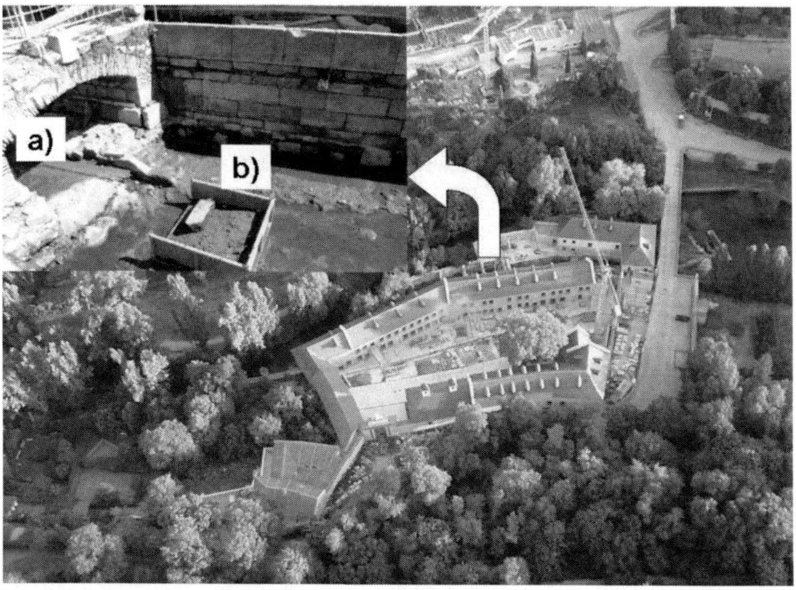

Figure 3. Recent aerial view of the Royal Old Mint of Segovia, with details of the archaeological reconstruction of the canals showing a) planks and b) one of the support blocks.

In [4] we presented the study of ten timber samples that were removed from their original position during the archaeological reconstruction of the canals of the Royal Old Mint. Later, we have had the opportunity to study three more samples. Consequently we present in this work the most recent analyzes of a total of six beams, three planks and four support blocks from the canal structure are presented (Table 1).

Table 1. Characteristics of timber samples from the Mint canal. Segment correlation: (intercorrelation is less than 0.10), in bold (intercorrelation exceeds the critical value of 0.32)

ID	*Type*	*State*	*Nº slices*	*Nº of sequences*	*Maximum radius (mm)*	*Maximum nº of tree rings*	*Average growth rings (mm)*	*Time span*	*Segment correlation*						
									1550 1599	1575 1624	1600 1649	1625 1674	1650 1699	1675 1724	1700 1749
CM1	Support block	Good	3	13	178	99	1.80±0.94	1578-1676		**.73**	**.71**	.12	----		
CM2	Beam	Good	6	30	161	106	1.52±0.55	1618-1723			.18	.18	**.48**	**.44**	
CM3	Beam	Good	2	10	192	161	1.19±0.82	1560-1720	**.54**	**.56**	**.61**	**.45**	**.33**	.24	
CM4	Beam	Poor	3	17	185	99	1.87±0.75	1561-1659	.31	**.41**	**.43**	.28			
CM5	Beam	Poor	3	16	186	135	1.37±0.63	1584-1718		**.53**	**.60**	**.54**	**.53**	**.46**	
CM6	Support block	Poor	2	11	166	104	1.59±1.02	1566-1669	**.47**	**.46**	**.52**	.27			
CM7	Support block	Poor	2	15	162	103	1.58±0.95	1622-1724			.24	.16	.31	.29	
CM8	Plank	Good	1	5	180	99	1.81±1.16	1558-1656	**.54**	**.66**	**.64**	**.47**			
CM9	Plank	Good	1	8	176	149	1.18±0.89	1580-1728		.29	.21	.18	**.37**	.25	.30
CM10	Plank	Poor	1	6	137	84	1.64±1.15	1612-1695			**.32**	**.47**	**.41**		
CM11	Beam	Good	1	6	211	127	1.67±1.10	1561-1687	**.57**	**.64**	**.66**	----	.15		
CM12	Beam	Poor	1	4	134	56	2.39±1.07	1558-1613	**.48**	**.47**					
CM13	Support block	Good	1	6	134	131	1.02±0.55	1590-1720		**.72**	**.70**	**.55**	**.43**	----	
PISY	Master chronology of living trees							1513-1995	**.46**	**.43**	**.49**	----	----	----	----
Average segment correlation									**.48**	**.54**	**.48**	.29	.29	.24	.17

Modified from Génova et al. (2011) with new data and results.

4. METHODS

The analysis of the living tree-ring chronologies and the timber samples was carried out by using dendrochronological methods ([19, 20, 21]).

The samples of the Royal Old Mint were sanded and polished (up to 400 grit) to facilitate recognition of the tree rings (Figure 4). Having selected for measurement by visual procedures at least four radii of each sample, ring widths of the timber samples were measured to an accuracy of 1/100 mm using a digital LINTAB positioning table connected to a stereomicroscope and TSAPWin software.

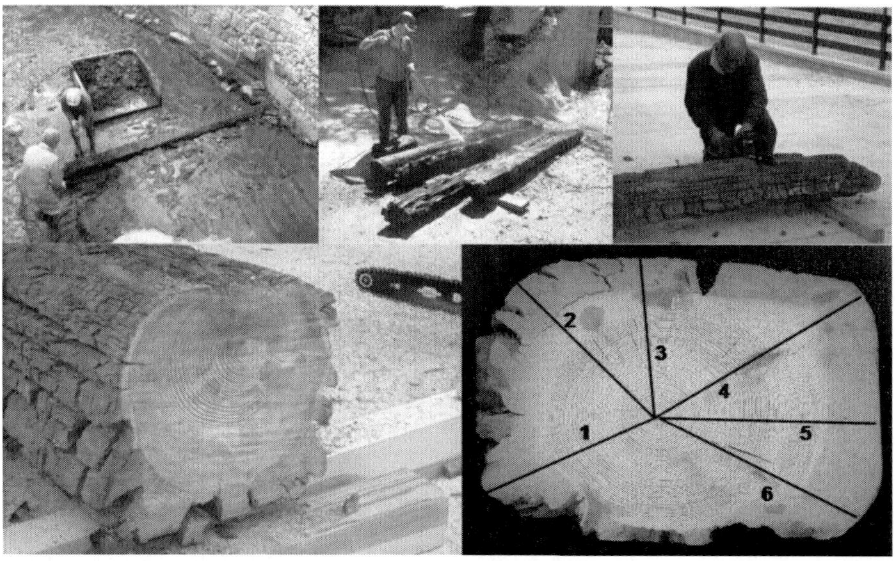

Figure 4. Timber samples of the Royal Old Mint were removed from their original position during the archaeological and historical reconstruction and were washed under pressure to remove existing sand and mud. Then the slices were cut with chainsaw and finally were polished. The pictures show the beam CM13 and the radii measured.

The measured tree-ring radii series were crossdated using TSAPWin software [22] and an average tree-ring series was elaborated for each piece. To ascertain the age of the timber samples from the Mint canal, documentary sources [16] and radiocarbon dating were used. On finding that the probable time span of the wood coming from the Mint canal matched the initial part of the *Pinus sylvestris* dendrochronological database of the Sierra de Guadarrama, the oldest tree-ring series (assembled in a master chronology) were selected to crossdate timber Mint, using specially the COFECHA program facilities [23].

The pointer years of these chronologies were also identified to support the correct dating [24, 2, 3], and to increase the information about extreme climate events. In accordance with the pointer year definition: "Concentration of cross-dated event years within a group of trees" [1], the decrease or the increase more than 20% of growth indices and one or more standard deviations from the chronological average were used to identify pointer years or pointer intervals [25].

5. RESULTS AND DISCUSSION

5.1. Chronologies of Royal Old Mint

The wooden deck that was covering the ancient rock canal (Juan de Herrera, ca. 1583–1590) and located under the upper canal (Sabatini, ca. 1771) ought to have had a felling date prior to the more recent canal [4]. The radiocarbon analysis of one of these timber samples (CM-2F, Centro Nacional de Aceleradores, Sevilla, España, 2012) indicates an age of 340 ± 40 BP, corresponding to 1463-1643 cal AD (2 sigma, 95% probability, according to [26]. Thus for both dating sources the temporal range was consistent. To obtain precise chronologies, the TSAPWin software and COFECHA program was step by step used and producing the final results as shown in table 1. The new samples analyzed in respect to [4] have increased the number (to 13) and the accuracy of the chronologies involved. Some individual sequences did not correlate statistically at certain periods (see Table I), and those periods were not used for further analysis.

5.2. Pointer years and events of special relevance

Extreme growth values and pointer years in individual chronologies, local chronologies and in the regional chronology of living trees of the Sierra de Guadarrama had been already identified [11]. Moreover, the pointer years were a significant support in the synchronization process between the chronologies of Old Royal Mint and the master chronology of Sierra de Guadarrama. The year 1601 was especially noteworthy, as it represented a very significant growth reduction [4].

The present review has determined that the Mint chronologies and the master chronology produced matches for the period 1558-1723, with 1600 and 1601 being recognized as common negative pointer years in the eleven series covering reaching that period. 1601 provides the minimum index in the regional chronology for the centre of Spain and this year coincides with many other anomalies documented in tree rings of Northern Hemisphere, indicating a global event that left its trace in the tree rings of woody plants [9]. And, according to [7], 1601 was the most severe short-term Northern Hemisphere cooling event of the past 600 years.

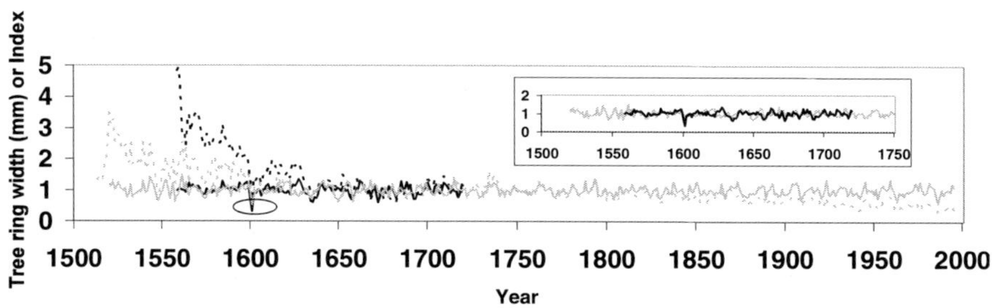

Figure 5. Raw and standardized chronologies from old living trees of the Sierra de Guadarrama (VI and VIArs) and of the Royal Old Mint (CM and CMArs). The period when VIArs and CMArs coincide is shown in detail; 1601 is noted as the most characteristic pointer year. Modified from Génova et al. (2011) with new data and results.

Continuing with an already long tradition that matches the major volcanic eruptions to growth reduction or other anomalies in tree rings (e.g., [5, 6, 12], among others), it has been inferred that the 1601 extreme pointer year was the effect of the eruption of Huaynaputina, which occurred in Peru at the beginning of 1600 AD [7]. It should be noted that taking into account these growth anomalies and other proxies, that this was the biggest eruption in the world in the last 600 years [7, 27, 9].

Our studies have demonstrated for the first time the effects of this eruption in the tree-ring records of Southern Europe, even if there has been no evidence of the effects of other more recent eruptions in the chronologies that have been analysed [11]. It needs to be emphasised, moreover, that the effects of this volcanic eruption were registered in the Sierra de Guadarrama as a pointer interval during a whole three years, from the starting year, 1600, until 1602.

While the authors who have analysed the 1601 macro-climatic event and its consequences for tree growth had attributed its effects to the severe cooling event [9, 7], some climatic reconstructions of the central Iberian Peninsula have also indicated that the start of the 17th century was very dry [28]. It could be that this volcanic eruption caused these climatic anomalies and its effects on tree growth or it could also be that they are related to the reduction of solar energy, due to the accumulation of ash in the atmosphere, and the consequent diminution of photosynthesis.

ACKNOWLEDGMENTS

I am very grateful to Begoña Martínez-Callejo who measured the timber samples of the Royal Old Mint, to Andrés Díez for your ongoing support, to Miguel Angel Moreno for your help in sampling and to Louis Ryan who reviewed the English version.

REFERENCES

[1] Schweingruber, F.H., Eckstein, D., Serre-Bachet, F., Bräker, O.U. Identification, presentation and interpretation of event years and pointer years in dendrochronology. *Dendrochronologia,* 1990, 8, 9–38.

[2] Schweingruber, F. H. Dendroecological information in pointer years and abrupt growth changes, in: *Methods of Dendrochronology: Applications in the Environmental Sciences, International Institute for Applied Systems Analysis,* Kluwer Academic. 1990.

[3] Querrec, L., Filion, L., Auger, R., Arseneault, D. Tree-ring analysis of white cedar (*Thuja occidentalis* L.) archaeological and historical wood in Quebec City (Quebec, Canada). *Dendrochronologia*, 2009, 27, 199–212.

[4] Génova, M., Ballesteros-Cánovas, J. A., Díez-Herrero, A., Martínez-Callejo, B. Historical Floods and Dencrochronological Dating of aWooden Deck in the Old Mint of Segovia, Spain. *Geoarchaelogy*, 2011, 26, 786–808. doi:10.1002/gea.20369.

[5] LaMarche, V. C., Hirschboeck, K. K. Frost rings in trees as records of major volcanic eruptions. *Nature,* 1984, 307, 121–126.

[6] Scuderi, L. C. Tree-ring evidence for climatically effective volcanic Eruptions. *Quaternary Research*, 1990, 34, 67–85.

[7] Briffa, K. R., Jones, P. D., Schweingruber, F. H., Osborn, T. J. Influence of volcanic eruptions on Northern Hemisphere summer temperatures over 600 years. *Nature,* 1998, 393, 450–455. doi:10.1038/30943.

[8] Knapp, P. A., Grissino-Mayer, H. D., Soule, P. T. Climate regionalization and the spatio-temporal occurrence of extreme single-year drought events (1500–1998) in the interior Pacific Northwest, USA, *Quaternary Research*, 2002, 58, 226–233. doi:10.1006/qres.2002.2376.

[9] Hantemirov, R. M., Gorlanova, L. A., Shiyatov, S. G. Extreme temperature events in summer in northwest Siberia since AD 742 inferred from tree rings. *Palaeogeography, Palaeoclimatology, Palaeoecology*, 2004, 209, 155–164. doi:10.1016/j.palaeo. 2003.12.023.

[10] Neuwirth, B., Schweingruber, F. H., Winiger, M. Spatial patterns of central European pointer years from 1901 to 1971. *Dendrochronologia*, 2007, 24, 79–89.

[11] Génova, M. Extreme pointer years in tree-ring records of Central Spain as evidence of climatic events and the eruption of the Huaynaputina Volcano (Peru, 1600 AD). *Climate of the Past,* 2012, 8, 751-764. doi: 0.5194/cp-8-751-2012.

[12] Jones, P. D., Briffa, K. R., Schweingruber, F. H. Tree-ring evidence of the widespread effects of explosive volcanic eruptions. *Geophysical Research Letters*, 1995, 22, 1333–1336.

[13] Bauer, E. Los Montes de España en la historia. Ministerio de Agricultura. Madrid, 1980.

[14] Rojo, A., Montero, G. El pino silvestre en la Sierra de Guadarrama. Ministerio de Agricultura, Pesca y Alimentación. Madrid, Spain, 1996.

[15] Martínez García, F., Costa, M. La interpretación de los bosques de *Pinus sylvestris* L. del sistema central español en la literatura geobotánica y forestal. Boletín de la Real Sociedad de Historia Natural. *Actas,* 2001, 96, 27–68.

[16] Murray, G.S. La historia del Real Ingenio de la Moneda de Segovia y el proyecto para su rehabilitación. Segovia, Fundación Real Ingenio de la Moneda de Segovia. 2006.

[17] Murray, G.S. El Real Ingenio de la Moneda de Segovia: Fábrica industrial más antigua, avanzada y completa que se conserva de la Humanidad. Razonamiento científico de la propuesta para su declaración como patrimonio de la humanidad. Segovia, Cámara de Comercio e Industria de Segovia. 2008.

[18] Murray, G.S., Izaga, J.M., Soler, J.M. El Real Ingenio de la Moneda de Segovia: Maravilla tecnológica del siglo XVI. Madrid, Fundación Juanelo Turriano. 2006.

[19] Fritts, H.C. Tree rings and climate. New York: Academic Press. 1976.

[20] Cook, E.R., Kairiukstis, L.A. *Methods of dendrochronology: Applications in the environmental sciences*. London, Kluwer. 1990.

[21] Vaganov, E.A., Hughes, M.K., Shashkin, A.V. *Growth dynamics of conifer tree rings: Images of past and future environments*. New York: Springer. 2006.

[22] Rinn, F. TSAPWin: time series analysis and presentation for dendrochronology and related applications, version 0.53: user reference. RinnTech, Heidelberg. 2003.

[23] Holmes, R. Users manual for Program Cofecha by Laboratory of Tree-Ring Research, University of Arizona, Tucson, Arizona. USA, 1999.

[24] Schweingruber, F.H. *Tree rings and environment*. Bern, Paul Haupt. 1996.

[25] Génova, M. Anillos de crecimiento y años característicos en el Sistema Central (España) durante los últimos cuatrocientos años. *Boletín de la Real Sociedad de Historia Natural,* 2000, 96, 33–42.

[26] Reimer, P. J., Baillie, M. G. L., Bard, E., Bayliss, A., Beck, J. W., Blackwell, P. G., Weyhenmeyer, C. E. Intcal09 and Marine09 radiocarbon age calibration curves, 0-50,000yeats cal BP. *Radiocarbon*, 2009, 51(4), 1111-1150.

[27] De Silva, S. L., Zielinski, G. A. Global influence of the AD1600 eruption of Huaynaputina, Peru. *Nature,* 1998, 393, 455–458.

[28] Domínguez-Castro, F., Santisteban, J. I., Barriendos, M., Mediavilla, R. Reconstruction of drought episodes for central Spain from rogation ceremonies recorded at Toledo Cathedral from 1506 to 1900: A methodological approach. *Global Planet Change*, 2008, 63, 230–242. doi:10.5194/cpd-6-1111-2010.

In: Volcanic Eruptions
Editor: Trent Milburn
ISBN: 978-1-63463-308-6

Chapter 4

THE SEISMIC SIGNATURES OF THE VOLCANIC CRISES: A REVIEW

Mauro Palo*
Deutsches GeoForschungsZentrum, Potsdam, Germany

Abstract

Volcano seismology is considered a good proxy of the internal conditions of the volcanic systems. In particular, the volcanic crises are anticipated by a loading process triggered by an overall upward magma migration inducing gas exsolution and stress build up within the feeding system and the hosting rocks. This process activates brittle failures within the volcanic edifice and pressurized magmatic fluids flowing through magma-filled cavities, generating the two end-members of the volcano seismicity: Volcano-Tectonic and Long-Period events, respectively. Volcano seismicity follows the disequilibrium conditions within the plumbing system preceding and accompanying the volcanic crises, exhibiting modifications of the source process in respect to the inter-eruptive phase in terms of wavefield properties and statistics of the earthquake occurrence. Although some common correlations between seismic activity and magma dynamics during the eruptive crises have been identified, a wide variability of behaviors appears as well, with a sharp dependence on the volcano and on the eruptive episode.

*E-mail address: mpalo@gfz-potsdam.de, mauro.palo79@gmail.com

Here I critically review the characteristics of the volcano seismicity before and during the volcanic crises, describing the source process of the volcanic earthquakes in terms of both the seismologic parameters and the statistical properties of the point process ruling their occurrence times and magnitude.

1. Introduction

The seismic monitoring of active volcanoes is one of the most powerful and diffused tool for the mitigation of the volcanic risk. Volcano seismicity is considered a good proxy of the internal stress of the volcanic system when critical conditions are approaching. Indeed an increase of the earthquake rate before the eruptions is often observed and is usually connected to a first approximation to an overall increase of the pressure in the shallow plumbing system (e.g., Lengliné et al., 2008).

However, behind this general correlation (even not always verified), the relationship between the observed seismicity and the approaching and/or ongoing eruption is not trivial, variable and time-dependent, thus making still difficult defining a common framework. This variability is the effect of several factors (often interacting one another) controlling the eruption timing and style, and the seismicity. These factors include (among the others) the nature of the magma and of the volcanic rock, the characteristics of the magma migration, the eruptive style, the capacity of the seismicity to accomodate the stress variations, the features of the seismic response.

In particular, the release of seismic energy displays a wide range of phenomena (see, e.g., Chouet and Matoza, 2012). Differently from the pure tectonic case where brittle failures dominate the seismicity, in volcanic areas different processes generate seismic signals. In particular, the presence of magmatic fluids flowing at shallow depths ($\lesssim$1-2km) produces another category of events besides the standard seismicity induced by brittle failures, displaying the two classes of phenomena different waveforms and spectra. Moreover, besides discrete releases of seismic energy, long-lasting tremor is also very common in volcanic areas and is imputed as well to nearly steady fluid flow.

Furthermore, the source of volcano seismicity is often localized within individual structures (magma-filled cavities) of the plumbing system without a self-similar network of faults characterizing the tectonic environment and the brittle response. These peculiar features of the volcano seismology make the release of stress by seismic radiation less efficient and complex in volcanic contexts, with strong elements of nonlinearity in the source mechanisms reflecting into feedback processes in the energy exchange between fluid and rock.

With the development of portable seismometers, the number of volcanoes monitored worldwide has been rapidly increased in the last decades, allowing to collect a large number of observations of the volcano seismicity, and in particular of the seismic response during the volcanic crises. Moreover, several volcanoes nowadays are very well seismically monitored, with dense permanent networks active for long periods. In this way, modifications of the seismic parameters during the inter-eruptive intervals are being monitored, and insights into the changes of the stress field inducing the seismic events and, thus, into the magma dynamics can be potentially inferred.

The basic parameters observed in the real-time seismic monitoring are the amplitude (magnitude) of the volcanic earthquakes and their rate, whose modifications are straightforwardly connected to an impending eruption. More complete volcano monitoring includes further variables such as the amplitude of the volcanic tremor, the frequency content of the seismicity, the hypocenters and the source mechanisms (stress and slip vectors and magnitude) of the volcanic earthquakes. A posteriori, powerful informations on the modifications of the source process of the volcano seismicity are also inferred from the frequency distributions of the occurrence times and of the magnitudes of the volcanic earthquakes, which often show an evolution of the statistical properties when the eruption is approaching.

Here I will critically review in individual sections different aspects of the volcano seismicity, reporting examples from different volcanoes and highlighting common elements and differences among the cases. In detail, in Section 3, I will define the statistical features of the point process ruling the volcanic earthquakes; in Section 4, I will look at the amplitude of the volcanic tremor; in Sections 5 and 6, the progression of the position and the physical mechanism of the source of the earthquakes is discussed. The results will be included in a framework of the magma dynamics accompanying the volcanic crises in Section 8, while possible future developments of the seismic monitoring in volcanic areas are proposed in Section 9.

Throughout the paper, I will refer to a volcanic crisis as a modification of the state of the volcano induced by magma activity. Thus, a volcanic crisis must be intended as the long-lasting "loading" process consisting in the migration of magma in the plumbing system inducing changes of physical and chemical parameters (such as earthquakes and infrasonic signals, surface deformation, gas flux variation, temperature increase at the vent, etc.), and possibly culminating in the external emission of material. Volcanic crises normally include an eruptive phase, which may have an effusive- or explosive-style lava emission. On the other hand, volcanic crises without lava emission can exist as well, for example in case of intrusive events.

2. The Variety of Seismic Signals at Volcanic Areas: Notes on the Nomenclature

The seismic energy in active volcanic areas can be released in a large variety of forms and source mechanisms, which in turn produces several types of waveforms. Some criteria have been more or less uniformly adopted from the scientific community to classify the signals (see McNutt (2002) for a definition). Such criteria are basically based on the frequency content of the signals. Broadly speaking, Volcano-Tectonic (VT) events are signals containing most of the energy at high frequencies ($\gtrsim$ 2Hz) with often a broad spectrum, while Long-Period (LP) events have narrower spectra displaying peaks at low frequencies ($\lesssim$ 2Hz). Nevertheless, the definition often depends on the author and this terminology can lead to ambigous classifications. In addition, hybrid events containing a mixture of the characteristics of both the events are very common.

In general, LP events are produced by the flowing of magmatic fluids throw cavities of the shallow plumbing system, with an active role of the fluids that generate feedback mechanisms and nonlinear signals, whereas the source mechanism of the VT events is dominated by brittle failures occurring within the volcanic edifice and potentially within the magma itself (Lavallée et al., 2008; Tuffen et al., 2008), in a way similar to the tectonic earthquakes (Burlini et al., 2007; Benson et al., 2010). Chouet et al. (1994) proposed that a key element distinguishing the two phenomena is the role of fluids, which in the LP events are actively involved in the generation of the elastic waves, while in the VT events do not partecipate in the source dynamics, although the magmatic processes are ultimately the source of energy for both the phenomena.

However, despite the quasi-universal waveform, LP signals can be triggered by a variety of processes such as non-stationary fluid movement (Julian, 1994), gas slug migration within two-phase fluids (Chouet et al., 2003), accelerated choked fluid flow (Chouet, 2003; De Lauro et al., 2008), etc. Moreover, LP events are generated also in silicic volcanoes, where very viscous magmas should inhibite fast fluid flow. For this reason, models involving interface waves and path effects have been proposed (Neuberg et al., 2000, 2006). Moreover, recently Bean et al. (2014) showed that seismic events with the characteristics of LP events can be generated also by stick-slip displacement, making even harder the definition of classes of events based only on the waveform.

On the other hand, due to the different source mechanism, LP and VT events are also mostly distinguished in the equivalent physical model reproducing the two phenomena. Specifically, LP events are produced by source mechanisms not (or scarcely) involving shear stresses, while VT events are well described by double-couple mechanisms and, in fact, often show P and S arrival in the waveforms. These classes must be considered as end-members, and processes involving both the mechanisms can exist, as verified recently also experimentally (Benson et al., 2010).

The two classes may coexist at individual volcanoes, with one class usually prevailing. The prevalent class depends on the chemical and rheological properties of the magma. In particular, the seismic energy release is tightly connected to the magma viscosity, which in turn affects the amount and the movement of the exsolved magmatic gases. Silicic volcanoes - such as andesitic-dacitic volcanoes - show high viscosity and magma density. The seismicity at these volcanoes is mostly produced by fracturing of the rock or of the magma itself (acting as brittle material) inducing VT or hybrid events (although LPs are generated in many cases, as well). Seismic release in this case is often cyclic and punctuate the growth of a magmatic dome and its following destruction by explosions and eruptions. Low-viscosity volcanoes - such as basaltic volcanoes - are rich in fluids and display a shallow plumbing system dominated by a magma-gas mixture. The seismicity is mostly induced by coherent gas slugs or pockets rising in the magma and interacting with the conduit walls. The size of these gas aggregates depends not trivially on the thermodinamical state of the magma and also on the geometry of the shallow conduit. The resulting seismicity is mostly composed of LP events, often with very stable source mechanisms.

Modifications of pressure and/or temperature within the feeding system - due, for instance, to uprising batches of magma prior to the eruptions - are firstly accomodated by thermodynamic changes of the magma-gas mixture. Thus, the properties of the seismicity at these volcanoes mostly reflect the dynamics of its fluid constituents.

Besides the waveforms and the source mechanism, the volcanic signals mostly define their nature on a statistical basis, displaying the source process a peculiar statistics of the amplitudes and occurrence times. It means that the proper definition of the volcanic signals should take into account not only the short time scales of the duration of a seismic event, but also its point process, that means a longer time scale suitable to define a meaningful statistical set of observations.

In the next section, I will explore in detail the statistical properties of the volcano seismicity. I will report several examples of the statistics of the rate and amplitude of the seismic events in volcanic areas, defining two main behaviors broadly associated with the VT and LP sources.

3. Statistics

In this section, I will review the statistical characteristics of the discrete seismic events occurring in volcanic contexts. The events are here considered as constituting a point process defined by a sequence of occurrence times and energies (or amplitudes).

The statistical features of the point process displays two major classes of behavior. One is mostly followed by VT events and reflects the self-similarity of the fault system in the crust, in strong analogy with the tectonic earthquakes (e.g., Grasso and Bachelery, 1995). For this class, the events are correlated in time and space, as an effect of the scale invariance of the source process (Collombet et al., 2003; Kilburn, 2003; Traversa and Grasso, 2010). On the other hand, the other class is mostly constituted by LP events, which normally do not show clear spatial and temporal correlations and activate one (or few) independent time and length scale (e.g., Benoit et al., 2003; Bottiglieri et al., 2005). In the following, I will describe separately the results for the two classes. I will refer to them as the class of the correlated events and of the independent events.

The different statistical features can be eventually imputed to the type of coupling between the stress field and the rigid structures of the plumbing system. In the case of correlated events, this coupling is very efficient and the seismic response of the rigid structures can be considered a good proxy of the stress conditions within the plumbing system. In this way, also the self-similarity of the system of dikes, joints, faults or other type of discontinuities present in the volcanic edifice (leading to the activation of a quasi-continuous set of length scales) is reflected into the produced discrete seismicity in the form of correlated events, whose macroscopic features (rate and magnitude) can display power law behavior. On the other hand, when the coupling is unefficient, the seismicity is no longer a direct proxy of the pressure conditions, while more complex relations can exist. In this case, the pressure dishomeneities are not straightforwardly transferred to the plumbing system activating branching networks of seismogenic structures, but they can only activate (under suitable thermodynamic and mechanical conditions) a certain source mechanism, mainly involving one (or few) length scale. The seismic events so generated appear mostly independent and are not organized into collective phenomena like those displaying power law behavior.

3.1. Correlated Events

3.1.1. Earthquake Rate

The most important and most adopted parameter to monitor an approaching eruption is the event rate, that is the number of volcanic earthquakes occurring in a fixed time interval. The event rate tightly mimics the changes of the mean stress within the volcanic structure (Dieterich et al., 2000); thus, following its time evolution is a good tool to monitor the progression of the internal conditions towards critical levels.

It has been verified with statistical tools that the event rate is larger during the eruptive episodes than the inter-eruptive periods. Grasso and Zaliapin (2004) reported that the mean duration of volcanic crises at Piton de la Fournaise (Reunion Island) is about 4 hours culminating with lava flow at the surface. The authors suggested that this phase could correspond to a possible outflow of the magma from the storage system. Moreover, they observed in this phase a very high and nearly constant VT event rate ($\sim$2500 ev/hour), two orders of magnitude larger than the values assumed few days prior to the eruption.

Similar results were found by Traversa and Grasso (2010) for Etna volcano (Sicily, Italy) during the eruptive crises of 2001 and 2002. The authors found a seismicity rate during the eruptive events about two orders of magnitude larger than the rate during the inter-eruptive intervals, but they could not establish whether uncorrelated events did exist due to the very high event rate during the crises. On the contrary, the correlation between the occurrence times of the events clearly emerged for the inter-eruptive periods for both the volcanoes Etna and Vesuvius.

Schmid and Grasso (2012) demonstrated a complete analogy between the tectonic and the volcanic seismicity, with a scaling law between the volcanic seismic rate and the eruption size (Volcanic Explosivity Index, VEI, Newhall and Self (1982)), in a way that the larger is the eruption, the sharper is the change of the event rate in respect to the background rate. The authors highlighted also a post-eruptive decaying behavior similar to the post-tectonic-mainshock Omori law, but with a slower damage relaxation, i.e. a longer decaying time scale after the eruption than that for the tectonic earthquakes.

A clear example of the relation between eruptive process and discrete seismicity was shown by Voight et al. (1999) for Soufriere Hills Volcano, Monteserrat. Voight et al. (1999) showed that a cyclic dome growth occurring in 1997 was sistematically accompained by an increase of earthquakes, especially of those classified as hybrid. The dome growth was produced by the build up of the pressure under the plug. Such pressure build up was the effect of the magma transport from the magma chamber towards the surface, with an additional contribution from the gaseous phase released during the magma upward migration. When the pressure reached a threshold, the earthquakes started to occur and increased until the plug reached critical mechanical conditions, above which a vulcanian explosion occurred. The explosion reduced quickly the pressure and consequently the earthquake rate, which dropped to zero at the end of the cycle.

A response of the seismicity to the eruptive activity on a longer time scale was reported by De la Cruz-Reyna et al. (2008) for Popocatepetl volcano, Mexico. The authors described the activation of the seismicity before the eruption of 1994, which followed a period of quiescence of about 70 years starting from the eruptive crisis of 1919-1927 (with the exception of a minor fumarolic event in 1947). The authors analyzed the reactivation of the volcano started in 1993 and culminated with a series of moderate ash explosions on 21 December 1994. Since then, Popocatepetl has been experiencing a series of explosions and its activity is still persisting. The authors found an increase of the VT seismicity starting from more than four years prior to the eruption, suggesting a very slow loading process, in line with the very long quiescence period. In particular, in the period from January 1993 till April 1994 a sharp increase of the event rate was detected, with peaks of $\sim$1 events/day. In the same period, the strongest events (magnitude$\sim$3.2) occurred. This rise of the seismic activity was accompained by a change of the external activity: an increase of the fumarolic activity and of the temperature of the small crater lake, and the progressive activation of new steam vents. In the period May 1994 - December 1994 the event rate reduced to $\sim$0.1-0.3 events/day with magnitude mostly lower than 2.5. At the surface, the temperature of the crater lake further increased, indicating an approaching of the magma to the surface, but without inducing stress change as strong as in the previous period.

A schematic diagram of the seismicity rate preceding the eruptions and of its possible causes is described by McNutt (2002) and closely mimics the eruptive history of the Popocatepetl volcano above reported. McNutt (2002, Fig. 18) qualitatively highlighted the strong increase of the high-frequency events (corresponding to VT events) before the eruption as the effect of the stress transfer between the uprising magma and the hosting rock. This increase of event rate is followed by a phase of relative quiescence, during which the circulation of magmatic gases (induced by the heat of the approaching magma) may produce LP activity and tremor of minor intensity. This last phase is generated in the shallowest 0-3 km of the plumbing system and is detectable only in the case in which the thermodynamic conditions of the upper volcanic system (possibly interacting with a hydrothermal system) allows an efficient gas release properly exciting the local rigid structures. As an effect, this last phase, even when detected, has a shorter duration than the previous one.

Whereas from a qualitatively point of view the increase of the event rate can be considered a good indication of an impelling eruption, in the framework of the volcanic risk mitigation it can be unsatisfactory without a mathematical model ruling the progression of the rate. With this aim, in the 80s a model successfully describing the behavior of materials in terminal stages of failure has been applied to the event rate prior to the eruptions. The model is known as Material Failure Forecast Method (FFM) and introduces a nonlinear second-order differential equation describing the time-evolution of a parameter representative of the stress status of the material or of the volcanic rock:

$$\ddot{\Omega} = A\dot{\Omega}^{\alpha} \tag{1}$$

where $\ddot{\Omega}$ and $\dot{\Omega}$ are the acceleration and rate of the parameter being monitored, respectively, and A and α are empirically determined constants. The coefficients A and α are inferred by regression of the logarithmic formulation of the Eq. 1. A depends on initial conditions, including the background event rate, and is thus variable from case to case. α is instead usually $\sim$2.

After integrating, Eq. 1 becomes (Collombet et al., 2003):

$$\dot{\Omega} \sim (t_e - t)^{\frac{-1}{\alpha-1}} \tag{2}$$

being t_e the eruption time. This espression is a special case of a general equation for time-to-failure laws that can be interpreted as resulting from collective critical phenomena (Sammis and Sornette, 2002), confirming that a class of seismic events is produced by volcanic processes involving a range of length scales mutually interacting.

From the point of view of the volcanic risk mitigation, the importance of Eq. 1 lays on the theoretical possibility to predict the time of the eruption. In fact, FFM predicts an eruption when Ω^{-1} goes to zero, which corresponds to an event rate approaching to infinite for times very close to the eruption.

Although this relation well fit the behavior of more than one observable, such as the strain rate or the seismic energy (e.g., Voight, 1988; Main, 1999; Lavallée et al., 2008), the best fit has been found applying the model to the event rate. The hypothesis behind the application of FFM to volcanic eruptions is that the magmatic pathway towards the surface is driven by rock failure in the volcanic plumbing system under sustained and near-constant loading induced by the stress transfer from migrating magma to the hosting rock (Chastin and Main, 2003), which implies that seismic activity well measures the stress status of the volcanic systems (Dieterich et al., 2000).

Several applications of FFM to volcanic contexts have been proposed. Here I report the main results obtained on three case-studies: Kilauea (Hawaii), Piton de la Fournaise (Reunion Island), Soufriere Hills (Montserrat).

Chastin and Main (2003) analyzed the volcano seismicity at Kilauea between 1959 and 2000 in relation with the eruption activity. They found that only about 50% of the eruptions (19 out of 35) showed a higher event rate in the day of the eruption than the background rate level. However, they found an increase of the event rate 10-15 days before the eruption stacking the time histories of the event rate preceding each eruption, moving back up to 100 days before the eruptions. This increase followed the FFM, with the event rate assuming values just before the eruptions one order of magnitude larger than the background level. The authors proposed that the event rate increase would be produced by a mean stress field, whose flucuations make this increase undetactable for some individual eruptions. On the other hand, only in about 15 % of the cases an event rate increase was followed by lava emission. The authors suggested that in the majority of the cases, the rate increase was produced by internal magmatic intrusion not reaching the surface. This would be in line with the results of Gudmundsson (2002), who claims that only about 10 % of dike injection leads to lava effusions.

Collombet et al. (2003) analyzed the VT events associated with 15 eruptions at Piton de la Fournaise in the period 1988-2001. They found an increase of the event rate following the Eq. 2 for the events occurring within about the two weeks preceding the eruptions, confirming the results of Chastin and Main (2003) and suggesting an universal validity of the FFM. Moreover, the authors suggested that two factors affect the event rate: the mean loading induced by migrating magma and the cascade of earthquake interactions, similar to the cascade of aftershocks following the main shock in tectonic environment. They proposed that the latter effect acts as a fluctuation of the main loading field, with the result that not every individual eruption is anticipated by an increase of the event rate, whereas this increase is only statistically detectable. In that sense, the former effect can be seen as a large scale effect, while the latter one acts on smaller scales (Grasso and Zaliapin, 2004).

Using the same data-set, Grasso and Zaliapin (2004) tried to define an alarm procedure on the basis of the increase of the VT event rate. They found that the best predictions are obtained reducing the observation period from the two weeks in which a rate increase is statistically detected to five days before the eruption. In this case, 65% of the eruptions were successfully predicted for an alarm duration less than 20% of the time considered.

Kilburn and Voight (1998) processed the seismic series preceding the breakout of lava in 1998 at Soufriere Hills volcano. They detected an increase of the rate of the seismic events prior to the eruption, from ~10 events/day to ~1400 events/day in the two weeks preceding the eruption of andesitic lava. Also in this case, the authors found that the rate increase is well fitted by FFM. In detail, they adopted both a linear and a nonlinear regression of data and found a preferred eruption time in the range 16-20/11, close to the actual eruption date (15/11). The estimated value of α for the nonlinear regression was 1.88, very close to the result of the linear case and to the most common value (~2).

Hammer and Neuberg (2009) analyzed the seismic rate at Soufriere Hills in 1997, before the dome collapse occurred in June of the same year. As reported also by other authors for the same volcano in other time periods (e.g., Voight et al., 1999), the seismic events at Soufriere are often time clustered in swarms, each swarm corresponding to a pressure loading in the plumbing system eventually culminating with a small eruption in the form of a vulcanian explosion or a pyroclastic flow. These seismic swarms puctuate at first the growth of the volcanic dome and then its removal. Hammer and Neuberg (2009) processed three days preceding the dome collapse, during which six swarms of LP events occurred. The authors remarked that, whereas during an individual swarm the event rate increased and then decreased, on longer time scales the event rate increased with time, moving from 0.5 ev/min to 2.5 ev/min. This increase was modelled by FFM and fitted by a linear regression (α ~2). The model predicted an eruption time in the range 11.45-14.45 of 25 June 1997, in good agreement with the actual dome collapse time, that occurred at 12.45 of the same day.

3.1.2. Amplitude Distribution

The self-similarity of the seismogenic structures of the volcanoes can lead to a spatial correlation between the volcanic earthquakes, in the sense that the seismogenic structures are mutually interacting elements of a multiscale faulting large system, as occurs for the tectonic seismicity (King, 1983). As an effect, the amplitudes of a class of volcanic earthquakes follows a power law, the well known Gutenberg-Richter (GR) distribution (Gutenberg and Richter, 1944):

$$log(N) = a - bM \tag{3}$$

where N is the cumulative number of earthquakes with magnitude larger than M, and a and b are constants. In particular, the parameter b is the slope of the GR distribution and gives the ratio between the frequency of large and small earthquakes. Moreover, it is inversely proportional to the average fault length that ruptures in an earthquake (Aki, 1965). b-values are normally close to 1 in the Earth's crust, but for the volcanic regions they assume values larger than 1, usually between 1 and 2 (Warren and Latham, 1970; Minakami, 1974). Moreover, within active volcanic areas heterogeneities of b-values has been detected, with higher values ($\sim$2) associated with magma-rich sectors (e.g., Wiemer et al., 1998; Murru et al., 2005).

The variations of the stress conditions before an eruption can affect the geometry of the network of the volcanic seismogenic sources (such as dikes or cracks). As a consequence, a possible modification of the b-value can be expected. Similar variations are predicted also in tectonic contexts and many authors have looked for it (Smith, 1986; Imoto, 1991; Enescu and Ito, 2001).

In fact, in many cases a change of the b-value prior to an eruption has been observed, consisting both in its increase and decrease, with the exact behavior of this parameter during the volcanic crises depending mostly on the case and on the volcano. Nevertheless, an increase of the b-value when the eruption is approaching has been more frequently observed at several volcanoes worldwide (McNutt, 2005).

At Etna volcano (Sicily, Italy), Murru et al. (2005) mapped the b-value in July-August 2001, during a lateral eruption. The authors analyzed separately the seismicity before and during the eruption and found two different b-value anomalies: b=1.84 at depths of $\sim$3 km and b=2.11 at depths of $\sim$1 km for the pre-erutive and co-eruptive phase, respectively. The authors interpreted this spatial-temporal change as an evidence of uprising magma ending with a high-velocity vertical dike emplacement, which in turn would promote the July-August volcanic crisis.

A higher b-value during the co- and post-erutive than the pre-eruptive phase at Etna volcano was detected also by Gresta and Patanè (1983) and De Natale et al. (1985) for the eruption of 17-23 March 1981. In this case, the b-value was $\sim$3 in Februar 1981, representing a sharp increase respect to the inter-eruptive seismicity that the authors associated with local changes of the stress field possibly imputed to a greater heterogeneity of the medium. Then, the b-value decreased to $\sim$2 few days before the eruption onset, while in the period 19-31 March it returned to values close to those assumed in Februar ($b \sim$3.3).

Different values was found by Vinciguerra (1999), who analyzed the time evolution of the scaling exponent D, defined aw $D = 2b$ before and during the flank eruption of Etna of September-October 1989. He found a general increase of D (from 1.6 to 2.6) since 9 months until 4 months before the eruption onset, an oscillatory behavior (between 1.5 and 2.6) between 4 months and one month before the onset, a steady value (around 1.6) during approximately the last month, followed by a drop (to about 1) when the eruption started. Few days after the eruption onset, D value increased again to about 1.8. As above, the increase of D (and therefore b-value) was imputed to a pressure build up in the volcanic edifice induced by pulses of fresh magma, with the net effect of a relative predomince of small cracks produced by an enhanced stress corrosion.

Wyss et al. (1997) analyzed the volcano seismicity at off-Ito volcano (Japan) between 1980 and 1996. The authors found an anomaluos high $b \sim$1.5 at depths of about 7 km or more, located below the coast south-east of Ito, whereas at shallower depths the b-value was around 1.7, suggesting a change of the physical state of the crust at depth $\sim$7 km. This anomaly coincided with the deeper end of the source (modelled as a tensile crack) of the surface deformation. On this basis, the authors surmised a magma chamber below 7 km feeding the eruptions of the volcano through a nearly vertical tensile crack. Moreover, the authors focused on the seismicity in the depth range corresponding to the presumed magma chamber (depth $\gtrsim$7 km) and found an increase of the b-value from 0.7 to 1.5 along the studied time interval. The same increase was also visible considering the seismicity during three eruptive phases included in the analyzed period (1989, 1993, 1995), indicating that this increase is induced by magma activity associated with the eruptions. In particular, the authors hypothesized a gradual enlargement of the crack network (leading to a higher heterogeneity of the medium) surrounding the magma chamber generated by the pressure exerted during the progression of the three intrusive episodes.

Wiemer et al. (1998) processed the seismicity of the Long Valley Caldera in the period 1982-1998. The authors found an increase of the b-value from $\sim$0.8 to $\sim$1.4 in 1989. This change appeared to be permanent or, at least, of long duration, as it was stable until the end of the analyzed period. Spatially, two high b-value (b$\sim$1.6-1.8) regions were located at depths of about 4-5 km and deeper than 7 km, with most of the seismicity nearly co-located with the shallowest anomaly, while in the other depth range b $\sim$1. The authors associated this change of b-value to an intrusion of magma and/or water beneath Mommouth Montain into a region corresponding to the shallow anomaly of 1989 altering the average distribution of cracks and/or locally increasing the pore pressure.

Novelo-Casanova et al. (2006) analyzed the seismic events at Popocatepetl volcano in the period January 1999 - June 2001, including a major eruptive activity in the period 11 December 2000 - 23 January 2001. In this case, the authors did not provide maps of the b-values and isolated the seismicity occurred in the depth range 2-8 km with magnitude between 1.9 and 3.3, thus the estimated b-values should be considered as mean values of the whole volcanic region. In the entire period preceding the eruption, the b-value was around 1.6, although large oscillations were superimposed and peaks of 1.3 and 2.3 were observed, as well. A relevant increase of the b-value was detected about 15 days before the eruption onset. In this phase, the b-value moved from about 1.6 to about 2.4. Values of 2.4-2.6 were assumed also during the first days of the eruption. Afterwards, it decreased sharply to about 1.5-1.6, that is the value assumed in the pre-eruptive period. Similarly to the other cases, the authors proposed that the b-value change was induced by a stress increase experienced by the shallow plumbing system, which in turn would be the effect of magma injection prior to the eruption.

Jolly and McNutt (1999) analyzed the seismicity at Matin-Mageik volcano complex (Alaska) in the period July 1996 - December 1997. They found a temporal increase of the b-value simultaneously to an increase of the maximum depth of the seismicity. In detail, during a shallow earthquake swarm beneath Mageik volcano in the period 16-25 October, the b-value increased to 1.59 (and remained nearly stable until April 1997) from the value of 1.01 assumed before the swarm. The authors modelled the results as the effect of a degassing intrusion acting at shallow depths and reducing the effective stress, while at greater depths the actual magma intrusion would increase the stress promoting the nucleation of deep seismicity. However, another shallow earthquake swarm occurred in November - December 1997 was not associated with any relevant change of the b-value.

Although the case of increase of the b-value when the eruption is approaching and eventually occurring is more common, some cases have been reported of a reduction of the *b*-value with the eruption occurrence, as well.

Klein (1982) analyzed the seismicity at Loihi Submarine Volcano (Hawaiian Hot Spot) during two seismic swarms occurred in 1971-1972 and 1975, presumibly associated with flank eruptions of the volcano. Differently from the background seismicity of the area that was located around the summit of the volcano edifice, during the 1971-1972 volcanic crisis the seismicity was mostly located on the flank of the volcano, with also a rise of the maximum amplitude. The seismicity located at the summit of the volcano showed a *b*-value of 2.13, whereas for the seismic clusters associated with flank eruption of 1971-1972 it dropped to 1.19. Similarly, the *b*-value calculated using the events of the 1975 volcanic crisis was 1.29. For this crisis, the events migrated towards North in respect to the location of the background seismicity rather than to the flank of the volcano, remaining confined to the Lohih's rift axis. To explain such a decrease of the *b*-value, the author proposed a change of the stress condition within the volcanic system, which during the eruptions would experience a diffused tectonic stress field rather than a more focused magma-induced stress (more active in the pre-eruptive stage).

Ibáñez et al. (2012) monitored the time evolution of the *b*-value during the 2011-2012 eruption of El Hierro volcano (Canary Islands). The eruption was a submarine volcanic event that began on 12 October, 2011, about 2 km off of the southern coast of El Hierro and was accompained by an intense seismic swarm started in July 2011. The seismicity was concentrated at depths between 10 km and 15 km in the pre-eruptive phase, with a deepening of the events starting about one month prior to the eruption onset, while in the co-eruptive phase the hypocentres were located at depths of about 15-20 km. Also the epicentres of the earthquakes evolved in time, with a location just underneath the island during about the first two months of the seismic swarm. Later on, in the time interval covering approximately the last month prior to the eruption onset, the epicentres moved southward, almost not overlapping with the location of the previous earthquakes. Finally, after the erution onset, the epicentres moved northward, falling in a region off-shore north of the island, even north of the epicentres of the first phase of the seismic swarm. For these three time intervals, the authors found *b*-values of 2.25, 1.34, 1.12, thus showing a general decrease moving towards the eruption onset and during the eruption itself. Similarly to Klein (1982), the authors proposed that the phase with high *b*-value have occurred during the magma intrusion from the upper mantle into the crust, whereas afterwards the volcano would have experienced a relaxation of the volcanic rocks at depths of 10-20 km (those hosting the seismicity) due to the draining of the magma reservoir that fed the eruption.

Besides the case of sharp variation of the b-value described above, it is worthy to mention also some cases in which the time evolution of the b-value is ambiguous and its possible variations do not emerge clearly. For example, Sanchez et al. (2004) processed the earthquakes occurred at Mount Pinatubo (Philippines) in the period June - August 1991, encompassing the cataclysmic eruption of the 15th of June, 1991. They found two prominent regions showing high b-values ($b \sim 1.7$), well correlated with low-velocity anomalies and associated with regions near magma bodies, but they did not detect relevant differences between the pre- and post-eruptive phases and thus concluded that the variations of b-value were mainly a function of space. Similarly, Murru et al. (2007) analyzed the volcanic seismicity at Etna between 1999 and 2005, including two flank eruptions occurred in 2001 and 2002-2003. They found two high b-value ($b \sim 1.82$-1.86) regions located at depths of 2 km and 6 km, which the authors associated with two magma storage zones. However, the authors also concluded that the b-value maps before and after the eruptions had not enough resolution to be compared and to highlight temporal variations.

As last example of the b-value behavior during a volcanic crisis, I report the results of Main (1987), who processed the seismicity before the explosive eruption of 18 May 1980 at Mount St. Helens (Washington). The author did not find a clear change of the b-value before the explosive eruption, but he detected a peak in the b-value ($b \sim 1.6$) before a phreatic eruption occurred on 17 March 1980 and a subsequent decrease during the phreatic event itself, reaching values in the range 0.6-0.8. Moreover, the frequency-magnitude distribution showed a double behaviuor: a power-law (following the GR relation suitable for the estimate of the b-value) for magnitudes below 4.4 and a Gaussian distribution for higher magnitudes. In addition, the earthquakes belonging to the two magnitude intervals displayed different frequency peaks (1 Hz and 2 Hz, respectively) and different characteristic source length ratios (2:1 and 6:1, respctively). The author associated this behavior with two different forms of energy release: low-magnitude events would be radiated by slipping faults, whereas LP events would generate high-magnitude events.

3.2. Independent Events

The last case study of the section 3.1 well introduces this part of the paper. Indeed, Main (1987) presented a volcano in which two classes of seismic energy release with different statistics coexisted, broadly matching the classes defined as correlated and independent seismicity in the section 3. While in the previous section I have described the properties of the events belonging to the first class, here the other class of events will be treated.

3.2.1. Inter-event Times

As already mentioned before, I have defined the independent events as induced by gas displacement, mostly produced in volcanoes with low-density magma. Specifically, these events are generated by the upward migration of coherent gas aggregation, such as slugs or pockets, within magma-filled structures of the plumbing systems, such as conduits or dikes, and its eventual bursting or exhalation at the free surface. When gas is entrapped in the form of slugs, the external bursting produces strombolian-like explosions. In these systems, the rising gases interact with the rigid structures producing the observed seismicity, which displays the features of the LP events.

The production of gas slugs is linked to the equilibrium conditions between the liquid and gasous phase of the magma-gas mixture, which is ruled by the complex thermo- and fluid-dynamic theory of the two-phase fluids (Chandrasekhar, 1943; Batchelor, 2000; Van Der Waals, 2004; Fagents et al., 2013). The effect is that for such volcanic systems, pressure variations due to new uprising magma batches may not reflect directly into the seismicity rate, which thus may be not a good proxy of the stress condition within the plumbing system and, as a consequence, FFM is mostly not suitable to model this class of seismicity.

The stationary phase (normally defining the inter-eruptive periods) of this seismic activity can be described by a point process with the features of a Poisson process (Bottiglieri et al., 2005; De Lauro et al., 2009b). In a Poisson process, the occurrence time of an event is independent of the occurrence times of the other events, and the distribution of the inter-event times follows a decreasing exponential function (Cox and Lewis, 1966):

$$f(\Delta t) = \lambda e^{-\lambda \Delta t} \quad (4)$$

where λ represents the rate of the process and Δt is the inter-event time.

Bottiglieri et al. (2005) analyzed the rate of the explosion-quakes (i.e. the seismic signal produced by gas slug bursting at the free surface with the features of LP events) at Stromboli volcano (Southern Italy) during a stationary phase of the volcano. They found that the explosive activity is well described by a Poisson process with an average inter-event time of 2.73 minutes. Similarly, De Lauro et al. (2009b) processed the occurrence times of the seismic events induced by gas bubbles bursting at the free surface of a lava lake at Erebus volcano (Antarctica). They found again a Poisson process ruling the occurrence times of the seismic events. In this case, the mean inter-event time was equal to 5.5 hours, suggesting that whereas the process driving the gas bursting is common, it can act on very different time scales depending on the magma composition, on its temperature and on the gas content.

A statistical parameter that is used to define the nature of point process is the variation coefficient C_v. It is defined as (Cox and Lewis, 1966):

$$C_v = \frac{\sigma_{\Delta t}}{\overline{\Delta t}} \quad (5)$$

where $\sigma_{\Delta t}$ is the standard deviation of the inter-event time series and $\overline{\Delta t}$ is the mean inter-event time. $C_v = 1$ for a Poissonian process, whereas $C_v > 1$ for a clustered process and $C_v = 0$ for a periodic one. The limit $C_v \to \infty$ indicates an uniform distribution of the inter-event times.

De Martino et al. (2011a,b) studied the behavior of the seismicity at Stromboli volcano during the volcanic crises of 2002-2003 and 2007, respectively. In both the cases, C_v was constantly close to one also after the crisis onset, that is during the lava emission, indicating that the explosive process inducing the observed LP seismicity at Stromboli is very stable.

Also at Mount St. Helens, Matoza and Chouet (2010) found a Poisson process ruling the LP activity during an aruption. Specifically, they found that the inter-event time distribution of a subset of the LP events (only those with amplitude below a threshold) followed Eq. 4 during the eruption of 2004-2008. The authors processed three disjoined time periods occurred in November 2004, July

2005 and October-December 2005, and found that $\frac{1}{\lambda} \simeq 90s, 112s, 250 - 500s$ for the three periods, respectively.

The stability of the source process is the effect of a non-destructive source mechanism, which is a feature of this type of volcanoes (e.g., Chouet et al., 2003). Such a stability makes difficult the detection of possible precursor phenomena emerging from the seismicity. In fact, the nature of the source mechanism of the seismic events (which is at the basis of the temporal and spatial independence of the discrete seismic events) inhibits escalating phenomena. On the contrary, any disequilibrium in the system tends to be masked in the seismicity. In that sense, McNutt (1996) commented that basaltic volcanoes do not show any precursory phenomena.

In line with this evidence, De Martino et al. (2011b) did not find any relevant increase of the seismic rate neither before nor during the eruption of Stromboli volcano of 2002-2003, which consisted in a lava effusion punctuated on 5 April 2003 by a major explosive events (paroxystic). In that case, the rate of the explosion-quakes during the non-eruptive phase was distributed following a Gaussian function with mean value corresponding to an inter-event time of about 250 s, and the values of the rate during the eruptive phase fell within this distribution.

Although the strombolian eruption does not affect the seismic event rate, De Martino et al. (2011b) highlighted an oscillatory behavior of the event rate with a period of about 3 days about three months before the eruption onset and lasting about 20 days. Similar behavior was observed also by De Martino et al. (2011a) during the eruption of Stromboli started on 27 Februar 2007 with an effusive phase and culminated on 15 March 2007 with a paroxystic explosion, thus mimicking the progression of the 2002-2003 eruptive crisis. The authors found a time interval of about 10 days (occurring about one month before the crisis onset), in which the amplitudes of the seismic events oscillated with a period of about 3 days. In this case, the signal was recorded also by a strainmeter, thus indicating that it comprehended also a deformative component. This signal introduced a phase of high-energy seismic events which, in turn, led to the eruption and was imputed to very slow oscillations of the volcanic conduit.

The strombolian eruption of 2007 showed also an increase of the event rate, differently from the case of 2002-2003. In that case, the rate moved from 0.004 ev/s (inter-event time of 5.5 min) of the non-eruptive phase to 0.009 ev/s (2 min) of the effusive phase. The event rate started to increase at the crisis onset and moved to the nearly stable value assumed during the eruptive phase in about ten days (De Martino et al., 2011a).

An increase of the event rate has been detected also at Ubinas volcano (Perú) by Traversa et al. (2011) before 143 explosive eruptions occurred between 2006 and 2008. The authors found that the LP events were temporarily clustered before each eruption, but without showing any correlation leading to a mainshock-aftershocks sequence. The increase of the event rate began about one day before the eruption, moving from about 60 events/day of the background level to about 200 events/day just before the eruption onset. Moreover, after the eruption, the event rate followed a relaxation process with the same features of the loading, thus in about one day the event rate moved from $\sim$250 events/day to $\sim$60 events/day.

An important element reflecting an instability within the shallow plumbing system of Stromboli volcano is the presence of LP swarms (De Martino et al., 2012). Swarms of events have been observed before and during the eruption of 2002-2003 (De Martino et al., 2011b), during the eruption of 2007 (De Martino et al., 2011a) and also in the inter-eruptive phase (De Martino et al., 2012). During the swarms, the event rate notably increase, moving from $\sim$0.005 ev/s up to $\sim$0.02 ev/s or more, and the C_v drops to $\sim$0.5, suggesting a more periodic process than during the stationary phase. Moreover, the events of the swarms: 1. are on average 0.5-1 orders of magnitude more energetic than the standard events; 2. have very shallow (and crater-pointing) polarization; 3. show a quasi-monochromatic spectral content with peak at about 3 Hz; 4. have very similar waveforms (De Martino et al., 2012).

The seismic swarms at Stromboli have been proposed to occur as a response to disequilibrium conditions in the magma-gas mixture at shallow depths (0.3-0.8 km) leading to a depressurization and an over-production of gas slugs, making them a proxy of a possible escalation of the disequilibrium to volcanic crises (De Martino et al., 2012). For example, during the eruption of 2002-2003 two long-lasting ($\sim$5-10 days) swarms occured about 40-50 days before the eruption onset (De Martino et al., 2011b). On the other hand, a series of swarms in 2010-2011 didn't lead to any relevant external activity of the volcano (De Martino et al., 2012).

3.2.2. Amplitude Distribution

Differently from the case of correlated events and as a consequence of the absence of multi-scale self-similar phenomena, the amplitude of these events does not follow a power law. On the contrary, the amplitude distribution is well described by a Gaussian function when the amplitude of the events is plotted on a logarithmic scale (log-normal distribution, hereafter).

De Martino et al. (2004) showed that the energy of the LP events at Stromboli volcano in the stationary phase is distributed in a log-normal way. Moreover, on the basis of the analysis of the trajectory space reconstructed with 580 hystories of the same process (the LP events), the authors concluded that all the events are generated by the same dynamical system. The log-normal distribution - with one most probable value of the amplitude of the LP events - is thus the effect of a stable and unique process generating the events.

The log-normal distribution of the amplitude at Stromboli was confirmed by De Martino et al. (2012) looking at a non-eruptive phase of the volcano in 2010-2011, indicating that this feature can be considered a time-independent evidence of the stationary strombolian activity. Moreover, it has been observed also at other volcanoes worldwide, suggesting that it could be a more general behavior common to a certain class of volcanoes.

As a "precursor" work (mentioned above), Main (1987) found at Mount St Helens a log-normal distribution of the seismic events with magnitude larger than 4.4. In that case, this distribution co-existed with a power-law distribution, thus potentially masking the complete shape of the log-normal behavior. Nevertheless, the author associated the log-normal distribution to a different form of "energy release" than the tectonic-loaded slipping faults, that are LP events induced by volcanic activity.

Rowe et al. (2000) analyzed the seismic signals induced by strombolian-like activity at Erebus volcano in the period 1994-1998 and found a peaked histogram of the size of the LP events occurred between October 1997 and July 1998. The authors interpreted the shape of the distribution as the effect of a preferred median size for bubble bursts, although they mentioned also the possible influence of catalog incompleteness or of two or more distinct populations of sources.

At the same volcano, similar results were found also by De Lauro et al. (2009b), who processed the LP seismicity of Erebus during 2005 and 2006. As in the case of Stromboli, they found a log-normal distribution of the event amplitudes. Specifically, the authors distinguished two classes of events on the basis of waveform, spectrum and polarization vector, with both the classes following a distinct log-normal amplitude distribution. Moreover, such a bi-modal log-normal distribution was associated with two independent processes, both belonging to the same class of events produced by gas slug upward migration and ruled by a Poisson process, but activating different energy scales. In that sense, the authors excluded effects (proposed by Rowe et al. (2000)) of catalog incompleteness, and associated the shape of the amplitude distribution with two preferential bubble sizes, thus validating the hypothesis of more than one population of sources.

Similarly, at Mount St. Helens (Washington), Matoza and Chouet (2010) found a bi-modal distribution on logarithmic scale of LP events occurring during the eruptive crises of 2004-2008. The authors associated the two Gaussians to two classes of LP events distinguished by the energy. Only the low-energy events (named *subevents*) were ruled by a Poisson process, whereas the other class displayed a peaked inter-event time distribution, indicating a quasi-period behavior.

Recently, Hurst et al. (2014) found a nearly log-normal distribution of the amplitudes of an earthquake swarm preceding the eruption of Tongariro volcano (New Zealand) occurred on 6 August 2012. In detail, the authors detected a frequency-magnitude relation for this swarm (occurred in July 2012) well different from the power law ruling the seismicity in the inter-eruptive period. The events of the swarm were distinguished into three families whose elements shared similar waveforms and spectra, with most energy contained around 2 Hz. In addition, the inter-event times between the events of the swarm showed a quasi-period behavior, with the most frequenty inter-event interval falling in the range 30-80 minutes (depending on the family). The reported features made this seismic swarm similar to the LP swarms observed at Stromboli by De Martino et al. (2011b,a, 2012).

The log-normal distribution emerged also during the effusive phase of the strombolian eruption of 2002-2003, that is in the period 28/12/2002-30/01/2003. In this case, the mean value of the distribution was very similar to that assumed in the non-eruptive phase, thus indicating that the emission of lava does not affect the process driving the background LP activity. The log-normal shape was mostly preserved also during the time-interval preceding the eruption onset (07/12/2002-28/12/2002), although the number of high-energy events was slightly higher than expected by the Gaussian distribution due to the presence of two long-lasting explosion swarms occurring in this phase. Moreover, the amplitude distribution of the time interval preceding the eruption onset showed also an increase of the mean value of about 76% respect to the previous phases (before 07/12/2002) (De Martino et al., 2011b).

Before the eruptive crises of 2007 of Stromboli, the amplitude distribution followed a log-normal shape, as well (De Martino et al., 2011a). Moreover, similarly to the 2002-2003 case, the mean amplitude in a one-month-long time interval preceding the eruption was larger than that assumed during the stationary activity (sampled in a period well before the eruption onset), with an increase of about 35%. However, after the eruption onset, the amplitude distribution was no longer fitted by a log-normal function, whereas it showed a nearly flat distribution encompassing both the amplitude peaks assumed during the pre-eruptive and the stationary phase, indicating a strong variability of the LP process during the eruption and, thus, a sharp escaping from the equilibrium conditions of the stationary phase (see also Buccheri et al. (2013) for a review of the seismicity at Stromboli during the eruptions of 2002-2003 and 2007).

Despite the seismic swarms of Stromboli are ruled by a point process different from that ruling the standard events, their amplitudes follow a log-normal shape too. Thus, although the events of the swarms are well distinguished from the standard seismic activity and could be considered as a sign of a disequilibrium of the magma-gas mixture at shallow depths, their amplitude is ruled by the same process, suggesting the existence of a common source mechanism (gas slug migration) (De Martino et al., 2012).

4. Volcanic Tremor and Continuous Signal

Besides the discrete seismic events introduced above, another powerful indication of the status of the volcano when an eruption is approaching is provided by the volcanic tremor. Volcanic tremor is a non-impulsive continuous or discontinuous low-energy seismic signal, that shares the same source mechanism and seismic wavefield of the LP events (Chouet, 2003; Konstantinou and Schlindwein, 2003; De Lauro et al., 2008). For this reason, it is often modelled as a sequence of LP events and is imputed to the interaction between the magma-gas mixture and the rock in the magma chamber or conduit (Chouet, 1985; Crosson and Bame, 1985; Julian, 1994; De Lauro et al., 2008).

Volcanic tremor is probably the most reliable precursor of the eruptions, as it has been observed in most cases associated with volcanic crises (see, e.g., McNutt, 1996, 2005). In particular, volcanic tremor seems to shortly precede the eruption onset, having thus a special role in terms of volcanic risk mitigation (McNutt, 1996). For example, analysing the reported precursory activity of 132 historical eruptions, Barberi et al. (1992) concluded that anomalous seismicity is the most frequent precursor and, in particular, the volcanic tremor is the most reported phenomenon anticipating the eruptions of a few hours. In a more quantitive way, looking for a relation between volcanic tremor and eruptions, McNutt (1992) analyzed 1100 episodes of tremor from 84 different volcanoes worldwide. He found that about 60% of the episodes accompained the eruptions. Moreover, in about 20% of the cases, the tremor was observed within 10 days before the eruption onset, while in $10 - 20\%$ it occurred in the 10 days following the eruption onset.

In more recent times, due to a general improvement of the seismic monitoring of active volcanoes all over the world, the occurrence of volcanic tremor before and during volcanic eruptions has been observed in several cases.

Kelut volcano (Java Island, Indonesia) erupted on February 10-12, 1990. Lesage et al. (1995) detected a sharp increase of low-energy volcano-tectonic events starting 24 hours before the eruption onset. The event rate gradually increased until becoming a continuous signal with the features of spasmodic volcanic tremor and eventually leading to the eruption. Before the appearence of volcanic tremor, the authors found an increase of the seismic activity starting three months before the eruption, with the occurrence of shallow VT events (often under the form of multiplets) with a rate of ~500-1000 events/day, whereas the background VT activity rate in the pre-eruptive stage was 8 events/day on average. The last three weeks before the eruption showed a scarce seismic activity, but in the day preceding the eruption the emergence of tremor anticipated the eruption onset.

Ruapehu volcano (New Zealand) erupted in 1995-1996. The eruption consisted of two stages of eruptive activity: Stage I: 17 September - early November 1995 and Stage II: 16 June - late July 1996. Bryan and Sherburn (1999) observed a persistent volcanic tremor with frequency content peaked around 7 Hz occurring one year before the onset of Stage I. In the same period, an intermittent volcanic tremor with spectral maximum around 2 Hz was observed. Differently from other cases, the rest of seismicity (such as VT events) displayed a rate in line with the inter-eruptive phase. During Stage I the volcanic tremor persisted, with the appearence of frequencies below 1 Hz in the first part (September 1995) and a wideband tremor later on (October 1995). During the last part of Stage I, an increase of discrete seismic activity was registered, as well, with a number of volcanic earthquakes up to $\sim$100 events/day. Between the two stages of the eruption, the 7-Hz tremor persisted continuously together with a relevant activity of shallow VT events ($\sim$100-200 events/day). When Stage II started, tremor was still observed, but its spectrum became wider. At the same time, VT activity ceased completely, while LP events occurred with a rate of $\sim$150 events/day. After the end of Stage II, the conditions slowly returned to those observed in the pre-erutive phase, with 7-Hz tremor dominating the seismicity.

The eruption of Etna volcano between 26 January and 24 June 2000 culminated in 64 lava fountain episodes, with an inter-episode time interval ranging between 3 hours and 10 days. Alparone et al. (2003) correlated the duration of the volcanic tremor with the eruptive activity and found that volcanic tremor occurred during each episode of lava fountain. In detail, they found a linear relation between the duration of tremor and the duration of lava fountain episode (both ranging in $\sim$30-600 seconds). Moreover, the authors detected a characteristic time-evolution of the tremor amplitude (measured by Reduced Displacement, described below) during an individual lava fountain episode. An individual eruptive episode consisted of an initial weak effusive activity followed by a Strombolian phase, a Fountaining phase and, in same case, a conclusive phase consisting of a sustained column, the whole eruptive episode lasting about 6 hours. Alparone et al. (2003) found that the tremor increased from the early stage of the eruption reaching a maximum during the phase of lava fountain or, if present, of sustained column. Moreover, the tremor amplitude scaled linearly with the lava funtain or sustained column height.

Aki and Ferrazzini (2000) analyzed the seismicity at Piton de la Fournaise before the eruption occurred between 9 March and 21 September 1998. The authors found volcanic tremor starting about 40 minutes before the eruption onset, superimposing on the background VT seismicity already announcing an impending eruption since about 1.5 days before the beginning of the eruption. The tremor showed a frequency content peaked at ~2 Hz and its source was located in a large area around the summit of the volcano, probably induced by an extended source region. Similar features were observed also for a class of LP events evidenced before the eruption onset. During the eruption, the tremor showed an oscillating behavior, with three main phases (lasting 10-15 days) of amplitude increase (up to five times the background value), that the authors associated with the intensity of the magma flow.

A sharp increase of the volcanic tremor was observed also at Anatahan volcano (Pacific Mariana Islands) by Pozgay et al. (2005) during the first historical eruption occurred on 10 May 2003. The authors showed that tremor amplitude basically increased after the eruption onset, reaching in the first ~3 hours of the eruption a value equal to about 15-20 times the pre-eruptive value of the background noise. Then, it assumed nearly constant high values for about two weeks; afterwards, its amplitude reduced drastically of about 90 %, but remaining well above the pre-eruptive background noise. On the other hand, VT activity started about 6 hours before the eruption onset and showed a rapid increase reaching ~80 events/day about one hour prior to the eruption onset.

Also at Bezymianny (Kamchatka) volcanic tremor precedes the eruptions. West (2013) examined the eruptions between 2006-2010. He found an increase of the tremor (by 2-3 orders of magnitude) 12-36 hours before the onset. Often the tremor energy increased gradually approaching the eruption and in a similar way it decreased after the end of the eruption. Moreover, for a class of eruptions (those emitting juvenile magmas) West (2013) found a linear relation between the cumulative moment magnitude of the released seismic energy and the repose time between successive eruptions, thus providing a tool for prediciting the energy of future eruptions.

At El Hierro volcano, although the first unrest of this (submarine) volcano was detected in July 2011 with the location of small-magnitude events underneath the main volcanic edifice (Ibáñez et al., 2012), volcanic tremor appeared only on 10 October 2011, that is about two days before the eruption onset. Volcanic tremor persisted for about two days, then it reduced to a value well above the pre-eruptive background level, probably induced by a variation of the magma flow rate produced by a change of the eruptive style, which evolved from a fissure to a central conduit emission (Ibáñez et al., 2012; Tárraga et al., 2014). During the eruption, Tárraga et al. (2014) detected two more increases of the tremor amplitude occurring on 3-7 and on 16-20 November 2011. The former increase coincides with an intensification of the eruption (announced by gas and stains on the sea surface), confirming the tight relation between tremor amplitude and flowing magma. The latter tremor increase was associated with the appearence of secondary vents on the volcano and with the origin of a corresponding stain appeared on the sea surface during the eruption (Tárraga et al., 2014). After the latter increase, tremor amplitude remained low until the end of the eruption (February 2012).

A sharp increase of the energy of the volcanic tremor was observed also by De Martino et al. (2011a) before the eruption of February-April 2007 of Stromboli. The authors found an enhancement of the tremor amplitude starting about two months before the eruption onset (February 27, 2007) and culminating just before the beginning of the lava effusion, when it reached an amplitude about ten times higher than the background signal. It is remarkable to note that, in the same two months, the rate of the explosion-quakes did not change, keeping the value assumed during the stationary activity.

In order to be able to compare the tremor amplitude recorded at different volcanoes, Aki and Koyanagi (1981) defined the "Reduced Displacement" (D_R), that is the tremor amplitude after normalizing for the instrument response and the geometrical spreading. For surface waves D_R it is defined as follows:

$$D_R = \frac{A}{2\sqrt{2}} \cdot \frac{r}{M} \tag{6}$$

where A is the peak-to-peak ground displacement, r is the source-sensor distance, and M is the instrument magnification. For body waves, the equation becomes:

$$D_R = \frac{A}{2\sqrt{2}} \cdot \frac{\sqrt{r\lambda}}{M} \tag{7}$$

where λ is the wavelength.

Di Grazia et al. (2009) monitored D_R before and during the eruption of Etna volcano occurred between 10 May 2008 and 6 July 2009, consisting of an initial Hawaiian activity followed by a later phase dominated by variable lava flows and strombolian activity. Starting from the second part of April (thus, more than one month before the eruption onset), the authors found a gradual increase of D_R, which moved from $\sim$2 cm^2 to $\sim$20 cm^2 just before the eruption onset. Afterwards, D_R dropped in about 10 days to $\sim$5 cm^2.

Thompson et al. (2002) analyzed D_R during the eruption of Shishaldin volcano (Alaska) of 1999. A seismic and thermal unrest of the volcano started in January-February 1999 and culminated in a sub-plinian phase occurred on 19 April 1999. The authors reported the appearance of low-energy tremor in January 1999. A sharp increase of D_R was detected on 7 April, when it reached 8 cm^2. However, a very strong increase of D_R occurred in correspondence of the sub-plinian event, when it assumed a value of $\sim$20 cm^2. Afterwards, D_R assumed similar values during the vigorous strombolian phases and the other eruptive phase occurred on 23 April 1999, thus punctuating the largest external activity of the volcano.

Benoit et al. (2003) evaluated D_R at eight volcanoes and one geothermal area and related it with the duration of the tremor. The authors found that the duration of the tremor episodes scales with D_R following an exponential function, differently from tectonic earthquakes, for which the relation between duration and magnitude is ruled by a power law. The formula is:

$$d(D_R) = d_t e^{-\lambda D_R} \tag{8}$$

where d is the duration of the tremor equal to or larger than a specific D_R, d_t is the total duration of the tremor, and λ^{-1} is a characteristic amplitude of the distribution. Benoit et al. (2003) found also that λ^{-1} is larger for tremor associated with eruptions than non-eruptive tremor, confirming a tight connection between tremor and eruption. Moreover, the authors found larger values of λ^{-1} for deep tremor and for tremor produced by magmatic eruptions (rather than by phreatic eruptions). The authors concluded that λ^{-1} is proportional to a geometric dimension of the source, implying that volcanic tremor is activated on a characteristic length scale, differently from the self-similar phenomena involved in the tectonic earthquakes.

McNutt (1994) determined D_R for 21 eruptions of 14 volcanoes occurring between 1964 to 1991 and found a linear relation between D_R and VEI. The author provided the following equation:

$$log_{10}(D_R) = 0.46 \times VEI + 0.08 \quad (9)$$

Moreover, the author found a similar relation also between D_R and the height of the ash cloud (ACH) produced by explosive eruptions:

$$log_{10}(D_R) = 1.80 \times log_{10}(ACH) - 0.08 \quad (10)$$

thus indicating that D_R is a good proxy for the eruption size. As an application, the author provided a D_R threshold above which aviation hazard must be taken into account (10 cm^2).

In a similar way, McNutt and Nishimura (2008) analyzed D_R and the temporal variation of the eruption tremor with geological data for 24 eruptive crises occurring from 1962 to 1994 at 18 volcanoes located worldwide. The authors found that D_R is roughly proportional to the square root of the cross sectional area of the vent. Moreover, they found that the eruption tremor shows basically three stages: an exponential increase at the first large external emission of the eruption, a maintenance at maximum level, an exponential decrease at the end of the eruptive sequence. The time constants of the exponential increase and decrease of the tremor amplitude changes from case to case from few minutes to several hours.

Another approach to seismically monitor active volcanoes looks at the continuous signal, without distinguishing between tremor and discrete seismic events. The Real-Time Seismic Measurement (RSAM) is commonly measured. RSAM is the amplitude of the seismic signal averaged over a moving time window (usually of some minutes), in order to infer the total seismic energy released in near real-time. A similar parameter is the Seismic Spectral Amplitude Measurement (SSAM), that is the seismic amplitude measured in different frequency ranges, thus allowing the evaluation of the contribution of individual frequency bands.

Chouet et al. (1994) inferred RSAM for the eruption of Redoubt volcano (Alaska) of December 1989 - April 1990. LP activity started about 23 hours before the eruption onset of 14 December 1989. LP rate increased in the following hours, until merging in a continuous tremor in the last 5 hours of the swarm. This increase of seismicity was visible as a gradual rise of RSAM, following the escalation of the seismic swarm and peaking at the onset of the eruption, when RSAM reached values about 4-6 times (depending on the station) larger than the background value. After the beginning of the eruptive phase, RSAM showed a systematic increase before each explosive eruptions punctuating the whole volcanic crisis, peaking in correspondence of the eruptive episodes at values up to 10 times larger than the background level.

RSAM and SSAM have been also adopted as parameter sensitive to the stress conditions of the volcano in FFM. Voight and Cornelius (1991) applied FFM to fit RSAM for two dome-growth episodes at Mount St. Helens in 1985 and 1986 and two explosive eruptions at Redoubt volcano in 1989-1990. The authors found a good fit of the model using RSAM and inferred values of the scaling parameter α ranging between 1.2 and 1.6 for Mount St. Helens, with the onset of the precursory RSAM acceleration observed 5-12 days before the eruption. The authors applied the model with good results to the case of Redoubt too. Moreover, they tried to predict the eruption of 2 January 1990, using only a subset of the available RSAM points, leaving out 1-6 days before the eruption. Fixing $\alpha = 2$, the model provided fair accurate eruption times also in this case, suggesting that RSAM can be a good proxy of the volcanic stress conditions alternative to the seismicity rate.

Redoubt eruption of 1989-1990 was analyzed by FFM also by Cornelius and Voight (1994) using RSAM and SSAM. In this case, the authors found a good fit to FFM of the points using both RSAM and SSAM for the dome-destroying eruption of 2 January 1990 (adopting $\alpha = 2$). On the other hand, for the rapid sequence of dome-collapse eruptions following the event of 2 January, signal amplitude diminished and RSAM signal-to-noise ratio decreased, with the effect that FFM was not well fitted anymore. Instead, eliminating the frequency bands dominated by noise and focusing on frequencies around 2 Hz, SSAM assumed a higher signal-to-noise ratio and FFM was successfully applied also to this sequence of eruptions.

Recently, Budi-Santoso et al. (2013) applied FFM using RSAM to the 2010 eruption of Merapi volcano (Java Island, Indonesia). The authors excluded from the analysis tectonic events and calculated RSAM in four disjoined frequency ranges spanning the interval 0.01-10 Hz and in the wider interval 1-15 Hz. The eruption started with an explosive event on 26 October 2010 and was preceded by about six weeks of an intense seismic activity. RSAM showed a relative maximum in correspondence of the eruption onset, but assumed its largest value in the period 3-10 November 2010, during intense pyroclastic flows. The authors predicted the eruption time by FFM with RSAM, with errors as small as ± 4 hours obtained within a 6-day lapse time before the eruption. Also when α was not fixed a-priori and was calculated by regression, it assumed values ~ 2. The best performances were obtained for the frequency band 3-5 Hz, which mostly hosted VT events, confirming that FFM well works with the class of correlated volcanic events.

5. Hypocenter Migration

Volcanic eruptions are sketched as an upward or lateral migration of magma possibly culminating in the external lava emission. As remarked above, magma movements transfer stress to the rigid structures of the plumbing system, which react releasing seismic radiation. In this scheme, the location of the seismicity preceding the eruptions can track the magma migration.

Although this scheme can be in some cases an oversimplification of the eruption dynamics, several cases of seismic foci migration before and during volcanic eruptions have been reported.

Klein (1982) analyzed a 13-month earthquake swarm occurring in 1971-1972 at Loihi volcano preceding a submarine eruption or an intrusion. The author found that the seismicity was located at depth of 20-50 km during the first month of the swarm, while later on it was concentrated at depths of 0-20 km, implying an upward migration of the seismicity possibly mimicking a similar magma dynamics.

Castellano et al. (1993) localized the seismicity nucleated at Etna volcano in the period 1988-1990, which included the eruption started on 11 September 1989. The authors found that the events occurring in 1988 (that is after the previous eruption occurred in 1986-1987) were located at depths of 7-25 km, with most of them in the depth range 15-25 km. Differently, the events of 1989 preceding the eruption had depths of 0-14 km, with most of them shallower than 8 km, thus indicating an approaching of the seismicity to the surface.

More recently, Di Grazia et al. (2009) analyzed the seismicity associated with the eruption of Etna of 13 May 2008. In this case, the location of the volcanic tremor showed a peculiar pattern, with a deepening of the source in the period 01/02/2008-15/03/2008, during which the source moved broadly from regions close to the summit of the volcano to points about 3 km below the summit. After the middle of March, the source of tremor moved sharply upward, being located at dephts of 0-2 km with a very scattered behavior. During about 8 days prior to the eruption onset, the source moved again to depths of $\sim$2 km. When the eruption started, the hypocentres moved upwards and concentrated in the uppermost $\sim$1.5 km of the volcanic edifice.

A migration of the source depth of seismicity has been observed also by Johnson et al. (2010) at Okmok volcano. In this case, the authors found a deep seismicity (earthquake foci as deep as 13 km) during the first days of the eruption occurred in the period 11 July - 15 August 2008. Afterwards, the earthquake hypocentres were always shallower than about 7 km, with an increase of the events nucleating at very shallow depths ($<$1 km) in the last 10 days of the eruption.

At Soufriere Hill volcano, Battaglia et al. (2005) found a clear upward and gradual migration of the earthquake hypocentres occurring during about 3 days prior to the eruption onset of 9 March 1998, that is during a seismic swarm preceding the eruption. In detail, the authors located 583 VT events with a maximum magnitude of 2.2 and found that at the onset of the seismic swarm the earthquakes nucleated at depths of about 8 km from the summit of the volcano. In the following times, the authors evidenced a monotonic shallowing of the source position, which moved to depths of about 7 km about 1.5 days before the eruption onset. Afterwards, the source shallowing became sharper, with also an increase of the event rate (from $\sim$1 to $\sim$6 events/min). In the few minutes preceding the eruption onset, the seismicity was located few hundred meters below the summit of the volcano, with the mean velocity of the upward source migration in the last 1.5 days equal to $\sim$0.1 m/min.

At the same volcano, Rowe et al. (2004) analyzed the earthquakes occurring in the period July 1995 - Februar 1996, that included a phreatic activity (abruptly began on 18 July 1995) and a subsequent series of steam and ash explosions, which continued for about 4 months and eventually led to an extended period of dome extrusion started in mid-November 1995. The authors found a series of families in the recordings, and relocated the events within the same family by a double-difference technique (Waldhauser and Ellsworth, 2000). The authors did not remark any systematic depth change during the analyzed period, although the source depth of the clusters was variable within about 2 km and a broadly bi-modal distribution of the hypocenter depths was highlighted, with the most frequent depths at ~3 km and ~1.5 km. Nevertheless, they remarked the existence of a slight decrease of the depth towards the end of some individual clusters, with a migration limited to few tens/hundreds of meters and possibly due to a change of pressure gradient within the plumbing system.

An indirect sign of migrating magma into the seismic signals was provided also by Aki and Ferrazzini (2000), who found a strong correlation between the duration of the precursory swarms of VT events and the elevation of the eruption sites at Piton de la Fournaise. The authors reported that precursory times are shorter than 1 hour for eruptions near the summit (at about 2.5 km) and longer than 6 hours for eruptions at elevations of about 1.8 km, suggesting that such a difference can be imputed to the different path lengths travelled by the magma before the eruption. On the other hand, LP events are absent in the precursory seismicity preceding the summit eruptions, while they appear prior to the flank eruptions occured near the caldera rim. On the basis of these evidences, the authors depicted two magma paths: the summit path and the rift zone path, whose seismic signatures are respectively VT and LP events. Moreover, LP events with different dominant frequency (1 Hz and 2 Hz) would track different stages of the flank eruptions, being the 1 Hz-LPs shallower than the 2 Hz-LPs.

More recently, at the same volcano De Barros et al. (2013) found a shallowing of the source position of the VT seismicity starting about 4 hours before the onset of the eruption occurred on 14 October 2010, and lasting about 1 hour, during which the source depth moved from values around the sea level to about 2 km a.s.l.. This migration coincided with an inflation, as measured by a GPS instrument nearby the summit of the volcano, thus reflecting an uprising magma movement. Afterwards, the VT hypocentres remained nearly stable at shallow depths even after the eruption onset. About one hour before the beginning of the eruption, a lateral migration of magma was punctuated by an increase of the GPS signal at a station on the south-eastern flank of the volcano and by VT events with larger energy released at very high frequencies (>10 Hz, HF events). HF events were generated by shallow failures in the area of the eruption and possibly reflected the dike propagation, which could create a pathway for the magma migration. The authors therefore suggested that these events were not directly induced by the magma movement but by the stress induced by this movement.

An indirect sign of magma migration is provided by b-value anomalies detected at different depths when measured at different times (e.g., Wiemer et al., 1998), indicating a modification of the stress conditions within the volcanic system. Uprising seismicity can also reflect ascending gas batches released from underlying magma, as in the case of Mammoth Mountain reported by Shelly and Hill (2011). On shorter time scales, Palo et al. (2009) detected a shallowing of the seismic source during the first ~10 s of the LP events preceding volcanic explosions at Colima volcano (Mexico) possibly generated by the upward migration (with velocity of ~300 m/s) of a pressure step potentially induced by gas aggregation or fluid displacement.

However, as remarked above, depicting the magma migration preceding the eruptions as a pure upward movement in most cases does not correspond to the real sources processes. Moreover, the seismic response due to magma movement is strongly nonlinear and only rarely produces a continuum of foci, whereas more often the seismic sources are spatially concentrated along faults and spatially clustered.

Harlow et al. (1996) looked at the seismicity before the catastrofic 1991 eruption of Mount Pinatubo, which started on 12 June with a strong explosion. The authors located the VT seismicity occurring between 8 May and the beginning of the eruption in two main spatially distinguished clusters, located beneath the summit of the volcano at depths of ~3 km and along the north-west flank at larger depths (~5 km). Whereas in May the earthquakes were mostly concentrated within the deeper cluster, during the first week of June a strong swarm populated the shallower cluster, extending moreover the cluster up to the surface and culminating in the extrusion of a lava dome. Then, in the days just before the eruption onset, the deeper seismicity sharply decreased remaining active the shallower cluster composed of events nucleated in the broad depth interval 0-3 km. Some years after the work of Harlow et al. (1996), Jones et al. (2001) refined the localization of the events composing the deeper cluster, which actually was elongated along a narrow, roughly linear structure, suggesting the activation of a pre-existing fault.

Similarly, Cerdeña et al. (2011) detected two clusters of VT events relocating the seismicity recorded at Tenerife in 2004-2005 during a reactivation of the volcano (not leading to an eruption, though). The clusters had a distance of about 10 km and formed two clouds of events centered at ~4 km and ~7 km (but extending up to depths of 10 km or more). The two clusters alternated their activity starting from January 2004, possibly as an effect of a pressure increase (induced by magma intrusion) activating two regions of the seismogenic crust below the volcano surface, both possibly connected to the main feeding conduit by branching of the plumbing system.

Gambino et al. (2004) found also two spatial trends along which the earthquakes occurred at Etna volcano from August 2001 till October 2002 (that is before the flank eruption begun on 27 October 2002) were aligned. The two alignements were roughly oriented in the directions NE-SW and NW-SE, well matching both the tectonic and volcanic seismogenic lineaments of Etna. Similarly, Ottemöller (2008) located the earthquakes of a swarm anticipating of a few days a dome collapse at Soufriere Hills volcano occurred on 12-13 July 2003, at shallow depths (<3 km) in a region with radius of ~ 150 m. The hypocentres did not show relevant time changes and the waveforms of the events of the swarm displayed high similarity, indicating a very stable source process.

6. Change of the Source Process: Focal Mechanisms

Several authors have also found changes of the focal mechanism (which depicts the moment tensor of the physical process describing the seismic source (Lay and Wallace, 1995)) of the earthquakes occurring during or after the volcanic crises. Time evolutions of the focal mechanisms are normally imputed to changes of the effective stress field in the volcanic region, where the stress state induced by magma displacement at depth combines with the regional nearly stationary tectonic stress field.

Roman et al. (2006, 2008) calculated the focal mechanisms of VT events recorded at Soufriere Hills volcano during the eruptive crisis started in July 1995. The authors found a change of the direction of the axis of maximum compressive stress in the weeks/months prior to each eruptive phase (and prior to a transition of the eruption style from effusive to explosive) in respect to the stress direction found during the inter-eruptive phases, with a discrepancy of about 90°. In detail, the direction of the p-axis (pressure axis, a proxy of the local principal stress axis) in the inter-eruptive phase (representative of the regional tectonic stress field) pointed towards NE-SW for the vast majority of the events, while during the eruptive phases solutions with p-axis pointing towards NE-SE appeared, as well. The authors indicated the inflation of a NE-SW oriented dike centered beneath the volcanic vent as a possible source of the observed rotation.

Similar results was found also by Roman et al. (2004) analysing VT events before and after three eruption of Crater Peak Vent at Mount Spurr (Alaska) in 1992. Prior to the eruptions (and also during 11 months in the post-eruptive phase), beneath Crater Peak the authors found a sub-horizontal p-axis different (rotated of $\sim 90°$on the horizontal plane) from that inferred when the regional tectonic setting dominated. At the same time, the p-axis beneath the summit of Mount Spurr was nearly vertical, thus different from both the previous p-axis directions. The authors imputed the change in p-axis beneath Crater Peak to an inflation of a dike system, whereas the slip occurring over a normal fault would have induced the p-axis direction observed beneath Mount Spurr.

Sarao et al. (2001) found a co-existence of focal mechanisms compatible with both the regional and the magma-induced stress fields analysing 28 earthquakes occurred at Etna in the period August 1990 - December 1991, that is before the eruption started on 15 December 1991. At depths lower than 10 km, the authors found focal mechanisms preferentially strike-slip imputed to a dike-induced stress field dominating at shallow depths and producing a continuous switch of the p- and t- (tensile) axes. At larger depths, normal focal mechanisms prevailed with alignment along the E-W direction, that is the direction of the main regional stress field. Moreover, the events occurring in the last months before the eruption onset showed a higher contribute of the CLVD (Compensated Linear Vector Dipole) component of the focal mechanisms, as well as a larger fraction of isotropic deformation (however mostly below $\sim 20\%$). A similar increase of number of events with high CLVD was found also before May 1991, when some explosive activity occurred at the volcano. The authors imputed the presence of non-DC (Double Couple) components to a depressurizing magma body and crack formation, leading in turn to magma injection towards shallower portions of the volcano.

Very similar results have been found also by Patanè and Privitera (2001) analysing the seismicity related to the 1989 and 1991-1993 eruptions of Etna. Defining the same two domains at different depth ranges, the authors found a deeper seismicity with dominant p-axis oriented NNW-SSE, that matched the direction of the regional stress field and was coherent with the stress field induced by the nearly N-S Africa-Eurasia slow collision. At small depths, the authors found a rotation of p- and t-axis of 45°-50°, which was imputed to upraising magma intruded in the upper crust generating a local different stress field modulating and overcoming the regional stress field.

A double depth-dependent behavior of focal mechanisms was found also at Mount St. Helen by Moran (1994), who analyzed the seismicity in the inter-eruptive period 1987-1992, that is after the eruption of October 1986. The author defined an *intermediate* (4-6.5 km) and a *deep* (6.5-10 km) depth interval. Intermediate earthquakes showed strike-slip focal mechanisms with p- and t-axis significantly misaligned with the regional tectonic stress field, indicating that the source of stress for events at these depths came from within the volcano, as supported also by the spatial clustering of the hypocentres. Focal mechanisms of deep earthquakes were also primarly strike-slip, but in this case they did not show a dominant axis orientation. However, the p-axis directions depicted a wheel-spoke pattern, radially pointing towards the center of the wheel, with the t-axes tangentially aligned. The wheel-spoke pattern enclosed an aseismic region west of the lava dome, interpreted by the author as a magma chamber experiencing a pressure increase due to the exsolution of volatile species during magma cooling. The represurization of the deep magma chamber could have produced also the pressurization of the shallow ($\lesssim$2 km) plumbing system, inducing in turn the intermediate seismicity as an effect of a "sealed" system no longer able to accomodate pressure steps through material transport and thus leading to plastic and brittle deformation of the surrounding rock. Besides the inter-eruptive period, the author analyzed also the post-18-May-1980 eruption phase. In this phase, on the opposite, the mechanisms of the deep earthquakes showed p-axes tangentially aligned with the center of the 1980 aseismic zone (broadly beneath the lava dome in the depth range 7-11 km and probably hosting a magma body) possibly induced by a pressure drop from within the aseismic zone as an effect of the draining of the magma chamber.

Ruppert et al. (2011) analyzed a seismic swarm started one month before the eruption of Kasatochi volcano (Alaska) started on 7 August 2008. The authors located the earthquakes in the depth range 5-10 km directly under the volcano and find p- and t-axis from the focal mechanisms consistent with the maximum and minimum regional stress orientation, suggesting a dominant component of the tectonic loading on the earthquake generation. On the other hand, a relevant CLVD component of the focal mechanisms and a N-S alignement of the hypocentres (that formed ~60°-70°with the p-axis direction) - besides an increasing earthquake magnitude, in line with the features of the volcano seismicity and in contrast with the mainshock-aftershock relation of the tectonic-loaded seismicity - indicated that a volcanic component (different from an intruding dike) to the source was active, as well. The authors proposed that the seismic cluster defined a region surrounding a magma diapir. A Mw 5.8 earthquake (occurred few hours before the eruption onset) introduced a change of the source region, which moved N-E of the previous hypocenter area, thus possibly reflecting the opening of a pathway for the fluids towards the surface.

7. Spectral Modifications

In some cases, explosive or eruptive episodes have effects also on the frequency content of the volcano seismicity. In particular, one of the most interesting phenomena is the so-called *gliding* effect, that is a gradual change of the spectral peaks, clearly visible in the spectrograms of the seismic signals.

Gliding effects have been found at Arenal volcano (Costa Rica) by Benoit and McNutt (1997) in the harmonic tremor following small eruptions. The authors analyzed the seismicity during two weeks in April 1994 belonging to a long phase of rewakening of the volcano started in 1968 and finished in 2010 and including lava extrusions, strombolian explosions and gas emissions at a nearly constant rate (Williams-Jones et al., 2001). Benoit and McNutt (1997) found a harmonic tremor developing just after the eruptions with fundamental frequency at about 2 Hz and overtones at ~4 Hz and ~6 Hz. The gliding phenomenon was observed during the 300-600 s following the eruption onset, when the fundamental frequency gradually increased up to 3.2-3.5 Hz and then suddenly stopped. The other frequency peaks showed the same increase, being preserved at every time the ratios between the frequencies of the spectral peaks. The authors modelled the harmonic tremor as the effect of the longitudinal resonance of a vertically-oriented fluid-filled cavity with size of 200-660m (assuming a "closed-closed" system), and the gliding effect as due to a change in the acoustic velocity in the magma-gas mixture filling the resonator, in turn produced by an increase of the fraction of the exsolved gas.

Lesage et al. (2006) gave a similar explanation to the frequency increase of the harmonic tremor observed in February 1997 at Arenal, although they remarked that harmonic tremor was visible also disconnected from the eruptions. The authors proposed that the increase of the gas content was induced by a change in the pressure within the plumbing system, which was connected to the surface through a fractured plug. Intermittent gas flow through the fractures would produce harmonic tremor if the period of the intermittency is stabilized by the resonance of the conduit (modelled as a pipe), otherwise broad-band tremor is generated. Moreover, the authors found two independent series of spectral peaks (and corresponding frequency shifts) associated with two different magmatic conduits independently producing tremor and/or explosions.

Differently from the previous authors, Almendros et al. (2012) modelled the harmonic tremor at Arenal as due to interference of waves produced, for instance, by multiple harmonic tremor sources, by a single tremor source with a scattered wavefield or by the seismic and acoustic wavefield radiated by a single tremor source.

A harmonic tremor was detected also by Mori et al. (1989) at Langila volcano (Papua Nuova Guinea) in the period 1977-1986, that is during an eruptive phase of the volcano following a reactivation occurred in 1954 and including strombolian and vulcanian explosions, lava ejections and flows and small pyroclastic flows. The authors found harmonic tremor with frequency maxima at 1 Hz, 2 Hz, 3 Hz (and in some cases 4 Hz) common to all the stations, suggesting the dominance of source effects. Moreover, they also observed a shift of the fundamental frequency from 1 Hz to 1.6 Hz in about two minutes. Similar to the case of Arenal, the authors modelled the source of the harmonic tremor as the resonance of a gas-filled cavity, while the gliding effect would be produced by changes of the size of the resonating structure (from $\sim$150 m to $\sim$100 m) and/or to a change of the volume of the gas fraction.

Harmonic tremor and gliding effects were observed at Soufriere Hills volcano by Neuberg et al. (2000) within the LP swarms accompanying the formation and collapse of the lava dome during the eruptive crisis of July 1995 - December 1997. Harmonic tremor was produced by merging of LP events occurring closer and closer in time, and showed a frequency content depending on the stations (thus suggesting a relevant contribute from path- and site-effects) and a number of overtones varying with the episode. However, in some cases, harmonic tremor was coherent across the array and displayed gliding effects lasting several minutes. Differently from the previous cases, here the authors modelled the harmonic tremor as the effect of repeating LP events occurring at very regular intervals for short times. In this scheme, the gliding effect is thus imputed to the increase of the rate of the LP events composing the events, rather to a change of the rheological properties of the medium.

At Semeru volcano (Indonesia) Schlindwein et al. (1995) found harmonic tremor analysing the seismicity recorded in October 1992, that is during an eruptive phase dominated by frequent steam explosions and a variety of acoustic events, among which a regular pumping sound. The authors detected about 40 episodes of harmonic tremor lasting between 40 s and 1000 s, with fundamental peak ranging between 0.5 Hz and 1.7 Hz and on average 4 to 6 overtones. Similarly to the other cases, a shift of the spectral peaks was observed, being the harmonic structure preserved, although the position of the frequency peaks was variable but not monotonically increasing, differently from above. The authors modelled the events as the effect of the oscillations of a gas-filled vertical dike (with size of about 500 m or less) bounded by a lava plug on top and a magma column at bottom. The shift of the spectral peaks was imputed to a change of the oscillation velocity of roughly 1.15 m/s.

Besides the harmonic tremor and the gliding effect, overall variations of the frequency content of volcanic tremor have been observed in several cases. For example, Tárraga et al. (2014) found a time-varying frequency content of the seismic signal before and during the submarine eruption of El Hierro occurred between 10 October 2011 and the end of February 2012. Specifically, the dominant frequency varied greatly before the eruption onset, with values in the range 0.4-4.5 Hz, while during the eruptive phase it was more stable between 0.5 Hz and 1.2 Hz, with sporadic phases showing spectral maximum around 2 Hz or more.

Analysing signals recorded in Februar 2012, Harris et al. (2005) detected a correlation between a convective magma motion beneath the lava lake of Erta volcano (Etiopia) and the frequency content of the seismic signal. In detail, periods of vigorous lava convection (high surface velocity, $\sim$0.1-0.4 m/s) - typically lasting tens to hundreds of minutes - produced seismic tremor with large content in high frequencies ($>$5 Hz), while during periods of sluggish (slow surface velocity, $\sim$0.01-0.08 m/s) the seismic signals had spectra with frequency mostly below 5 Hz.

Also Carniel et al. (2003) found time variable properties of the volcanic tremor at Ambrym volcano (Vanuatu archipelago), with a ground state with low energy and stable spectra and phases of high energy and different spectral content, often triggered by large (M>4) tectonic events. High-energy phases were composed of discrete events (lasting one or few hours) without P- and S- arrivals, showing broad spectra roughly contained in the range 2-8 Hz, differently from the ground state of the tremor, which displayed few well defined maxima in the spectra mostly below 4 Hz. As above, the authors associated such a variable tremor to a time-dependent activity of a lava lake, which in turn was affected by a variable feeding of gas-rich magma batches from deeper regions towards the surface.

Besides the continuous volcanic tremor, time-dependent frequency content has been observed also for LP events associated with volcanic eruptions or explosions.

Lesage et al. (1995) found a change of the frequency content of LP events preceding the eruption of Keluk volcano (Java Island, Indonesia) of 10-12 February, 1990. In detail, the authors detected an increase of the seismicity starting about three months before the eruption onset mostly composed of very shallow (∼150-750 m below the crater summit) VT events, often occurring in multiplets. Besides this seismicity, they found also a class of monochromatic LP events with frequency peak ranging between 5.8 Hz and 6.2 Hz before 3 January, while in the period 3-6 January the dominant frequency moved to about 5.2 Hz. The authors modelled these events as due to the resonance of fluid-filled cavities and suggested a change of the fluid properties and/or of the surrounding rock as causing such a spectral modification.

Bryan and Sherburn (2003) detected a change of the frequency content of the seismicity prior to and after the eruption of Ruapehu volcano of 1995-1996 (September-November 1995; June-July 1996). In detail, the authors compared the frequency content of the seismicity recorded during 6.5 weeks in the pre-eruptive phase (1994) and six months in the post-eruptive stage (1998). They found that the dominant frequency of both tremor and volcanic earthquakes was ∼2 Hz in the pre-eruptive stage, while in the post-eruptive stage this frequency was still present but subordinated to frequencies in the range 0.8-1.4 Hz. The same scheme was observed also in 1999 in the spectra of recordings from a permanent seismic sensor. The authors attributed the spectral changes to structural modifications of the volcanic plumbing system resulting from the 1995-1996 eruption.

Looking at the same eruption, Bryan and Sherburn (1999) detected a change of the spectra of the volcanic tremor at the onset of the eruption. Specifically, they found the appearance of a peak around 1 Hz just few days before the eruption onset (17 September), modifying the stable spectra with maxima around 2 Hz and presumibly reflecting the opening of new pathways created by magma intrusion. Moreover, during the eruption the spectra of tremor (and earthquakes) became wideband (2-10 Hz) punctuating a change in the eruptive style from phreatomagmatic to magmatic.

At Colima volcano, De Lauro et al. (2012) reported that the spectra of the LP events preceding the vulcanian-style eruptions had a monotonically decreasing envelope with fundamental frequency peaked at $\sim$0.5 Hz and secondary maxima at integer multiples (whereas the background signal is characterized by spectral peaks at $\sim$0.15 Hz and $\sim$0.3 Hz (Palo and Cusano, 2013)). Moreover, the individual spectral peaks were associated to different nearly monochromatic independent signals extracted through a decomposing numerical technique working in the time domain (Independent Component Analysis). The authors modelled the observed spectra as the effect of the superposition of four vibration modes of a fluid-filled cavity with cylindrical symmetry.

Lokmer et al. (2008) analyzed the LP (and VLP) seismicity at Etna since November till August 2005, thus encompassing the effusive eruption of September 2004 - March 2005. They found families of events after filtering the waveforms in the band 0.3-1.5 Hz and detected a change of the dominant frequency from about 0.4 Hz to about 0.6 Hz moving from the pre-eruptive to the post-eruptive phase. Moreover, in this transition the authors highlighted also an increase of the quality factor (Q) and a change of the polarization direction, which moved from predominantly transversal to pure radial motion. The authors proposed a model in which LP events are generated by gas slugs injected into a cavity filled with either magmatic or hydrothermal fluids. Moreover, they attrubuted the frequency and Q changes to a re-establishment of the pressure balance occurring at the end of the effusive eruption, thus as an effect of a modification of the velocity and attenuation properties of the medium, while the polarization changes would be induced by a new stress regime established after the eruption affecting the direction along which the cavity (modelled as a crack) discharges.

A pressure drop was proposed also by De Martino et al. (2011b) to explain the different spectra of the explosion quakes before and during the eruption of Stromboli of December 2002. The authors detected a change of the dominant frequency of the explosion quakes induced by the strombolian-like explosions (persistent also during the lava effusion), as well as of the envelope of the spectra. In fact, in the pre-eruptive phase the spectra showed a bell shape with dominant frequency falling between 2 Hz and 3 Hz, while in the eruptive stage the spectra had a monotonically decreasing envelope with maximum at $\sim$3 Hz. The authors modelled the spectral change as due to a modification of the geometry of the vibrating volcanic structure, which passed from a conical to a cylindrical symmetry.

Similarly, a depressurization of the shallow plumbing system at Stromboli volcano was proposed also by De Martino et al. (2012) to model the source of the monochromatic swarms of explosion quakes observed in 2002-2003, 2007 and 2010-2011. The authors assigned to the swarms the role of a proxy of a temporary escape from equilibrium conditions of the thermodynamic state of the magma-gas mixture. Supporting this interpretation, they highlighted also a persistent change of the spectra of the standard explosion quakes when the first swarm occurred in the period 2010-2011, confirming that the swarms can be considered an effect of a structural modification of the conditions within the plumbing system.

8. The Magma Dynamics and the Seismic Response: A Framework

Although several models have been proposed to connect the individual features of the volcano seismicity with the magma behavior, a common framework assumes that the release of seismic energy is induced by variations of the internal conditions of the volcanic system before the eruptions, which in turn are schematically depicted as the final stage of an upward migration of magma from regions where it accumulates (magma chambers) towards the surface.

In this scheme, the principal effect of the magma migration is a stress increase mostly promoted by the magmatic gases exsolved at shallow depths and especially effective at closed-conduit volcanoes. Stress transfer is efficiently accomodated by the emission of seismic radiation, which therefore represents a good proxy for detecting changes of the internal conditions of the volcanic edifice and of the plumbing system. As remarked above, seismic energy is released with a variety of waveforms and source mechanisms including continuous volcanic tremor, Volcano-Tectonic and Long-Period events. VT events are brittle releases of accumulated stress along pre-formed or new seismogenic discontinuities of the volcanic edifice, in analogy with the tectonic-loaded case. For gas-rich magmas, stress excess can induce also unsteady flow of magmatic gases interacting with fluid-filled cavities producing LP events. In this case, the features of the seismic radiation in time and frequency domains are constrained by the geometry and the filling of the volcanic cavities. LP events can be considered the constituents of the volcanic tremor, which has been modelled as just the continuous generation of LP events. However, LP events have been also modelled as due to seismic waves trapped wihin the conduit between a plastic and a brittle frictional regime or, recently, as slow-rupture earthquakes produced by the deformation of the volcanic edifice with a strong imprinting of path effects, indicating that the mechanisms of stress release in volcanic contexts are probably multiple and not yet completely understood.

Often the stress perturbation propagates upward and induces the nucleation of earthquakes at shallower and shallower depths prior to the eruption (Castellano et al., 1993; Battaglia et al., 2005), thus somehow allowing to infer the migration of the stress wavefront and thus of the uprising magma. Together with this upward migration, the magma migration leads also to an increase of the stress transfer with time, with the effect of an escalating nucleation of earthquakes, by which the volcanic system releases the enhancing transferred stress. The increase of the event rate has been modelled as due to an enlargement of the seismogenic discontinuities by extension and coalescence of close cracks embedded in the volcanic edifice (Kilburn, 2003), although an interaction between the events similar to the mainshock-aftershocks relation of the tectonic seismicity contributes to the observed escalating process, as well (Collombet et al., 2003).

The increasing earthquake rate is mostly observed for VT events for silicic volcanoes, which display high density magmas and a dominance of brittle failures, thus a spatio-temporal correlation between the events is not surprising and reflects into the distribution of the VT earthquake magnitudes, which follows the Gutenberg-Richter law. Moreover, the time variations of the stress conditions before and during the eruptions can modify the scaling properties of the distribution, that is the b-value, which decreases when the stress increases. Changes of the b-value imply also variations of the relations of self-similarity of the fault network, which acts as a whole self-organized system modifying the ratio between the frequency of large and small earthquakes. Indeed, the b-value is connected to the fractal dimensions of the network and thus to its geometry (Wyss et al., 1997). Besides the stress change, rising magma can affect the b-value also by the thermal gradient generated in the plumbing system, with larger thermal gradients leading to higher b-values (Warren and Latham, 1970). The overall stress increase before the eruptions can lead both to a decrease of the b-value (Klein, 1982; Ibáñez et al., 2012), as well as to an increase (Wyss et al., 1997; Novelo-Casanova et al., 2006), being the latter case more common. The increase of the b-value has been imputed to secondary effects of the rising magma, such as a rise of the pore pressure induced by the exsolution of volatilies that locally promote the faulting mechanisms or the expansion of the fault network by creation of new cracks (Wyss et al., 1997; Wiemer et al., 1998; Vinciguerra, 1999).

On the contrary, for basaltic volcanoes, where LP seismicity dominates, the events are mostly independent (Bottiglieri et al., 2005; De Lauro et al., 2009b) and an event rate rise is seldom observed and imputed to an increase of the magma degassing before the eruption (De Martino et al., 2011a). The increase of degassing prior to the eruption is a quite common feature and is produced by the upward migration of new magma from deeper parts of the plumbing system, with release of the gasous fraction above depths of about 1-3 km mostly due to the reduction of the hydrostatic pressure (McNutt, 1996). Moreover, the interaction between high-temperature magma and shallow hydrothermal systems can promote the release of water in gasous phase. In addition, a further source of the pressure reduction favouring the gas exsolution is the opening of fractures connecting the plumbing system and the surface (producing, in turn, seismicity), mostly effective in closed-conduit volcanoes. In this way, the magmatic gases are decoupled from the rest of the magma and go ahead of it, reflecting into the appearance of sustained volcanic tremor short before the eruption onset (McNutt, 1996).

The seismic energy released during the pre- and co-eruptive phase has an imprinting of the stress field produced by the magma dynamics. Indeed, the focal mechanisms describing the source process generating the volcano seismicity show that these events accomodate an excess of stress acting along directions often different from those along which the regional tectonic loading acts (Roman et al., 2006, 2008). Moreover, even for VT events, for which an approximation of the source with a double-couple force system is normally suitable, a relevant isotropic or CLVD component of the moment tensor solutions is often detected, probably reflecting an important role in the source mechanism of fluids, which would reduce the efficiency of the shear stress favouring volumetric expansion/contraction and mass transportation (flowing fluids) (Sarao et al., 2001).

The stress increase produced before the eruptions affects also the equilibrium conditions of the magma-gas mixture composing the shallow plumbing system. One effect of this change is the variation of the seismic and acoustic velocity of the medium, which reflects into a modification of the spectra of the earthquakes, often accompanied by a gliding effect, that is a gradual increase of spectral peaks composing nearly harmonic spectra (Benoit and McNutt, 1997). Recently, changes in the medium properties (velocity and/or rheology) prior to the eruptions have been detected also auto-correlating the seismic noise (Brenguier et al., 2008). Time-variable thermodynamic conditions throughout the volcanic crises produce also a migration of the nucleation location of the coherent gas aggregates generating the LP seismicity, often leading also to a variation of the spectral content of the seismicity as an effect of a change of the structures trapping and self-sustaining the seismic energy (Giudicepietro et al., 2009; De Martino et al., 2011b,a).

9. Perspectives

In the last decades, volcano seismology has led to a strong improvement in the knowledge of the geometry of the volcanic plumbing systems and of the dynamics of the magma before and during the eruptive crises. Nevertheless, the seismic observations are still mostly blind to low-energy and deep signals. For example, in recent years, a class of events named Deep Low-Frequency (DLF) events has been observed at some Japanese volcanoes (Nakamichi et al., 2003; Ukawa, 2005). DLF events have been located at middle/deep-crust or at the uppermost mantle and have been associated to a seismic response of the magma movements at the roots of the feeding system, thus potentially representing a powerful tool for mitigating the volcanic risk and enlighting the onset of the magma migration. Similarly, small transient magma-triggered slow-slip events have been recently observed at Kilauea (Brooks et al., 2008), suggesting the existence of a further silent form of stress release in volcanic areas, in analogy with the tectonic context of the subduction interfaces (Schwartz and Rokosky, 2007). However, the detection of these events is still very limited presumibly for an inadeguate seismic monitoring at most volcanoes.

The increase of the detection capability of the volcano seismicity should be achieved both by a more sensitive seismic monitoring and by an refinement of the numerical techniques adopted for the analysis of the seismic signals. Strainmeters and tilmeters in borehole have been installed in some volcanic areas usually at depths of some hundred meters. These instruments can reveal deformations of less than one part per billion, thus being potentially able to detect even deep magma movement. Promising results have been found in some cases (Dzurisin et al., 1983; Guo et al., 1993; Voight et al., 1998, 2010; De Martino et al., 2011b, 2012), although the elevated costs of the installation there limit a large employment. Recently, encouraging results have been also obtained by measuring the volcanic deformation by Interferometric Synthetic Aperture radar (InSAR), based on electromagnetic radiation emitted from satellites (see, e.g. Dzurisin, 2003; Lu et al., 2005; Pedersen and Sigmundsson, 2006). Looking at the numerical techniques, Independent Component Analysis (ICA) has been in the last decade successfully applied to the seismicity of several volcanoes, allowing to isolate low-energy seismic signals within the recordings of earthquakes and tremor (e.g. De Lauro et al., 2008; De Martino et al., 2011b; De Lauro et al., 2012; Palo and Cusano, 2013; Carniel, 2014). Differently from the standard seismological technique reconstructing the seismic wavefield (f.i., f-k method) ICA decomposes the signals in the time domain estimating the distribution of the signal amplitude, and detects the basic constituents of the traces looking for statistically independent (non-normally distributed) signals hidden in the recordings.

At the same time, as volcanoes are complex systems, the definition of volcanic earthquakes with the usual parameters borrowed from the tectonic seismology (magnitude and location) could be unsuitable. Especially for the volcanic events involving fluid-solid interactions, a more complete characterization should include, for example, the definition of the dynamical system generating the signals in terms of effective degrees of freedom and fundamental signals. Recent applications of this approach have shown that the volcanic signals can be described as the superposition of few nonlinear vibration modes of the main shallow plumbing system underlying as many low-dimension independent dynamical systems (De Lauro et al., 2009a, 2012; Palo and Cusano, 2013). At the same time, the definition of classes of events based on the waveforms or spectrum can be inaccurate, while a more meaningful distinction of the events should look at the statistics of the occurrences of the events, at the physics of the source process and at the hypocentres as a whole, and should aim to clarify the role of the volcanic earthquakes in releasing the stress.

Moreover, future directions in the study of the volcanic signals should take into account the interaction with external sources. From that point of view, volcanoes can no longer be considered as isolated systems, but as belonging to a larger system with several components mutually interacting. Studies developing this view have highlighted the existence of statistically relevant correlations between the volcanic activity and external forcing, such as large tectonic earthquakes and tides (Linde and Sacks, 1998; Neuberg et al., 2000; Manga and Brodsky, 2006; De Lauro et al., 2013).

10. Conclusion

In this article I have revised the properties of the volcano seismicity during the eruptive crises. In particular, I have analyzed how the seismicity changes when an eruption is approaching and evolving in respect to the stationary or quiescent state.

The principal element affecting the features of the volcanic seismicity is the variation of stress experienced by the rigid structures of the volcanic edifice, which reacts releasing the accumulated elastic energy in the form of earthquakes. The stress increase can be broadly imputed to the magma rising from deeper regions of the crust towards the surface, alimented by the gasous fraction exsolved at shallow depths promoting an escalating process. The seismic reaction of the volcano reflects the evolution of the internal state towards critical conditions, the individual earthquakes displaying time-variable hypocentres, focal mechanism, frequency content, besides an overall increase of the earthquake rate and often the appearance of volcanic tremor. On the other hand, the seismicity preceding and accompanying the eruptions has also an imprinting of multi-scale phenomena reflecting into a variation of the statistical properties of the earthquake rate and of the amplitude distribution, which behave similarly to the tectonic-induced earthquakes. However, while this scheme applies to source mechanism dominated by brittle failures, another class of volcanoes - for which seismicity is dominated by fluid-induced events - on the contrary shows a preferential time and length scale. For this class there is a less effective coupling between stress transfer and seismic release, with the effect that the seismic precursors of the eruptions are more variable and dependent on the case study and ultimately less reliable.

References

Aki, K., 1965. Maximum likelihood estimate of b in the formula logn= a-bm and its confidence limits. *Bull. Earthq. Res. Inst.* 43, 237–239.

Aki, K., Ferrazzini, V., 2000. Seismic monitoring and modeling of an active volcano for prediction. *Journal of Geophysical Research* 105, B7, 16617–16640.

Aki, K., Koyanagi, R., 1981. Deep volcanic tremor and magma ascent mechanism under Kilauea, Hawaii. *Journal of Geophysical Research: Solid Earth* (1978–2012) 86, B8, 7095–7109.

Almendros, J., Abella, R., Mora, M., Lesage, P., 2012. Time-dependent spatial amplitude patterns of harmonic tremor at Arenal volcano, Costa Rica: Seismic-wave interferences? *Bulletin of the Seismological Society of America* 102, 6, 2378–2391.

Alparone, S., Andronico, D., Lodato, L., Sgroi, T., 2003. Relationship between tremor and volcanic activity during the southeast crater eruption on mount Etna in early 2000. *Journal of Geophysical Research* 108, B5, 2241.

Barberi, F., Bertagnini, A., Landi, P., Principe, C., 1992. A review on phreatic eruptions and their precursors. *Journal of Volcanology and Geothermal Research* 52, 4, 231–246.

Batchelor, G.K., 2000. *An introduction to fluid dynamics*. Cambridge university press.

Battaglia, J., Ferrazzini, V., Staudacher, T., Aki, K., Cheminée, J.L., 2005. Pre-eruptive migration of earthquakes at the Piton de la Fournaise volcano (Réunion Island). *Geophysical Journal International* 161, 2, 549–558.

Bean, C.J., De Barros, L., Lokmer, I., Métaxian, J.P., O'Brien, G., Murphy, S., 2014. Long-period seismicity in the shallow volcanic edifice formed from slow-rupture earthquakes. *Nature geoscience* 7, 1, 71–75.

Benoit, J.P., McNutt, S.R., 1997. New constraints on source processes of volcanic tremor at Arenal volcano, Costa Rica, using broadband seismic data. *Geophysical Research Letters* 24, 449–452.

Benoit, J.P., McNutt, S.R., Barboza, V., 2003. Duration-amplitude distribution of volcanic tremor. *Journal of Geophysical Research: Solid Earth* (1978–2012) 108, B3.

Benson, P.M., Vinciguerra, S., Meredith, P.G., Young, R.P., 2010. Spatio-temporal evolution of volcano seismicity: A laboratory study. *Earth and Planetary Science Letters* 297, 1, 315–323.

Bottiglieri, M., De Martino, S., Falanga, M., Godano, C., Palo, M., 2005. Statistics of inter-time of strombolian explosion-quakes. *EPL (Europhysics Letters)* 72, 3, 493–498.

Brenguier, F., Shapiro, N.M., Campillo, M., Ferrazzini, V., Duputel, Z., Coutant, O., Nercessian, A., 2008. Towards forecasting volcanic eruptions using seismic noise. *Nature Geoscience* 1,2, 126–130.

Brooks, B.A., Foster, J., Sandwell, D., Wolfe, C.J., Okubo, P., Poland, M., Myer, D., 2008. Magmatically triggered slow slip at Kilauea volcano, hawaii. *Science* 321,5893, 1177–1177.

Bryan, C., Sherburn, S., 1999. Seismicity associated with the 1995–1996 eruptions of Ruapehu volcano, New Zealand: narrative and insights into physical processes. *Journal of Volcanology and Geothermal Research* 90, 1, 1–18.

Bryan, C.J., Sherburn, S., 2003. Eruption-induced modifications to volcanic seismicity at Ruapehu, New Zealand, and its implications for eruption forecasting. *Bulletin of Volcanology* 65,1, 30–42.

Buccheri, G., De Lauro, E., De Martino, S., Falanga, M., Palo, M., 2013. From the standard strombolian activity to the volcanic crises at Stromboli (Italy): An overview of the seismic signatures, in: *Complex Monitoring of Volcanic Activity: Methods and Results*. Nova Publishers, pp. 93–110.

Budi-Santoso, A., Lesage, P., Dwiyono, S., Sumarti, S., Jousset, P., Metaxian, J.P., et al., 261, 153–170, 2013. Analysis of the seismic activity associated with the 2010 eruption of Merapi volcano, Java. *Journal of Volcanology and Geothermal Research* .

Burlini, L., Vinciguerra, S., Di Toro, G., De Natale, G., Meredith, P., Burg, J.P., 2007. Seismicity preceding volcanic eruptions: New experimental insights. *Geology* 35,2 183–186.

Carniel, R., 2014. Characterization of volcanic regimes and identification of significant transitions using geophysical data: a review. *Bulletin of Volcanology* 76,8 1–22.

Carniel, R., Di Cecca, M., Rouland, D., 2003. Ambrym, Vanuatu (july–august 2000): spectral and dynamical transitions on the hours-to-days timescale. *Journal of Volcanology and Geothermal Research* 128, 1, 1–13.

Castellano, M., Ferrucci, F., Godano, C., Imposa, S., Milano, G., 1993. Upwards migration of seismic focii: A forerunner of the 1989 eruption of Mt Etna (Italy). *Bulletin of Volcanology* 55,5 357–361.

Cerdeña, I.D., Del Fresno, C., Rivera, L., 2011. New insight on the increasing seismicity during Tenerife's 2004 volcanic reactivation. *Journal of Volcanology and Geothermal Research* 206, 1, 15–29.

Chandrasekhar, S., 1943. Stochastic problems in physics and astronomy. *Reviews of Modern Physics* 15, 1.

Chastin, S.F., Main, I.G., 2003. Statistical analysis of daily seismic event rate as a precursor to volcanic eruptions. *Geophysical research letters* 30, 13, 1671.

Chouet, B., 1985. Excitation of a buried magmatic pipe: a seismic source model for volcanic tremor. *Journal of Geophysical Research: Solid Earth* (1978–2012) 90, B2, 1881–1893.

Chouet, B., 2003. Volcano seismology. *Pure and Applied Geophysics* 160,3–4 739–788.

Chouet, B., Dawson, P., Ohminato, T., Martini, M., Saccorotti, G., Giudicepietro, F., De Luca, G., Milana, G., Scarpa, R., 2003. Source mechanisms of explosions at Stromboli volcano, Italy, determined from moment-tensor inversions of very-long-period data. *Journal of Geophysical Research: Solid Earth* (1978–2012) 108, B1, 2019.

Chouet, B.A., Matoza, R.S.,251, 108–175, 2013. A multi-decadal view of seismic methods for detecting precursors of magma movement and eruption. *Journal of Volcanology and Geothermal Research* .

Chouet, B.A., Page, R.A., Stephens, C.D., Lahr, J.C., Power, J.A., 1994. Precursory swarms of long-period events at Redoubt volcano (1989–1990), Alaska: Their origin and use as a forecasting tool. *Journal of Volcanology and Geothermal Research* 62, 1, 95–135.

Collombet, M., Grasso, J.R., Ferrazzini, V., 2003. Seismicity rate before eruptions on Piton de la Fournaise volcano: Implications for eruption dynamics. *Geophysical Research Letters* 30, 21.

Cornelius, R.R., Voight, B., 1994. Seismological aspects of the 1989–1990 eruption at Redoubt volcano, Alaska: The materials failure forecast method (FFM) with RSAM and SSAM seismic data. *Journal of Volcanology and Geothermal Research* 62, 1, 469–498.

Cox, D.R., Lewis, P.A., 1966. The statistical analysis of series of events. *Monographs on Applied Probability and Statistics* 1.

Crosson, R., Bame, D., 1985. A spherical source model for low frequency volcanic earthquakes. *Journal of Geophysical Research: Solid Earth* (1978–2012) 90, B12, 10237–10247.

De la Cruz-Reyna, S., Yokoyama, I., Martínez-Bringas, A., Ramos, E., 2008. Precursory seismicity of the 1994 eruption of Popocatépetl volcano, central Mexico. *Bulletin of Volcanology* 70,6 753–767.

De Barros, L., Bean, C.J., Zecevic, M., Brenguier, F., Peltier, A., 2013. Eruptive fracture location forecasts from high-frequency events on Piton de la Fournaise volcano. *Geophysical Research Letters* 40,17 4599–4603.

De Lauro, E., De Martino, S., Del Pezzo, E., Falanga, M., Palo, M., Scarpa, R., 2008. Model for high-frequency strombolian tremor inferred by wavefield decomposition and reconstruction of asymptotic dynamics. *Journal of Geophysical Research: Solid Earth* (1978–2012) 113,B02302.

De Lauro, E., De Martino, S., Falanga, M., Palo, M., 2009a. Decomposition of high-frequency seismic wavefield of the strombolian-like explosions at Erebus volcano by Independent Component Analysis. *Geophysical Journal International* 177, 3, 1399–1406.

De Lauro, E., De Martino, S., Falanga, M., Palo, M., 2009b. Modelling the macroscopic behavior of strombolian explosions at Erebus volcano. *Physics of the Earth and Planetary Interiors* 176, 3, 174–186.

De Lauro, E., De Martino, S., Palo, M., Ibañez, J., 2012. Self-sustained oscillations at Volcán de Colima (México) inferred by Independent Component Analysis. *Bulletin of Volcanology* 74, 279–292.

De Lauro, E., De Martino, S., Falanga, M., Petrosino, S., 2013. Synchronization between tides and sustained oscillations of the hydrothermal system of campi flegrei (italy). *Geochemistry, Geophysics, Geosystems* 14, 8, 2628–2637.

De Martino, S., Errico, A., Palo, M., Cimini, G., 2012. Explosion swarms at Stromboli volcano: A proxy for nonequilibrium conditions in the shallow plumbing system. *Geochemistry, Geophysics, Geosystems* 13, 3, Q03012.

De Martino, S., Falanga, M., Godano, C., 2004. Dynamical similarity of explosions at Stromboli volcano. *Geophysical Journal International* 157, 3, 1247–1254.

De Martino, S., Falanga, M., Palo, M., Montalto, P., Patanè, D., 2011a. Statistical analysis of the volcano seismicity during the 2007 crisis of Stromboli, Italy. *Journal of Geophysical Research* 116, B9, B09312.

De Martino, S., Palo, M., Cimini, G., 2011b. A statistical study of the Stromboli volcano explosion quakes before and during 2002–2003 eruptive crisis. *Journal of Geophysical Research: Solid Earth* (1978–2012) 116, B04303.

De Natale, G., Gresta, S., Patané, G., Zollo, A., 1985. Statistical analysis of earthquake activity at Etna volcano (march 1981 eruption). *Pure and Applied Geophysics* 123,5, 697–705.

Di Grazia, G., Cannata, A., Montalto, P., Patanè, D., Privitera, E., Zuccarello, L., Boschi, E., 2009. A multiparameter approach to volcano monitoring based on 4d analyses of seismo-volcanic and acoustic signals: The 2008 mt. Etna eruption. *Geophysical Research Letters* 36, 18, 307.

Dieterich, J., Cayol, V., Okubo, P., 2000. The use of earthquake rate changes as a stress meter at Kilauea volcano. *Nature* 408,6811, 457–460.

Dzurisin, D., 2003. A comprehensive approach to monitoring volcano deformation as a window on the eruption cycle. *Reviews of Geophysics* 41, 1001.

Dzurisin, D., Westphal, J.A., Johnson, D.J., 1983. Eruption prediction aided by electronic tiltmeter data at Mount St. Helens. *Science* 221,4618, 1381–1383.

Enescu, B., Ito, K., 2001. Some premonitory phenomena of the 1995 Hyogo-Ken nanbu (Kobe) earthquake: seismicity, b-value and fractal dimension. *Tectonophysics* 338,3, 297–314.

Fagents, S.A., Gregg, T.K., Lopes, R.M., 2013. *Modeling Volcanic Processes: The Physics and Mathematics of Volcanism*. Cambridge University Press.

Gambino, S., Mostaccio, A., Patanè, D., Scarfì, L., Ursino, A., 2004. High-precision locations of the microseismicity preceding the 2002–2003 Mt. Etna eruption. *Geophysical Research Letters* 31,18, L18604–1.

Giudicepietro, F., D'Auria, L., Martini, M., Caputo, T., Peluso, R., De Cesare, W., Orazi, M., Scarpato, G., 2009. Changes in the VLP seismic source during the 2007 Stromboli eruption. *Journal of Volcanology and Geothermal Research* 182, 3,162–171.

Grasso, J., Bachelery, P., 1995. Hierarchical organization as a diagnostic approach to volcano mechanics: Validation on Piton de la Fournaise. *Geophysical Research Letters* 22,21 2897–2900.

Grasso, J.R., Zaliapin, I., 2004. Predictability of volcano eruption: Lessons from a basaltic effusive volcano. *Geophysical research letters* 31, 5,L05602-1.

Gresta, S., Patanè, G., 1983. Variation of b-values before the etnean eruption of march 1981. *Pure and Applied Geophysics* 121,2, 287–295.

Gudmundsson, A., 2002. Emplacement and arrest of sheets and dykes in central volcanoes. *Journal of Volcanology and Geothermal Research* 116, 3,279–298.

Guo, Y., Karasawa, N., Goddard, W., 1993. Mechanism of the 1991 eruption of Hekla from continuous borehole strain monitoring. *Nature* 365, 21.

Gutenberg, B., Richter, C.F., 1944. Frequency of earthquakes in california. *Bulletin of the Seismological Society of America* 34, 185–188.

Hammer, C., Neuberg, J., 2009. On the dynamical behaviour of low-frequency earthquake swarms prior to a dome collapse of Soufrière Hill volcano, montserrat. *Geophysical Research Letters* 36, 6, L06305.

Harlow, D.H., Power, J.A., Laguerta, E.P., Ambubuyog, G., White, R.A., Hoblitt, R.P., 1996. Precursory seismicity and forecasting of the June 15, 1991, eruption of Mount Pinatubo, in: *Fire and Mud, Eruptions and Lahars of Mount Pinatubo*, Philippines, pp. 285–306.

Harris, A.J., Carniel, R., Jones, J., 2005. Identification of variable convective regimes at Erta Ale lava lake. *Journal of Volcanology and Geothermal Research* 142, 3, 207–223.

Hurst, T., Jolly, A.D., Sherburn, S., in press, 2014. Precursory characteristics of the seismicity before the 6 august 2012 eruption of Tongariro volcano, North island, New Zealand. *Journal of Volcanology and Geothermal Research* .

Ibáñez, J., De Angelis, S., Díaz-Moreno, A., Hernández, P., Alguacil, G., Posadas, A., Pérez, N., 2012. Insights into the 2011–2012 submarine eruption off the coast of El Hierro (Canary Islands, Spain) from statistical analyses of earthquake activity. *Geophysical Journal International* 191, 2, 659–670.

Imoto, M., 1991. Changes in the magnitude–frequency b-value prior to large (M>6.0) earthquakes in Japan. *Tectonophysics* 193,4 311–325.

Johnson, J.H., Prejean, S., Savage, M.K., Townend, J., 2010. Anisotropy, repeating earthquakes, and seismicity associated with the 2008 eruption of Okmok volcano, Alaska. *Journal of Geophysical Research: Solid Earth* (1978–2012) 115, B9, 6991.

Jolly, A.D., McNutt, S.R., 1999. Seismicity at the volcanoes of Katmai National Park, Alaska; July 1995–December 1997. *Journal of Volcanology and Geothermal Research* 93, 3, 173–190.

Jones, J.P., Thurber, C.H., Lutter, W.J., 2001. High-precision location of pre-eruption seismicity at Mount Pinatubo, Philippines, 30 may–3 june, 1991. *Physics of the Earth and Planetary Interiors* 123, 2, 221–232.

Julian, B.R., 1994. Volcanic tremor: Nonlinear excitation by fluid flow. *Journal of Geophysical Research: Solid Earth* (1978–2012) 99, B6, 11859–11877.

Kilburn, C.R., 2003. Multiscale fracturing as a key to forecasting volcanic eruptions. *Journal of Volcanology and Geothermal Research* 125, 3, 271–289.

Kilburn, C.R., Voight, B., 1998. Slow rock fracture as eruption precursor at Soufriere Hills volcano, Montserrat. *Geophysical Research Letters* 25,19 3665–3668.

King, G., 1983. The accommodation of large strains in the upper lithosphere of the earth and other solids by self-similar fault systems: the geometrical origin of b-value. *Pure and Applied Geophysics* 121,5–6, 761–815.

Klein, F.W., 1982. Earthquakes at Loihi submarine volcano and the Hawaiian hot spot. *Journal of Geophysical Research: Solid Earth* (1978–2012) 87, B9, 7719–7726.

Konstantinou, K.I., Schlindwein, V., 2003. Nature, wavefield properties and source mechanism of volcanic tremor: a review. *Journal of Volcanology and Geothermal Research* 119, 1, 161–187.

Lavallée, Y., Meredith, P., Dingwell, D., Hess, K.U., Wassermann, J., Cordonnier, B., Gerik, A., Kruhl, J., 2008. Seismogenic lavas and explosive eruption forecasting. *Nature* 453,7194, 507–510.

Lay, T., Wallace, T.C., 1995. *Modern global seismology*. volume 58. Academic press.

Lengliné, O., Marsan, D., Got, J.L., Pinel, V., Ferrazzini, V., Okubo, P., 2008. Seismicity and deformation induced by magma accumulation at three basaltic volcanoes. *Journal of Geophysical Research: Solid Earth* (1978–2012) 113, B12, B12305.

Lesage, P., Mora, M.M., Alvarado, G.E., Pacheco, J., Métaxian, J.P., 2006. Complex behavior and source model of the tremor at Arenal volcano, Costa Rica. *Journal of Volcanology and Geothermal Research* 157, 1, 49–59.

Lesage, P., et al., 1995. Seismic precursors of the February 10, 1990 eruption of Kelut volcano, Java. *Journal of volcanology and geothermal research* 65, 1, 135–146.

Linde, A.T., Sacks, I.S., 1998. Triggering of volcanic eruptions. *Nature* 395,6705, 888–890.

Lokmer, I., Saccorotti, G., Di Lieto, B., Bean, C.J., 2008. Temporal evolution of long-period seismicity at Etna volcano, Italy, and its relationships with the 2004–2005 eruption. *Earth and Planetary Science Letters* 266, 1, 205–220.

Lu, Z., Masterlark, T., Dzurisin, D., 2005. Interferometric synthetic aperture radar study of Okmok volcano, Alaska, 1992–2003: Magma supply dynamics and postemplacement lava flow deformation. *Journal of Geophysical Research: Solid Earth* (1978–2012) 110, B02403.

Main, I.G., 1987. A characteristic earthquake model of the seismicity preceding the eruption of Mount St. Helens on 18 may 1980. *Physics of the Earth and Planetary Interiors* 49, 3,283–293.

Main, I.G., 1999. Applicability of time-to-failure analysis to accelerated strain before earthquakes and volcanic eruptions. *Geophysical Journal International* 139, 3, F1–F6.

Manga, M., Brodsky, E., 2006. Seismic triggering of eruptions in the far field: volcanoes and geysers. *Annu. Rev. Earth Planet. Sci* 34, 263–291.

Matoza, R.S., Chouet, B.A., 2010. Subevents of long-period seismicity: Implications for hydrothermal dynamics during the 2004–2008 eruption of Mount St. Helens. *Journal of Geophysical Research: Solid Earth* (1978–2012) 115, B14, 12206.

McNutt, S.R., 1992. Volcanic tremor, in: *Encyclopedia of earth system science*. volume 4, pp. 417–425.

McNutt, S.R., 1994. Volcanic tremor amplitude correlated with the volcano explosivity index and its potential use in determining ash hazards to aviation. *Acta Vulcanol.* 5, 193.

McNutt, S.R., 1996. Seismic monitoring and eruption forecasting of volcanoes: a review of the state-of-the-art and case histories, in: *Monitoring and mitigation of volcano hazards*. Springer, pp. 99–146.

McNutt, S.R., 2002. Volcano seismology and monitoring for eruptions. *INTERNATIONAL GEOPHYSICS SERIES* 81, 383–406.

McNutt, S.R., 2005. Volcanic seismology. *Annu. Rev. Earth planet. Sci.* 32, 461–491.

McNutt, S.R., Nishimura, T., 2008. Volcanic tremor during eruptions: Temporal characteristics, scaling and constraints on conduit size and processes. *Journal of Volcanology and Geothermal Research* 178, 10–18.

Minakami, T., 1974. Seismology of volcanoes in Japan. *Physical Volcanology* 6, 1–27.

Moran, S.C., 1994. Seismicity at Mount St. Helens, 1987–1992: Evidence for repressurization of an active magmatic system. *Journal of Geophysical Research: Solid Earth* (1978–2012) 99, B3, 4341–4354.

Mori, J., Patia, H., McKee, C., Itikarai, I., Lowenstein, P., De Saint Ours, P., Talai, B., 1989. Seismicity associated with eruptive activity at Langila volcano, Papua New Guinea. *Journal of Volcanology and Geothermal Research* 38, 3, 243–255.

Murru, M., Console, R., Falcone, G., Montuori, C., Sgroi, T., 2007. Spatial mapping of the b-value at Mount Etna, Italy, using earthquake data recorded from 1999 to 2005. *Journal of Geophysical Research: Solid Earth* (1978–2012) 112, B11, 12303.

Murru, M., Montuori, C., Console, R., Lisi, A., 2005. Mapping of the b-value anomalies beneath Mt. Etna, Italy, during July–August 2001 lateral eruption. *Geophysical Research Letters* 32, 5, L05309–1.

Nakamichi, H., Hamaguchi, H., Tanaka, S., Ueki, S., Nishimura, T., Hasegawa, A., 2003. Source mechanisms of deep and intermediate-depth low-frequency earthquakes beneath Iwate volcano, Northeastern Japan. *Geophysical Journal International* 154, 3,811–828.

Neuberg, J., Luckett, R., Baptie, B., Olsen, K., 2000. Models of tremor and low-frequency earthquake swarms on Montserrat. *Journal of Volcanology and Geothermal Research* 101, 83–104.

Neuberg, J.W., Tuffen, H., Collier, L., Green, D., Powell, T., Dingwell, D., 2006. The trigger mechanism of low-frequency earthquakes on Montserrat. *Journal of Volcanology and Geothermal Research* 153, 37–50.

Newhall, C.G., Self, S., 1982. The volcanic explosivity index (VEI) an estimate of explosive magnitude for historical volcanism. *Journal of Geophysical Research: Oceans* (1978–2012) 87, C2, 1231–1238.

Novelo-Casanova, D., Martinez-Bringas, A., Valdés-González, C., 2006. Temporal variations of Q_c^{-1} and b-values associated to the December 2000–January 2001 volcanic activity at the Popocatepetl volcano, Mexico. *Journal of Volcanology and Geothermal Research* 152, 3,347–358.

Ottemöller, L., 2008. Seismic hybrid swarm precursory to a major lava dome collapse: 9–12 July 2003, Soufriere Hills volcano, Montserrat. *Journal of Volcanology and Geothermal Research* 177, 4,903–910.

Palo, M., Cusano, P., 2013. Wavefield decomposition and phase space dynamics of the seismic noise at Volcàn de Colima, Mexico: evidence of a two-state source process. *Nonlinear Processes in Geophysics* 20, 71–84.

Palo, M., Ibáñez, J., Cisneros, M., Bretón, M., Del Pezzo, E., Ocaña, E., Orozco-Rojas, J., Posadas, A., 2009. Analysis of the seismic wavefield properties of volcanic explosions at Volcán de Colima, México: Insights into the source mechanism. *Geophysical Journal International* 177, 3,1383–1398.

Patanè, D., Privitera, E., 2001. Seismicity related to 1989 and 1991–93 Mt. Etna (Italy) eruptions: Kinematic constraints by fault plane solution analysis. *Journal of Volcanology and Geothermal Research* 109, 77–98.

Pedersen, R., Sigmundsson, F., 2006. Temporal development of the 1999 intrusive episode in the Eyjafjallaj ökull volcano, Iceland, derived from insar images. *Bulletin of Volcanology* 68,4, 377–393.

Pozgay, S.H., White, R.A., Wiens, D.A., Shore, P.J., Sauter, A.W., Kaipat, J.L., 2005. Seismicity and tilt associated with the 2003 Anatahan eruption sequence. *Journal of Volcanology and Geothermal Research* 146, 60–76.

Roman, D., De Angelis, S., Latchman, J., White, R., 2008. Patterns of volcano-tectonic seismicity and stress during the ongoing eruption of the Soufri`ere Hills volcano, Montserrat (1995–2007). *Journal of Volcanology and Geothermal Research* 173, 3,230–244.

Roman, D., Neuberg, J., Luckett, R., 2006. Assessing the likelihood of volcanic eruption through analysis of volcano-tectonic earthquake fault–plane solutions. *Earth and Planetary Science Letters* 248, 244–252.

Roman, D.C., Moran, S.C., Power, J.A., Cashman, K.V., 2004. Temporal and spatial variation of local stress fields before and after the 1992 eruptions of crater peak vent, Mount Spurr volcano, Alaska. *Bulletin of the Seismological Society of America* 94, 6, 2366–2379.

Rowe, C., Aster, R. C., Kyle, P. R., Dibble, R. R., Schlue, J. W., 2000. Seismic and acoustic observations at Mount Erebus Volcano, Ross Island, Antarctica, 1994–1998. *Journal of Volcanology and Geothermal Research* 101, 1, 105–128.

Rowe, C., Thurber, C., White, R., 2004. Dome growth behavior at Soufriere Hills volcano, Montserrat, revealed by relocation of volcanic event swarms, 1995–1996. *Journal of Volcanology and Geothermal Research* 134, 3,199–221.

Ruppert, N.A., Prejean, S., Hansen, R.A., 2011. Seismic swarm associated with the 2008 eruption of Kasatochi volcano, Alaska: Earthquake locations and source parameters. *Journal of Geophysical Research: Solid Earth* (1978–2012) 116, B2, 7435.

Sammis, C., Sornette, D., 2002. Positive feedback, memory, and the predictability of earthquakes. *Proceedings of the National Academy of Sciences* 99, 1, 2501–2508.

Sanchez, J., McNutt, S.R., Power, J., Wyss, M., 2004. Spatial variations in the frequency-magnitude distribution of earthquakes at Mount Pinatubo volcano. *Bulletin of the Seismological Society of America* 94, 2, 430–438.

Sarao, A., Panza, G., Privitera, E., Cocina, O., 2001. Non-double-couple mechanisms in the seismicity preceding the 1991–1993 Etna volcano eruption. *Geophysical Journal International* 145, 2, 319–335.

Schlindwein, V., Wassermann, J., Scherbaum, F., 1995. Spectral analysis of harmonic tremor signals at Mt. Semeru volcano, Indonesia. *Geophysical Research Letters* 22,13, 1685–1688.

Schmid, A., Grasso, J.R., 2012. Omori law for eruption foreshocks and aftershocks. *Journal of Geophysical Research: Solid Earth* (1978–2012) 117, B07, 7307.

Schwartz, S.Y., Rokosky, J.M., 2007. Slow slip events and seismic tremor at circum-pacific subduction zones. *Reviews of Geophysics* 45, 3, 3004.

Shelly, D.R., Hill, D.P., 2011. Migrating swarms of brittle-failure earthquakes in the lower crust beneath Mammoth Mountain, California. *Geophysical Research Letters* 38, 20, 20307.

Smith, W.D., 1986. Evidence for precursory changes in the frequency-magnitude b-value. *Geophysical Journal International* 86, 3,815–838.

Tárraga, M., Martí, J., Abella, R., Carniel, R., López, C., 2014. Volcanic tremors: Good indicators of change in plumbing systems during volcanic eruptions. *Journal of Volcanology and Geothermal Research* 273, 33–40.

Thompson, G., McNutt, S.R., Tytgat, G., 2002. Three distinct regimes of volcanic tremor associated with the eruption of Shishaldin volcano, Alaska 1999. *Bulletin of Volcanology* 64,8 535–547.

Traversa, P., Grasso, J.R., 2010. How is volcano seismicity different from tectonic seismicity? *Bulletin of the Seismological Society of America* 100, 4,1755–1769.

Traversa, P., Lengliné, O., Macedo, O., Métaxian, J.P., Grasso, J.R., Inza, A., Taipe, E., 2011. Short term forecasting of explosions at Ubinas volcano, Perú. *Journal of Geophysical Research: Solid Earth* (1978–2012) 116, B11, 11301.

Tuffen, H., Smith, R., Sammonds, P.R., 2008. Evidence for seismogenic fracture of silicic magma. *Nature* 453, 511–514.

Ukawa, M., 2005. Deep low-frequency earthquake swarm in the mid crust beneath Mount Fuji (Japan) in 2000 and 2001. *Bulletin of Volcanology* 68, 47–56.

Van Der Waals, J.D., 2004. *On the continuity of the gaseous and liquid states* . Courier Dover Publications.

Vinciguerra, S., 1999. Seismic scaling exponents as a tool in detecting stress corrosion crack growth leading to the september–october 1989 flank eruption at Mt. Etna volcano. *Geophysical Research Letters* 26,24 3685–3688.

Voight, B., 1988. A method for prediction of volcanic eruptions. *Nature* 332, 125–130.

Voight, B., Cornelius, R.R., 1991. Prospects for eruption prediction in near real-time. *Nature* 350,6320, 695–698.

Voight, B., Hidayat, D., Sacks, S., Linde, A., Chardot, L., Clarke, A., Elsworth, D., Foroozan, R., Malin, P., Mattioli, G., et al., 2010. Unique strainmeter observations of vulcanian explosions, Soufri`ere Hills volcano, Montserrat, July 2003. *Geophysical Research Letters* 37, L00E18.

Voight, B., Hoblitt, R., Clarke, A., Lockhart, A., Miller, A., Lynch, L., McMahon, J., 1998. Remarkable cyclic ground deformation monitored in real-time on Montserrat, and its use in eruption forecasting. *Geophysical Research Letters* 25,18 3405–3408.

Voight, B., Sparks, R., Miller, A., Stewart, R., Hoblitt, R., Clarke, A., Ewart, J., Aspinall, W., Baptie, B., Calder, E., et al., 1999. Magma flow instability and cyclic activity at Soufrière Hills volcano, Montserrat, British West Indies. *Science* 283,5405, 1138–1142.

Waldhauser, F., Ellsworth, W.L., 2000. A double-difference earthquake location algorithm: Method and application to the Northern Hayward Fault, California. *Bulletin of the Seismological Society of America* 90, 6,1353–1368.

Warren, N.W., Latham, G.V., 1970. An experimental study of thermally induced microfracturing and its relation to volcanic seismicity. *Journal of Geophysical Research* 75, 23,4455–4464.

West, M.E., 2013. Recent eruptions at Bezymianny volcanoa seismological comparison. *Journal of Volcanology and Geothermal Research* 263, 42–57.

Wiemer, S., McNutt, S.R., Wyss, M., 1998. Temporal and three-dimensional spatial analyses of the frequencymagnitude distribution near Long Valley caldera, California. *Geophysical Journal International* 134, 2,409–421.

Williams-Jones, G., Stix, J., Heiligmann, M., Barquero, J., Fernandez, E., Gonzalez, E., 2001. A model of degassing and seismicity at Arenal volcano, Costa Rica. *Journal of Volcanology and Geothermal Research* 108, 121–139.

Wyss, M., Shimazaki, K., Wiemer, S., 1997. Mapping active magma chambers by b-values beneath the Off-Ito volcano, Japan. *Journal of Geophysical Research: Solid Earth* (1978–2012) 102, B9,20413–20422.

In: Volcanic Eruptions
Editor: Trent Milburn
ISBN: 978-1-63463-308-6

Chapter 5

EFFECT OF VOLCANIC ERUPTIONS ON STRATOSPHERIC OZONE AND IRRADIANCE

***Susana B. Diaz*[1,*] *and Alejandro A. Paladini*[1]**
[1]INGEBI/CONICET, Instituto de Genética y Biología Molecular (INGEBI), Argentina
CONICET, Vuelta de Obligado, Buenos Aires, Argentina

ABSTRACT

Major volcanic eruptions can inject large amounts of sulfur into the stratosphere, increasing the stratospheric aerosol layer for several years. In the last decades, this effect was observed after the eruptions of El Chichón, in 1982, and Mt. Pinatubo, in 1991, which had a considerable contribution to ozone depletion. The natural variability of atmospheric ozone occurs in time scales ranging from day to day, to decadal. Atmospheric circulation, chemistry, and radiative processes play important roles in the variability of ozone. Large volcanic eruptions reaching the stratosphere could cause significant temporary changes. The effect of a volcanic eruption on stratospheric ozone is largest when large chlorine and bromine levels are present in the atmosphere. How past volcanic eruptions have changed stratospheric ozone was studied using models. It was concluded that eruptions of El Chichon and Pinatubo resulted in globally total ozone losses and severe ozone depletion in the

* E-mail: diazsusanab@gmail.com.

lower stratosphere. Earlier eruptions (Krakatau, Santa Maria and Agung) resulted in globally total ozone increases and almost no ozone changes in the stratosphere. This difference in ozone response was caused by the amount of ozone depleting substances present in the atmosphere, which increased the availability of chlorine and caused a change in the chemistry, during the last decades. In the mid-1990s, a maximum in stratospheric ozone depletion was observed, as consequence of ozone response to volcanic aerosols from Mt. Pinatubo, superimposed to the depletion produced by halocarbons.

One of the reasons that make stratospheric ozone important is the attenuation of solar ultraviolet (UV) radiation while it trespasses the atmosphere. Radiation reaching the Earth's surface is influenced by scattering and absorption processes in the atmosphere and the ground. Sun-Earth distance, atmospheric gases and aerosols, solar zenith angle (SZA), clouds and surface albedo are the main factors that determine radiation at ground-level. The effect of volcanic eruptions on UV radiation is complex. On one side, depletion of stratospheric ozone results in an increase in UV radiation. In addition, volcanic eruptions increase the aerosol amount and change aerosol size composition, producing important variation in optical properties of the atmosphere. As a result, a decrease is usually observed in direct UV radiation, due to absorption produced by the emitted particles. At the same time, an increase in the diffuse radiation may be experienced, resulting from scattering increase. As consequence of these two processes the effect on global UV radiation is difficult to anticipate.

In this chapter, we present a review of the effect of major volcanic eruptions on the ozone layer and UV radiation. We also introduce our own results on the effect of Puyehue-Cordon Caulle volcanic complex eruption, in 2011, which did not affect globally the ozone layer but produced a large regional impact on aerosols and UV radiation.

1. Volcanic Eruptions and Ozone

1.1. Ozone

Ozone is a trace gas mostly present in the stratosphere. It has had an important roll on the evolution of life on Earth since it absorbs solar UV-B radiation, which is harmful to living systems. The total amount of ozone in the atmosphere is extremely small. Near 90% of the total ozone in the atmosphere is located in the stratosphere, and the rest, in the troposphere [1].

Ozone is constantly being formed and destroyed in the atmosphere. Its concentration in the stratosphere varies with altitude, reaching a maximum at about the middle of the layer. Ozone is created by an interaction between oxygen and sunlight, and it is destroyed through a series of processes which involve sunlight, oxygen, nitrogen and hydrogen. It has also been observed that large volcanic eruptions and some anthropogenic chemical compounds may affect the ozone layer [2].The total ozone column is measured in Dobson Units (DU). One DU corresponds to an average concentration of approximately 1 part per billion per volume.

Natural variability of atmospheric ozone exhibits both temporal and geographical variations. They occur as consequence of atmospheric circulation, chemistry, and radiative processes [3, 4]. Total ozone column varies with latitude, between 230 and 500 DU, with a world average of around 300 DU [1]. Larger total ozone column is typically observed at higher latitudes and lower values in the tropical regions. Temporal variations include a seasonal cycle, which presents a maximum in spring and a minimum in autumn [1], day to day variations and a diurnal cycle, with larger values in the morning decreasing toward the evening [5]. In addition, temporal changes related to the 11 year sun spot cycle, the quasi-biennial oscillation (QBO), regional El Niño/La Niña effects and the 27 days sun rotation, are observed.

Depletion in stratospheric ozone has been occurring since the mid-1970's [6, 7] both as a small worldwide depletion and as a severe seasonal depletion localized over Antarctica and, to some extend, the Arctic. The depletion centered over Antarctica and surrounding regions is known as the "ozone hole". It starts at late winter or early spring and persists until late spring. During this process more than 50% of the regional stratospheric ozone is destroyed. This phenomenon results from the coincidence of three factors: high altitude ice crystals clouds (Polar Stratospheric Clouds), isolation produced by the Antarctic polar vortex and the presence of halocarbons in the stratosphere, which has been found to have a strong anthropogenic component [7, 3, 8].

1.2. Effect of Volcanoes on Ozone

Volcanic eruptions produce changes in the atmosphere, which may affect several parameters, i.e., aerosol optical depth, aerosol size and composition, stratospheric and trophospheric ozone amounts, Ultraviolet (UV) radiation direct and diffuse components. Eruptions consist of a mixture of gases, aerosol, and silicate particles. Ash and sulfate aerosols in the lower atmosphere have short time effects on the atmosphere and climate, while volcanic aerosols injected high into the stratosphere produce significant radiative/chemical and dynamical effects, which may influence over longer time-scales [9-13].

In the atmosphere, a layer of sulfuric acid (SO_2) aerosol is found near 15-25 km altitude, which is important for stratospheric ozone chemistry [14]. Although the stratospheric SO_2 is less than 0.1% of the present in the troposphere, this small amount is important since the lifetime in the stratosphere is much longer than in the troposphere, due to the lack of precipitation. During volcanically quiescent periods, the main source of this aerosol layer is thought to be the product of the oxidation of a biogenic gas, carbonyl sulfide, which presents an atmospheric lifetime long enough to penetrate the stratosphere in the form of sulfur dioxide (SO_2) [15, 8]. Large volcanic eruptions are a major source of sulfur to the stratosphere, injecting large amounts of this compound and increasing the stratospheric aerosol layer. The effect may last for several years and can be observed at sites far from the source. The contribution to the aerosols optical depth (AOD) from residual stratospheric aerosols resulting from the eruption of Mt. Pinatubo, in 1991, was detected in the Russian Arctic, in 1993 [16] and in Oklahoma, until 1995 [17].

Volcanic aerosols affect stratospheric circulation and temperature, and provide surfaces for chemical heterogeneous reactions, leading to ozone depletion [11]. Two large volcanic eruptions were present between 1980 and 1995, which affected the ozone layer (El Chichon and Mt Pinatubo) [13, 18]. Minimum total ozone, around 5.5% below the 1964–1980 average, was observed in the mid-1990s. Simulations by Chemical Circulation Models (CCMs) exhibited good agreement with measurements, and indicated that this minimum was caused by the ozone response to volcanic aerosols from the eruption of Mt. Pinatubo (June 1991) superimposed to the effect of ozone depleting substances (ODSs) [8]. It is estimated that, enhanced stratospheric aerosols were also present throughout much of the decade of the 1980s due to earlier volcanic eruptions (i.e., El Chichon), increasing the existing downward trend in ozone, consequence of ODSs [2].

Several studies were carried out in order to quantify the impact of major volcanic eruptions on the ozone layer. Since the eruptions of El Chichon (1982) and Mt Pinatubo (1991) occurred at almost the same time with solar maxima, it is difficult to separate the effect of solar cycle and these eruptions [8]. Angell [19] evaluated the impact of three major volcanic events on global and regional total ozone after adjusting for the QBO. He reported that the ozone deficiency, which can be attributed to the volcanoes, ranged between 2 and 4%, at the equatorial latitudes, lasting for several months after the eruption. Observed negative ozone anomalies following the Mt. Pinatubo event were larger (up to 5%) over the Northern Hemisphere, in winter and at high latitudes. Similar results were obtained by Brunner et al. [20], McCormack et al. [21], Robock et al. [22] and Zerefos et al. [23, 24], between others.

A variety of tools were used to explain these seasonal and geographical differences in the anomalies. A study with two-dimensional model simulations [25] found that the inter-annual dynamical variability reinforced the ozone perturbation in the NH mid-latitudes, while in the SH the circulation mitigated or even canceled the aerosol-induced chemical ozone reactions. Telford et al. [26], using a nudged CCM (UK Chemistry and Aerosols (UKCA)) simulation, concluded that the depletion of stratospheric ozone due Mt Pinatubo was mainly the result of photochemical changes produced by heterogeneous reactions, but with some evidence of dynamically induced ozone reduction, especially in the NH mid-latitudes. These two results confirmed the conclusions of Hadjinicolaou et al. [27], which showed the existence of a large dynamical effect on ozone following the eruption.

Polar ozone depletion also showed to be affected by volcanic eruptions. Rex et al. [28] and Tilmes et al. [29] observed enhanced polar ozone loss in the Arctic winter 1991/1992, due to the presence of Mt. Pinatubo aerosols, although their quantitative estimates of the effect differed. Portmann et al. [12] reported that Antarctic ozone depletion in the 1980s and early 1990s was influenced by enhanced sulfate aerosol from El Chichón and some earlier minor eruptions. Also, there were several attempts to discern the effects of volcanic aerosol perturbations on Polar Stratospheric Clouds characteristics [30-32], but the results were inconclusive.

Different models have been used to determine the chemical and dynamical effects of volcanic aerosols in polar regions (e.g., [33-37]. They have shown that the polar vortex strengthens in the NH after a volcanic eruption, as consequence of changes in the equator-to-pole temperature gradient in the lower stratosphere. Since stronger polar vortex increases the probability of formation of polar stratospheric clouds, the rate of heterogeneous chemical destruction of stratospheric ozone increases.

Some studies have concluded that the effect of volcanic eruptions on stratospheric ozone depletion is largest when chlorine and bromine levels are highest [38]. Since the eruptions of El Chichon and Mt Pinatubo occurred during a period of high chlorine abundance in the stratosphere, Tie et al. [34] suggested that the impact of these major volcanic eruptions would have been smaller or they would even have produced an increase in ozone, in the presence of lower chlorine levels in the atmosphere. Using a version of the GFDL CCM, Austin et al. [39] determined that, while the most recent major eruptions (El Chichon and Pinatubo) resulted in globally averaged total ozone losses and severe ozone depletion in the lower stratosphere, earlier eruptions (Krakatau, Santa Maria and Agung), resulted in globally averaged total ozone increases and almost no ozone changes in the stratosphere. It was concluded that, the observed difference in ozone response was caused by the change in the chemistry, due to the increased availability of chlorine during more recent eruptions. From these studies, it may be inferred that, as stratospheric chlorine decreases, as consequence of the Montreal Protocol, the impact of future major volcanic eruptions on ozone would decrease. But, since halogen levels are still high in the stratosphere, significant ozone depletion could occur, in the event of large volcanic eruptions in the next few decades, interrupting temporarily the future recovery of the ozone layer [8].

Although there have not been any major volcanic eruptions in the first decade of the twenty first century, changes in background stratospheric aerosols have been observed. Hofmann et al. [40], analyzing ground-based measurements, detected an increase in aerosols since 2002. They attributed this effect to an increase in the SO_2 emissions resulting from an enhancement in global coal consumption, mainly in China. They also concluded that, the contributions from minor volcanic activity and from increased tropical up-welling, due to changes in the Brewer-Dobson circulation, were not significant. However, other study performed from the Cloud-Aerosol Lidar with Orthogonal Polarization (CALIOP) [41] concluded that small volcanic eruptions may have played a role.

Aircraft measurements in the volcanic plume of the Hekla, Iceland, showed that minor volcanic eruptions can also deplete ozone [42], although the effect would be regional and of short residence [8]. In April 2010, the volcano Eyjafjallajökull (Iceland) was active producing a dramatic amount of ash, for several days, which affected Europe [43-46]. Nevertheless, geologically, this eruption was very modest, with limited sulfur emissions and its impact was mainly restricted to the regional troposphere [47].

2. VOLCANIC ERUPTIONS AND UV RADIATION

2.1. UV Radiation

Solar UV radiation reaching the Earth's surface is affected by scattering and absorption processes while trespassing the atmosphere and reflecting on the ground.

Scattering may take place by reflection, refraction, or diffraction of a radiation beam and it gets a maximum value for particle radius of the order of the wavelength of the radiation [14]. Larger particles also scatter radiation efficiently, while smaller particles are not efficient scatterers [14].

The flux in the UV portion of the spectrum is a very small percentage of the total UV and visible radiation (usually less than 1%) [1]. However, UV is responsible for important beneficial and harmful effects on ecosystems and human life (DNA damage, Vitamin D photoproduction, erythema, etch) . Each effect presents distinctive wavelength dependence. The function that represents that dependence is called "action spectrum" [48] and the spectral irradiance weighted by the corresponding action spectrum and integrated in wavelength is named with the effect (for example: erythemal irradiance).

UV radiation at ground level presents large natural variation and most of it may be accounted for the geometry of the Earth-Sun system. The distance between the Earth and the Sun and the Solar Zenith Angle (SZA) are the main geometric factors that govern changes in intensity of solar radiation with time of the day, latitude and season, and the dependence of irradiances on these parameters is well established [49, 50].

Other parameters influencing UV are atmospheric factors such as gases present in the atmosphere, clouds and aerosols. The ground albedo, which causes solar radiation to bounce between the surface and the atmosphere, also determine ambient UV radiation. As a result of the above-mentioned parameters, UV radiation shows also a variation with altitude, usually increasing with this factor [51-53].

Total ozone column is the most important atmospheric gas affecting ground-level UV-B irradiance. Its efficiency in absorbing the radiation is better at lower wavelengths in the UV-B than at larger [1].

In the troposphere, absorbers of UV radiation include ozone, sulfur dioxide, nitrogen oxides, bromine and chlorine compounds and the Oxygen dimmer [54, 55], different types of aldehydes, acetone, peroxyacetyl nitrate (PAN), propanal, glioxal, nitrated aromatics, certain organic acids, and others

[54-56]. Nevertheless, the abundance of most of these compounds in the troposphere is usually small to produce measurable effects on surface UV, except during natural hazards, like forest fires and volcanic eruptions or near the source of emission, in polluted areas [8].

The presence of clouds may be responsible for large changes in the irradiance. They usually attenuate the UV radiation, although under broken cloud conditions, an increase, relative to clear sky values, may be observed [57-60].

Surface reflectivity (albedo) in the UV, is usually less than 0.1 but, in the presence of snow, it increases considerably, reaching values closed to 1, varying with snow type and age. Blumthaler and Haferi [52] observed that, in the alpine region, the albedo decreased from 0.8 in winter to 0.45 in spring. In surfaces covered by fresh pure snow, albedo closed to unity was reported [61]. Observed enhancements in surface irradiance at 324 nm, as consequence of the presence of snow, were between 8% and 39%, with larger increases reported at Arctic sites surrounded by uniform snow cover, and smaller at urban sites or sites near open water [62].

The effect of atmospheric aerosols on surface UV radiation depends on the total atmospheric loading and their optical and microphysical properties. Several studies have shown long- and short-term effects of aerosols on irradiances [63-67]. Large differences have been observed in irradiance between urban and rural locations, or between rather polluted sites in the Northern Hemisphere and cleaner sites in the Southern Hemisphere [68].

In a global scale, scattering of solar radiation by aerosols increases the Earth's albedo because a fraction of the scattered light is reflected back to space. This cooling of the Earth’s surface is observed following large volcanic eruptions. After Mt Pinatubo eruption, in 1991, a decrease in mean surface temperatures was observed for the following two years [69].

2.2. Effect of Volcanoes on UV Radiation

Ozone depletion, resulting from volcanic eruptions would lead to an increase in UV Radiation. In addition, the optical properties of the atmosphere are affected by eruptions since they modify aerosols loading and size distribution, by injecting coarse (ash) and fine (sulfate) particles [45]. While, direct radiation at ground level decreases as a result of eruptions, due to absorption by some of the emitted particles, the effect on the total radiation is difficult to predict, since other particles from the eruption may lead to an increase of the diffuse [2].

It has been observed that the increase of SO_2 over areas affected by high volcanic activity or over regions close to coal burning industries, may result in an attenuation of erythemal irradiance between 2 and 5% [70, 71] and, at some UV wavelengths, the reduction can exceed 20% [71]. A survey of 13 locations in Canada and Japan indicated only two sites where SO_2 was important for the reduction of UV irradiance [72]. These cities were Kagoshima, Japan, located at about 10 km from a volcano, and Toronto, Canada, exhibiting local pollution sources.

With the aims of analyzing in more detail the effect of volcanic eruptions on UV irradiance, we present a case study.

2.3. Case Study: Puyehue-Cordon Caulle Eruption

On June 4th, 2011, after a period of low activity, a fissure opened in the Puyehue-Cordon Caulle volcanic complex (40°35′25″S 72°07′02″W, Chile) (Figure 1), sending ash 45,000 feet into the atmosphere [73, 74]. Cordón Caulle is one of the most active in Southern Andes and the previous event was in 1960. Both eruptions occurred through a fissure in the section of the Cordón Caulle while the stratocone of the Puyehue volcano remained dormant. In the 2011 event, ash, sand and pumice were ejected. While the ash emission was blown east, heavier material was falling out of the ash cloud and finer particles remained suspended in the atmosphere. A layer of material, around 30 centimeters deep, covered the ground near the town of San Carlos de Bariloche (Figure 1). The plume reached the Atlantic Ocean and turned around the world, affecting downwind regions of the Southern Hemisphere, for a few months, and forcing flight cancellations at several airports [73, 74]. In September 2011, the airport of San Carlos de Bariloche was still not operative.

The ash plume was captured by several NASA satellites. MODIS (Moderate Resolution Imaging Spectroradiometer), Terra and Aqua satellites was one of the instruments that provided daily imagery of the plume [75]. Figure 2a shows the image for June 6th, a couple of days after the eruption started, Figure 2b and 2c, correspond to September 17th and November 16th, respectively, when the activity still continued, with a plume much smaller than during the opening phase. During the activity period, high atmospheric winds were carrying the ash away and, depending on wind intensity, it went as far as 120–250 kilometers from the vent.

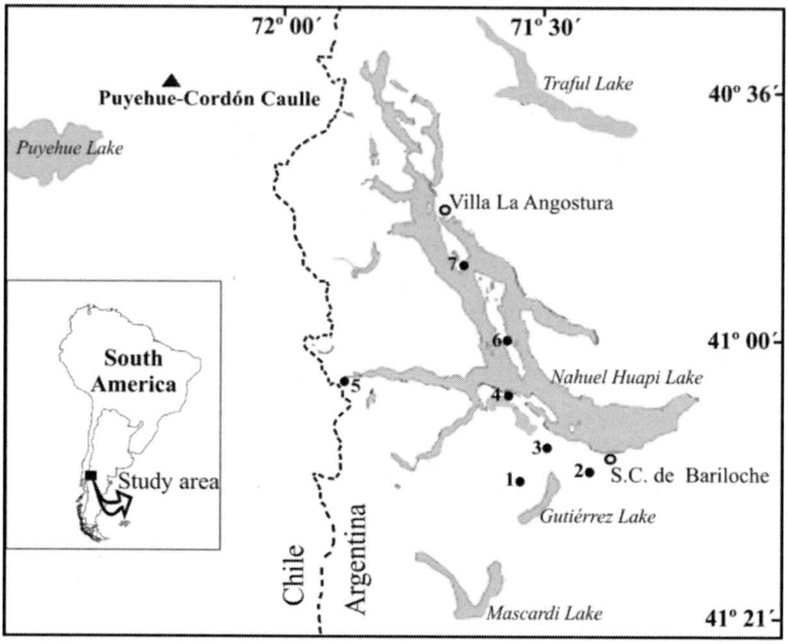

Figure 1. Area of Study: 1) Mt Catedral, 2) Mt Otto, 3) Laboratory of Photobioloy, 4) Port Pañuelo and San Eduardo Chapel, 5) Port Blest, 6) Victoria Island – Port Anchorena and 7) Quetrihue Penninsula - Arrayanes Forest.

This eruption did not affect the ozone layer, but it produced changes in irradiances and regional aerosols. With the aims of quantifying the effect, we have performed a study of direct and global UV irradiance and Aerosols Optical Dpeth (AOD), at different sites inside Nahuel Huapi National Park (NHNP) [76].

The NHNP is comprised the geological province of "Nordpatagonian Cordillera" (Patagonian Andes) and encompasses different ecological units: a) Altoandina which is above 1600 m.s.l, and occupies ~19% of the Park area, b) Forest that develops in ~76% of the park area, encompassing a humid forest in the western part changing to a transitional forest to the east according to a steep W-E precipitation gradient, and, c) Steppe [77]. Our study was performed at the Altoandina and Forest units of the park.

Our main site of study was the Laboratory of Photobiology (LPh), located at the west of San Carlos de Bariloche, on a derivation of the road to Catedral Village.

San Carlos de Bariloche is a town with near 80,000 inhabitants and about 20,000 ha, included in the Nahuel Huapi National Park (NHNP) (Figure 1).

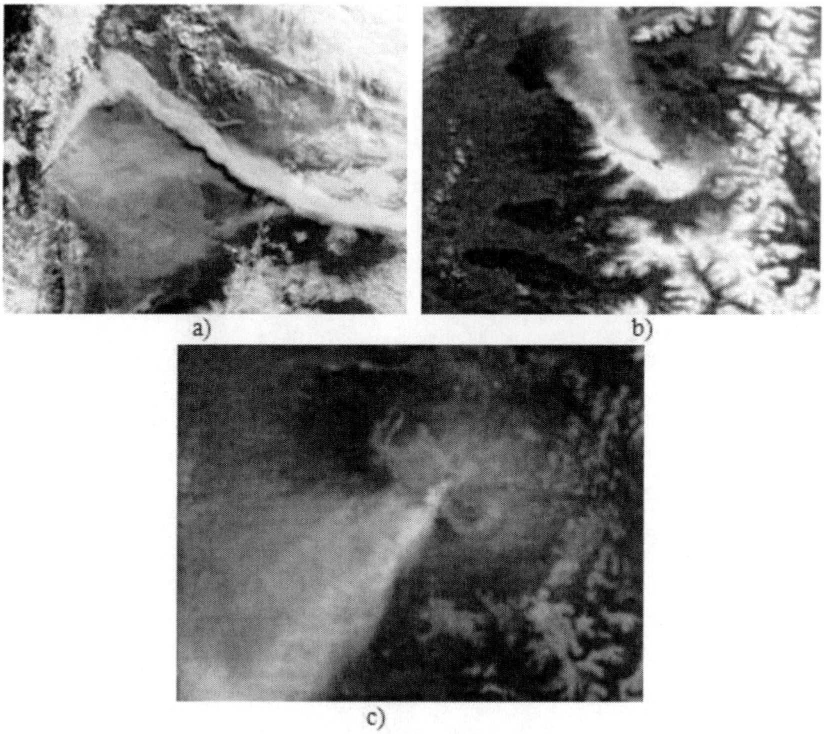

Figure 2. Images for the eruption of the Puyheue-Cordon Caulle volcanic complex: a) June 6th, 2011 (NASA Goddard/MODIS Rapid Response Team), b) September 17th (NASA image courtesy Jeff Schmaltz MODIS Rapid Response Team, NASA-GSFC) and c) November 16th (NASA image courtesy Jeff Schmaltz, LANCE/EOSDIS MODIS Rapid Response Team at NASA GSFC).

The city is surrounded by a mixed Nothofagus forest, the ground is snow covered during part of the winter and the weather is highly variable due to the strong westerly winds. The LPh is surrounded by a planted field of non-native pine tree species, spotted with native trees and shrubs. The site lacks neighbors, except for a small research laboratory. To complete the study, we analyzed data collected during short campaigns at Mt Otto and Mt Cathedral (Figure 1).

Mt Otto is situated at ~4 km southwest from San Carlos de Bariloche. It is a tourist point with a lift that reaches the top at 1386 m.s.l, where our mobile station was sited. Mt Catedral is a ski resort, and our station was set up at Mountain Refuge Lynch, located at 1930 m.s.l. While we performed our campaigns, in September 2010 and 2011, the snow was present at all the sites;

however, the snow pack was lower at lower altitude sites. At this type of locations, aerosols, are likely biogenic, contributed by the forest and soil and coarse particles are produced by soil dust, fungal spores, pollen and microorganisms [78].

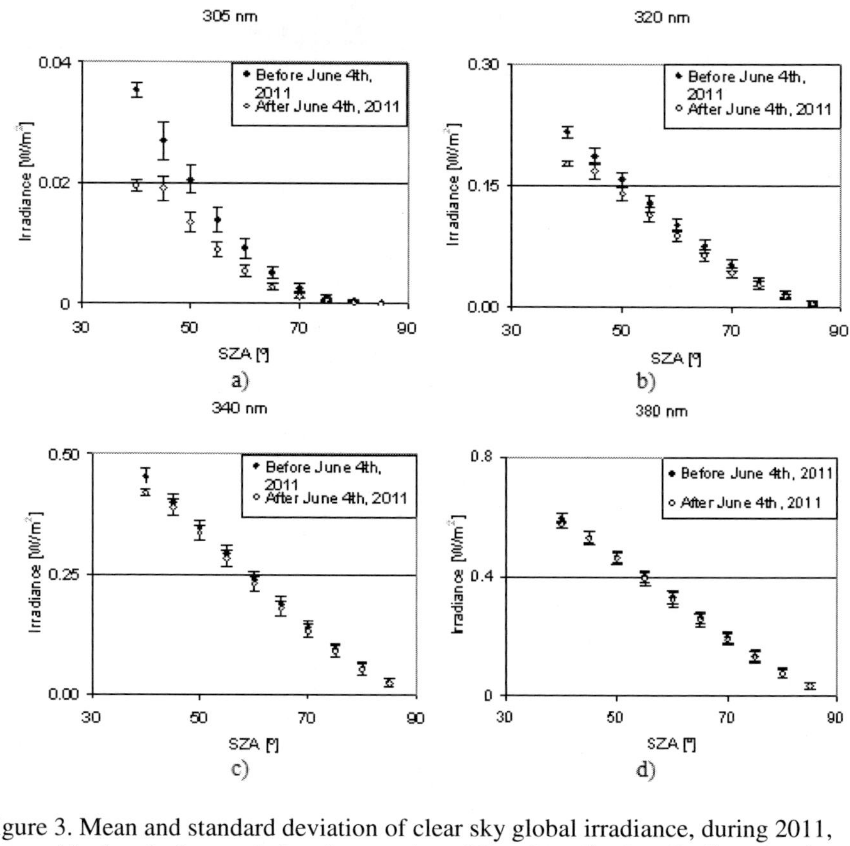

Figure 3. Mean and standard deviation of clear sky global irradiance, during 2011, grouped in days before and after the eruption of Puyehue-Cordon Caulle volcanic complex (June 4th, 2011).

Global irradiance has been permanently measured at the Laboratory of Photobiology (LPh), INIBIOMA, Universidad Nacional del Comahue (LPh) (41.13°S, 71.42°W, 804m.s.l.) since 1998 [79].

In order to determine the effect of the volcano on global irradiance, data collected during 2011, before and after the eruption, and in 1999, as reference year, were used. In addition, in our campaigns during September 2010 and September 2011, we measured global irradiance, aerosol optical depth (AOD) and direct radiation simultaneously at LPh and Mt Otto (41.15°S, 71.38°W,

1386m.s.l.) or Mt Catedral (41.17°S, 71.48°W, 1930m.s.l.). Multi-channel radiometers were used to collect global irradiance. A GUV 511 served at the fixed station and a BIC 250 at the mobile station.

Aerosols optical depth (AOD) and direct radiation were obtained by means of two handheld Microtops II sun-photometers [76].

Global irradiance obtained for clear days, in 2011, were separated in two groups, before and after the eruption (date June 4th) and mean and standard deviation were calculated for each of them.

In Figure 3, it may be observed that, while there was almost no difference between values before and after the eruption, at 340 and 380 nm (Figure 3c and d), at 305 and 320 nm (Figure 3 a and b), irradiance after the eruption exhibited a decrease, which was more pronounced at the lowest wavelength (around 40%, at SZA 45°).

To probe the hypothesis that the observed results were a consequence of the eruption and there was not significant effect of other factors, for example albedo, year 1999 was considered, when no eruption or any other major event occurred. In this case, similar results to 2011 were observed for 340 and 380 nm, probing that, the results observed for 2011, were not the consequence of compensation between the effect of albedo and the eruption. At 305 nm, the difference between both groups was smaller for 1999 than for 2011 and, at 320 nm, no significant difference was detected, in 1999.

Since, 305 nm is a wavelengths affected by ozone, we selected pair of days, one before and one after June 4th, with equal ozone and compared them. In addition, with the aims of increasing the size of our sample, we modeled the global irradiance for clear days in 1999 and 2011, applying a disort model [80], with no aerosol load. Then, we calculated the difference in irradiance consequence only of ozone changes, in pair of days with one of them before and one after June 4th.

$$\Delta Irr_{Oz} = \left(I_{0i} - I_{0j}\right) \tag{1}$$

where ΔIrr_{Oz} is difference in modeled global irradiance due to ozone changes, I_{0i} is modeled irradiance for day i, after the eruption, i=1 to m, and I_{0j} is modeled irradiance for day j, before the eruption, j=1 to n, in both cases calculated with aerosol load equal zero.

Also, The difference between measured values after and before the eruption, at the same SZA, are the result of ozone and AOD variations:

$$\Delta Irr_{Oz+AOD} = (I_i - I_j) \quad (2)$$

where ΔIrr_{Oz+AOD} is difference in measured global irradiance due to ozone and aerosols changes, I_i is measured irradiance at day i, after the eruption, i=1 to m, and I_j is measured irradiance at day j, before the eruption, j=1 to n.

Finally, we calculated the irradiance variation due to the volcano eruption as the difference between (2) and (1) [76]:

$$\Delta Irr_{AOD} = \Delta Irr_{Oz+AOD} - \Delta Irr_{Oz} \quad (3)$$

The results, comparing days before and after June 4th, in 1999 and 2011, are summarized in Table I. It was observed that, for 1999, the difference between clear days of both groups was not statistically significant, at any wavelength, but, as reflected by the standard deviation, less variability was exhibited during 1999 than in 2011, when, in addition, 12% decrease (SZA < 60°) was observed in the group of days after the eruption, at 320 nm and 18%, at 305 nm. The results observed at 305 nm, were similar for pair of days with equal ozone and for the rest of the days after applying ozone correction.

Table I. Mean and standard deviation for global irradiance before and after June 4th, SZA < 60°

	305 nm	320 nm	340 nm	380 nm
1999	-2.3 +/- 3.8	-3.1 +/- 3.1	2.7 +/- 2.7	-0.5 +/- 2.1
2011	-18.0 +/- 8.8	-12.1 +/- 9.1	-3.1 +/- 5.4	-1.6 +/- 4.5

Figure 4 shows AOD and Angstrom exponent [81] obtained during the campaigns, for the three sites, at 380 nm [76]. From the few clear sky days we had during the 2011 campaign, two exhibited AOD similar to 2010, and only one much larger value [Figure 4a]. This observation would explain the large variability observed in global irradiance after the eruption. In addition, an inverse relation was observed between AOD and the Angstrom exponent (Figures 4 a & b respectively), indicating that increases in AOD would correspond to an increase in coarse particles.

When comparing direct irradiance measured during the campaigns 2010 and 2011, we observed a more pronounced effect of the eruption than in the global irradiance [76]. These would be expected since the increase in the amount of particles in the atmosphere would result in a decrease of the direct irradiance, but, also, an increase in the diffuse. In our study, we also observed that irradiance at sites at lower altitude was more affected by the eruption than those at higher altitude; as a consequence of coarser particles being present at lower altitudes. In addition, we observed a decrease in global irradiance at 305 nm, even those days when AOD, at 380 nm, were similar in 2010 and 2011; this would be a consequence of the presence of fine particles (SO_2).

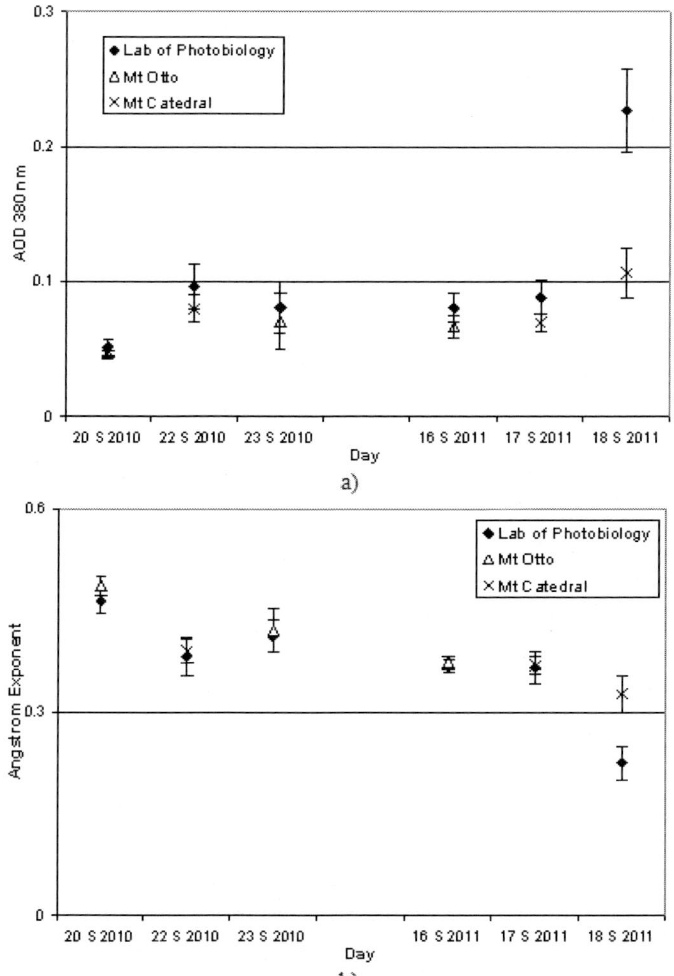

Figure 4. Aerosol optical depth and Angstrom exponent derived from measurements performed in September 2010 and 2011.

As a result of the eruption, ecosystems might have been affected by the decrease in irradiance for several months. The observed spectral dependence in the decrease of global irradiance would result in more pronounced effect on those biological functions more sensitive to lower wavelengths, as vitamin D photoconversion [82], than on those exhibiting a flatter action spectrum (i.e., phytoplanction production [83]). Also, ecosystems living at lower altitude would have resulted more affected than those at higher altitude.

ACKNOWLEDGMENTS

This chapter was performed at INGEBI, Argentina. It was supported by the Agencia Nacional de Promocion Cientifica y Tecnologica (ANPCyT), Argentina (PICT2007 N00377). Additional fundings for data collection and analysis was provided by Argentina's Consejo Nacional de Investigaciones Cientificas y Tecnicas (CONICET). The authors are thankful to NASA, Jeff Schmaltz and Holli Riebeek, LANCE/EOSDIS MODIS Rapid Response Team at NASA GSFC, for MODIS images. We also thank to Mrs Mariana Reissig for drawing the zonal map from a satellite image. The authors wish to thank Mr. Rocky Booth, Mr. Jim Ehramjian and the UV group (Biospherical Instruments Inc.) for the calibration of the reference GUV. We also want to thank the technical and scientific bureau of Nahuel Huapi National Park, who granted the permissions for the measurements inside different areas of the Park; Alta Patagonia, Refugio Lynch and their personnel, who provided the logistics required during the campaigns performed at Mount Catedral; and Fundación S.M. Furhman and their personnel, who made possible the transportation and measurements at Mount Otto. We are grateful to Laboratory of Photobiology (INIBIOMA, Universidad Nacional del Comahue) and its personnel, for their support during data collection.

REFERENCES

[1] Diaz, S. B., C. R. Booth, J. Morrow. (2000) Chapter 1: UV Optics and Physics. The effects of UV Radiation on Marine Ecosystems. Editores Serge Demers, Stephen De Mora y María Vernet. Cambridge University Press.

[2] WMO (1998). Scientific Assessment of Ozone Depletion: 1998. United Nations Environmental Program, World Meteorological Organization.

Global Ozone Research and Monitoring Project - Report No 44 WMO, Geneva.

[3] WMO (1990) Report of the International Ozone Trends Panel: 1988, Global Ozone Research and Monitoring Project Report No. 18, WMO, Geneva.

[4] WMO (1995) Scientific Assessment of Ozone Depletion: I994, Global Ozone Research and Monitoring Project-Report No. 37, WMO, Geneva.

[5] Koller, L. R. (1965) Solar Radiation. Ultraviolet Radiation. Ed. John Wiley & Sons Inc. New York, 2nd ed.

[6] Farman, J. C., B. G. Gardiner and J. D. Shanklin (1985) Large losses of Total Ozone in Antarctica reveals seasonal ClOx/NOx interaction. *Nature,* 315, 207-210.

[7] Molina, M. J. and F. S. Rowland (1974) Stratospheric sink of chlorofluormethanes: chlorine atom-catalysed destruction of ozone. *Nature,* 249, 810-812.

[8] WMO (2010). Scientific Assessment of Ozone Depletion: 2010. United Nations Environmental Program, World Meteorological Organization. Global Ozone Research and Monitoring Project - Report No 52 WMO, Geneva.

[9] Brasseur, G., and C. Granier (1992) Mount Pinatubo aerosols, chlorofluocarbons, and ozone depletion. *Science,* 257, 1239- 1242.

[10] Durant, A., Bonadonna, C., and Horwell, C. (2010) Atmospheric and Environmental Impacts of Volcanic Particulates. Elements, Vol. 6, 1811-5209/10/0006-0235$2.50 DOI: 10.2113/ gselements.6.4.235, 235-240.

[11] Hofmann, D. J., and S. Solomon (1989) Ozone destruction through heterogeneous chemistry following the eruption of El Chichon. *J. Geophys. Res*., 94, 5029-5041.

[12] Portmann, R. W., S. Solomon, R. R. Garcia, L. W. Thomason, L. R. Poole, and M. P. McCormick (1996) Role of aerosol variations in anthropogenic ozone depletion in the polar regions. *J. Geophys. Res.,* 101, 22991 -23006.

[13] Solomon, S., R. W. Portmann, R. R. Garcia, L. W. Thomason, L. R. Poole, and M. P. McCormick (1996) The role of aerosol trends and variability in anthropogenic ozone depletion at northern midlatitudes. *J. Geophys. Res.,* 101, 6713 -6727.

[14] Seinfeld, J. H., and S. N. Pandis (1986) Atmospheric Chemistry and Physics of Air Pollution, Wiley. Aerosol microphysics: nucleation, condensation, coagulation, deposition.

[15] SPARC (Stratospheric Processes And their Role in Climate) (2006) Assessment of Stratospheric Aerosols Properties, edited by L. Thomason and Th. Peter, SPARC Report No. 4, WCRP-124, WMO/TD- No. 1295.

[16] Skouratov, S. (1997) Influence of the Pinatubo eruption on the aerosol optical depth in the Arctic in the summer of 1993. *Atmospheric Research*, 44, 125-132.

[17] Michalsky, J., F. Denn, C. Flynn, G. Hodges, P. Kiedron, A. Koontz, J. Schlemmer, and S. E. Schwartz (2010), Climatology of aerosol optical depth in north and central Oklahoma: 1992–2008. *J. Geophys. Res.,* 115, D07203, doi:10.1029/2009JD012197.

[18] Jackman, C. H., E. L. F. l. eming, S. Chandra, D. B. Considine, and J. E. Rosenfield. (1996) Past, present and future modeled ozone trends with comparisons to observed trends. *J. Geophys. Res*., 101, 28753 – 28767.

[19] Angell, J. K. (1997) Estimated impacts of Agung, El Chichon, and Pinatubo volcanic eruptions on global and regional total ozone after adjustment for the QB. *Geophys. Res. Lett.*, 24, 647-650.

[20] Brunner, D., J. Stachelin, J. A. Maeder, I. Wohltmann, and G. E. Bodeker (2006) Variability and trends in total and vertically resolved stratospheric ozone based on the CATO ozone data set. *Atmos. Chem. Phys*., 6 (12), 4985-5008, doi: 10.5194/acp-6-4985-2006.

[21] McCormack, J. P., and L. L. Hood (1997) The frequency and size of ozone "mini-hole" events at northern midlatitudes in February. *Geophys. Res. Lett.,* 24, 2647-2650.

[22] Robock, A., T. Adams, M. Moore, L. Oman, G. Stenchikov (2007) Southern Hemisphere atmospheric circulation effects of the 1991 Mount Pinatubo eruption. *Geophys. Res. Lett.,* 34, L23710, doi: 10.1029/2007GL031403.

[23] Zerefos, C. S., K. Tourpali, and A. F. Bais (1994) Further studies on possible volcanic signal to the ozone layer. *J. Geophys. Res.,* 99, 25741 - 25746.

[24] Zerefos, C. S., K. Tourpali, and A. F. Bais (1996) Recent volcanic signals in the ozone layer, in The Mount Pinatubo Eruption: Effect on the Atmosphere and Climate, NATO ASI Series I, Vol. 142, edited by G. Fiocco, D. Fua, and G. Visconti, 211 -216, SpringerVerlag, Berlin.

[25] Fleming, E. L., C. H. Jackman, D. K. Weisenstein, and M. K. W. Ko (2007) The impact of interannual variability on multidecadal total ozone simulations. *J. Geophys. Res.,* 112, D10310, doi: 10.1029/2006 JD007953.

[26] Telford, P., P. Braesicke, O. Morgenstern, and J. Pyle (2009) Re-assessment of causes of ozone column variability following the eruption of Mount Pinatubo using a nudged CCM. *Atmos. Chem. Phys.*, 9 (13), 4251-4260, doi: 10.5194/acp-9-4251-2009.

[27] Hadjinicolaou, P., J. A. Pyle, M. P. Chipperfield, and J. A. Kettleborough (1997) Effect of interannual meteorological variability on mid-latitude O3, *Geophys. Res. Lett.*, 24 (23), 2993-2996.

[28] Rex, M., R. J. Salawitch, P. von der Gathen, N. R. P. Harris, M. P. Chipperfield, and B. Naujokat (2004) Arctic ozone loss and climate change. *Geophys. Res. Lett.*, 31, L04116, doi: 10.1029/2003GL018844.

[29] Tilmes, S., R. Müller, R. J. Salawitch, U. Schmidt, C. R. Webster, H. Oelhaf, C. C. Camy-Peyret, and J. M. Russell I. I. I. (2008) Chemical ozone loss in the Arctic winter 1991–1992. *Atmos. Chem. Phys.,* 8 (7), 1897-1910, doi: 10.5194/acp-8-1897-2008.

[30] Deshler, T., B. J. Johnson, and W. R. Rozier. (1994) Changes in the character of polar stratospheric clouds over Antarctica in 1992 due to the Pinatubo volcanic aerosol. *Geophys. Res. Lett.,* 21 (4), 273-276.

[31] David, C., S. Bekki, S. Godin, G. Mégie, and M. P. Chipperfield (1998) Polar stratospheric clouds climatology over Dumont d'Urville between 1989 and 1993 and the influence of volcanic aerosols on their formation. *J. Geophys. Res.*, 103, 22163-22180.

[32] Fromm, M., J. Alfred, and M. Pitts (2003) A unified, long-term, high-latitude stratospheric aerosol and cloud database using SAM II, SAGE II, and POAM II/III data: Algorithm description, database definition, and climatology. *J. Geophys. Res.,* 108 (D12), 4366, doi: 10.1029/2002JD002772.

[33] Zhao, J., R. P. Turco, and O. B. Toon (1995) A model simulation of Pinatubo volcanic aerosols in the stratosphere. *J. Geophys. Res.*, 100 (D4), 7315-7328.

[34] Tie, X. X., G. P. Brasseur, B. Briegleb, and C. Granier (1994) Two-dimensional simulation of Pinatubo aerosol and its effect on stratospheric ozone, *J. Geophys. Res.,* 99 (D10), 20545-20562.

[35] Stenchikov, G., A. Robock, V. Ramaswamy, M. D. Schwarzkopf, K. Hamilton, and S. Ramachandran (2002) Arctic Oscillation response to the 1991 Mount Pinatubo eruption: Effects of volcanic aerosols and ozone depletion. *J. Geophys. Res.,* 107 (D24), 4803, doi: 10.1029/2002JD002090.

[36] Stolarski, R. S., A. R. Douglass, S. Steenrod, and S. Pawson (2006) Trends in stratospheric ozone: Lessons learned from a 3D Chemical Transport Model. *J. Atmos. Sci.*, 63 (3), 1028-1041.

[37] Tabazadeh, A., Y. S. Djikaev, P. Hamill, and H. Reiss (2002) Laboratory evidence for surface nucleation of solid polar stratospheric cloud particles. *J. Phys. Chem. A,* 106, 10238-10246.

[38] Tie, X. X., and G. P. Brasseur (1995) The response of stratospheric ozone to volcanic eruptions: Sensitivity to atmospheric chlorine loading. *Geophys. Res. Lett.,* 22 (22), 3035-3038.

[39] Austin, J., L. W. Horowitz, M. D. Schwarzkopf, R. J. Wilson, and H. Levy I. I. (2013) Stratospheric ozone and temperature simulated from the preindustrial era to the present day. *J. Clim.*, 26, doi: 10.1175/JCLI-D-12-00162.1, 3528-3543.

[40] Hofmann, D., J. Barnes, M. O'Neill, M. Trudeau, and R. Neely (2009) Increase in background stratospheric aerosol observed with lidar at Mauna Loa Observatory and Boulder, Colorado. *Geophys. Res. Lett*., 36, L15808, doi: 10.1029/2009GL039008.

[41] Vernier, J. P., J. P. Pommereau, A. Garnier, J. Pelon, N. Larsen, J. Nielsen, T. Christensen, F. Cairo, L. W. Thomason, T. Leblanc, and I. S. McDermid (2009) Tropical stratospheric aerosol layer from CALIPSO lidar observations. *J. Geophys. Res.,* 114, D00H10, doi: 10.1029/2009JD011946.

[42] Millard, G. A., T. A. Mather, D. M. Pyle, W. I. Rose, and B. Thornton (2006) Halogen emissions from a small volcanic eruption: Modeling the peak concentrations dispersion, and volcanically induced ozone loss in the stratosphere. *Geophys. Res. Lett.,* 33, L19815, doi: 10.1029/2006GL026959.

[43] Flentje, H., Claude, H., Elste, T., Gilge, S., K¨ohler, U., Plass-D¨ulmer, C., Steinbrecht, W., Thomas, W., Werner, A., and Fricke, W. (2010) The Eyjafjallaj¨okull eruption in April 2010 – detection of volcanic plume using in-situ measurements, ozone sondes and lidar-ceilometer profiles, *Atmos. Chem. Phys*., 10, 10085–10092, doi:10.5194/acp-10-10085-2010.

[44] Harrison, R. G., K. A. Nicoll, Z. Ulanowski, and T. A. Mather (2010), Selfcharging of the Eyjafjallajökull volcanic ash plume. *Environ. Res. Lett.,* 5, 024004, doi:10.1088/ 1748-9326/5/2/024004.

[45] Ansmann, A., et al. (2011), Ash and fine mode particle mass profiles from EARLINET-AERONET observations over central Europe after the eruptions of the Eyjafjallajökull volcano in 2010. *J. Geophys. Res.,* 116, D00U02. doi:10.1029/2010JD015567.

[46] Stohl, A., Prata, A. J., Eckhardt, S., Clarisse, L., Durant, A., Henne, S., Kristiansen, N. I., Minikin, A., Schumann, U., Seibert, P., Stebel, K., Thomas, H. E., Thorsteinsson, T., Tørseth, K., and Weinzierl, B. (2011) Determination of time- and height-resolved volcanic ash emissions and their use for quantitative ash dispersion modeling: the 2010 Eyjafjallaj¨okull eruption. *Atmos. Chem. Phys.,* 11, 4333–4351, doi:10.5194/acp-11-4333-2011.

[47] Thomas, H. E. and Prata, A. J. (2011) Sulphur dioxide as a volcanic ash proxy during the April–May 2010 eruption of Eyjafjallaj ¨okull Volcano. *Iceland, Atmos. Chem. Phys.,* 11, 6871–6880, doi:10.5194/acp-11-6871-2011.

[48] Nobel, P. S. (1983). Light, Biophysical Plant Physiology and Ecology. NewYork, Freeman and Co.

[49] Frölich, C. (1987) Variability of the solar "constant" on time scales of minutes to years. *Journal of Geophysical Research*, 92, (D1), 796-800.

[50] Madronich, S. (1993) The Atmosphere and UV-B Radiation at Ground Level, in Environmental UV Photobiology. Edited by R. Young et al. Plenum Press, New York.

[51] Blumthaler, M., W. Ambach, and R. Ellinger. (1997) Increases in solar UV nadiation, with altitude. *J. Photochem. Photobiol. B. Biol.,* 39, 130-134.

[52] Blumthaler, M., and D. Haferi. (1999) Effects of albedo on spectral UV irradiance in high mountains. *EGS, Geophys. Res. Abs.,* 1(2), 1029-7006.

[53] Dahlback, A., N. Gelsor, J. J. Stamnes, Y. Gjessing. (2007) UV measurements in the 3000–5000 m altitude region in Tibet. *J. Geophys. Res.*, vol. 112, D09308, doi:10.1029/ 2006JD007700.

[54] Atkinson, R., D. L. Baulch, R. A. Cox, R. F. Hampson Jr., J. A. Kerr, M. J. Rossi, and J. Troe (1997) Evaluated kinetic, photochemical and heterogeneous data for atmospheric chemistry: Supplement V. IUPAC Subcommittee on Gas Kinetic Data Evaluation for Atmospheric Chemistry. *J. Phys. Chem. Ref. Data*, 26 (3), 521-1011.

[55] Sander, S. P., R. R. Friedl, D. M. Golden, M. J. Kurylo, R. E. Huie, V. L. Orkin, G. K. Moortgat, A. R. Ravishankara, C. E. Kolb, M. J. Molina, and B. J. Finlayson-Pitts (2003) Chemical Kinetics and Photochemical Data for Use in Atmospheric Studies: Evaluation Number 14, JPL Publication 02-25, Jet Propulsion Laboratory, Pasadena, Calif.

[56] Jacobson, M. Z. (1998) Isolating the causes and effects of large ultraviolet reductions in Los Angeles. *J. Aerosol Sci.*, 29, S655–S656.

[57] Bais, A. F., Zerefos, C. S., Meleti, C., Ziomas, I. C., and Tourpali, K. (1993) Spectral measurements of solar UVB radiation and its relations to total ozone, SO2, and clouds, *J. Geophys. Res.*, 98, 5199–5204.

[58] Frederick, J. and H. Steele (1995) The transmission of sunlight through cloudy skies: An analysis based on standard meteorological information, *J. Appl. Meteorol.*, 34, 2755-2761.

[59] Estupinan, J. G., S. Raman, G. H. Crescenti, J. J. Streitcher, and W. F. Barnard (1996) The effects of clouds and haze on UV-B radiation. *Journal of Geophysical Research*, 101, (16), 807-816.

[60] Chubarova, N. Y., N. A: Krotkov, I. V. Geogdzhaev, T. K. Kondranin, and V. U. Khattatov (1997) Spectral UV Irradiance: the Effects of Ozone, Cloudiness and Surface Albedo. Proceedings IRS'96 Current problems in Atmospheric Radiation. Smith and Stamnes (Eds) A Deepak Publishing, Hampton Meeting, Fairbanks.

[61] Meinander, O., A. Kontu, K. Lakkala, A. Heikkilä, L. Ylianttila, and M. Toikka. (2008) Diurnal variations in the UV albedo of arctic snow. *Atmos. Chem. Phys.*, 8 (21), 6551-6563, doi: 10.5194/acp-8-6551-2008.

[62] Fioletov, V. E., J. B. Kerr, D. I. Wardle, N. Krotkov, and J. R. Herman (2002) Comparison of Brewer ultraviolet irradiance measurements with Total Ozone Mapping Spectrometer satellite retrievals, *Opt. Eng.,* 41, 3051-3061.

[63] Chubarova, N. Y., A. Y. Yurova, N. Krotkov, J. Herman, and P. K. Bhartia (2002) Comparisons between ground measurements of broadband ultraviolet irradiance (300-380 nm) and Total Ozone Mapping Spectrometer ultraviolet estimates at Moscow from 1979 to 2000. *Opt. Eng.*, 41, 3070-3081.

[64] Jaroslawski, J. P., and J. W. Krzy´scin (2005) Importance of aerosol variations for surface UV-B level: Analysis of ground-based data taken at Belsk, Poland, 1992- 2004. *J. Geophys. Res.,* 110, D16201, doi: 10.1029/2005JD005951.

[65] Kambezidis, H. D., A. D. Adamopoulos, and D. Zevgolis (2005) Spectral aerosol transmittance in the ultraviolet and visible spectra in Athens, Greece. *Pure Appl. Geophys.,* 162 (3), 625-647.

[66] Meloni, D., A. di Sarra, J. DeLuisi, T. Di Iorio, G. Fiocco, W. Junkermann, and G. Pace (2003) Tropospheric aerosols in the Mediterranean: 2. Radiative effects through model simulations and measurements. *J. Geophys. Res.,* 108 (D10), 4317, doi: 10.1029/2002-JD002807.

[67] Meloni, D., F. Marenco, and A. di Sarra (2003) Ultraviolet radiation and aerosol monitoring at Lampedusa, Italy. *Ann. Geophys.*, 46 (2), 373-383.

[68] McKenzie, R., G. Bodeker, G. Scott, J. Slusser, and K. Lantz (2006) Geographical differences in erythemally-weighted UV measured at mid-latitude USDA sites. Photochem. *Photobiol. Sci.,* 5 (3), 343-352, doi: 10.1039/B510943D.

[69] IPCC (Intergovernmental Panel on Climate Change) (1995) Radiative Forcing of Climate Change. In Climate Change 1994 (Edited by Houghton, J. T., Meira Filho, L. G., Bruce, J., Lee, H., Callander, B. A., Haites, E., Harris, N. and Maskell, K.), pp. 1-231. Cambridge University Press, Cambridge.

[70] Tsitas, S .R., and Y. L. Yung (1996) The effect of volcanic aerosols on ultraviolet radiation in Antarctica. *Geophys. Res. Lett.*, 23, 157- 160.

[71] McKenzie, R. L., C. Weinreis, P. V. Johnston, B. Liley, H. Shiona, M. Kotkamp, D. Smale, N. Takegawa, and Y. Kondo, (2008) Effects of urban pollution on UV spectral irradiances. *Atmos. Chem. Phys.*, 8 (18), 5683-5697, doi: 10.5194/acp-8-5683-2008.

[72] Fioletov, V. E., E. Griffioen, J. B. Kerr, D. I. Wardle, and O. Uchino (1998) Influence of volcanic sulfur dioxide on spectral UV irradiance as measured by Brewer spectrophotometers. *Geophys. Res. Lett.*, 25, 1665-1668.

[73] NASA (2013). Online, available from http://www.nasa.gov/topics/earth /features/ 20110615-volcano.html

[74] SERNAGEOMIN (2013) Reporte Especial de Actividad Volcánica No 122 Complejo Volcánico Puyehue—Cordón Caulle. Online available from: http:// www.sernageomin.cl/volcan.php?pagina=6&iId=38].

[75] NASA (2013) Online available from: Image courtesy Jeff Schmaltz, LANCE/EOSDIS MODIS Rapid Response Team at NASA GSFC. Caption by Holli Riebeek.

[76] Diaz, S. B., A. A. Paladini, H. G. Braile, M. C. Dieguez, G. A. Deferrari, M. Vernet and J. Vrsalovic (2014) Global and direct UV irradiance variation in the Nahuel Huapi Nacional Park (Patagonia,Argentina) alter the eruption of Puyehue-Cordon Caulle (Chile). *Journal of Atmospheric and Solar-Terrestrial Physics*, 112(2014) 47–56.

[77] Mermoz, M., Ubeda, C., Grigera, D., brión, C., Martín, C., Bianchi, E. and Planas, H. (2009) E. l. Parque Nacional Nahuel Huapi. Sus características ecológicas y estado de conservación. APN Ed. Parque Nacional Nahuel Huapi, San Carlos de Bariloche Argentina., 80pp.

[78] Matthias-Maser, S. and Jaenicke, R (1995) Size distribution of primary biological aerosol particles with radii _0.2μm. *Atmos. Res.,* 39, 279–286.

[79] Diaz, S., C. Camilion, G. Deferrari, H. Fuenzalida, R. Armstrong, C. Booth, A. Paladini, S. Cabrera, C. Casiccia, C. Lovengreen, J. Pedroni, A. Rosales, H. Zagarese and M. Vernet (2006) Ozone and UV radiation over southern South America: Climatology and anomalies, *Photochem. Photobiol.*, 2006, 82, 834-843.

[80] Stamnes, K., S. C. Tsay, W. Wiscombe, and K. Jayaweera (1990) Numerically stable algorithm for discrete-ordinate-method radiative transfer in multiple scattering and emitting layered media. *Appl. Opt.,* 27, 2502-2509.

[81] Angstrom,A. (1929) On the atmospheric transmission of Sun radiation and on dust in the air. *Geogr. Ann.,* 12, 130-159.

[82] Bouillon, R., J. Eisman, M. Garabedian, M. Holick, J. Kleinschmidt, T. Suda, I. Terenetskaya and A. Webb (2006) Action Spectrum for the Production of Previtamin D3 in Human Skin. UDC: 612.014.481-06, CIE, Vienna.

[83] Neale, P. J. and D. J. Kieber (2000) Assessing biological and chemical effects of UV in the marine environment: spectral weighting functions in Causes and Environmental Implications of Increased UV-B Radiation, ed. R. E. Hester and R. M. Harrison, Royal Society of Chemistry, Cambridge, 61-84.

In: Volcanic Eruptions
Editor: Trent Milburn

ISBN: 978-1-63463-308-6

Chapter 6

VOLCANIC COMPLEX PUYEHUE-CORDÓN CAULLE: IMPACT OF VOLCANIC ASH ON INSECTS IN PATAGONIA, ARGENTINA

V. Fernández-Arhex[1*], A. L. Pietrantuono[1], M. E. Amadio[2] and O. Bruzzone[1]

[1]CONICET-INTA EEA-Bariloche, Bariloche, Río Negro, Argentina
[2]CONICET- INIBIOMA, Lab. Ecotono, Bariloche, Río Negro, Argentina

ABSTRACT

In June 4th 2011, there was a major volcanic eruption of the Puyehue-Caulle complex (PCC) in southern Andean range near the Argentina-Chile border. This event covered with ashes over 7.5 million hectares in Argentinean Patagonia during for a year and affecting the flora and fauna, including the insect. On this chapter we present different case studies which evaluated the effect of volcanic ash on survival, motivation and use of habitat in different species of insects. Laboratory bioassays results have shown that the ash does not affect the species studied in the same way, and also there are differences between guilds of phytophagous insects. Phloem-sucking insects are not strongly affected, actively choose their habitats for living and are capable of discriminate unfavorable habitats (i.e., presence of volcanic ash). On the other hand on orthopteran species, the volcanic ash has a strong aversive and insecticidal effect

* Correspondence author: fernandezarhex.v@inta.gob.ar

similar to that of inert dust. In this case the volcanic ash could potentially have a protective effect against insect pests, reducing the damage they can cause to grasslands and pastures. The impact of the ashes from PCC on the insect community may be radical in the acute deposition phase, with substantial qualitative effects in the chronic phase of exposure. The recovery of populations affected by ash in desert areas where dry ash persists will be slower, and this will have tangible and long-term consequences for insect host plants, and on the development of populations of vertebrate insectivores. By contrast, the presence of ash in humid regions will impact the ecosystem by the addition of nutrients, which in combination with water retention by the ash will lead to a qualitative and quantitative recovery of the populations under favorable conditions. Therefore, we propose that the ash can generate two types of responses on insects: direct (on individuals) or indirect (on individual-environment interactions).

Keywords: Herbivory, Inert dust, Insecticide

INTRODUCTION

Impact of Volcanic Ash on the Ecosystem

Natural catastrophic events such as volcano eruptions have greatly affected environments in wide regions around the world. Ash and gases impelled by these eruptions into the atmosphere carry large volumes of particles of different sizes (nanometer and ultrafine) that are scattered around the earth (NASA 2011). However, the greater accumulation of different grain size was observed in the range of 10 kilometers from the center of the volcano, causing devastating effect (Sparks et al. 1997). The most important consequences of this type of event are loss of habitats for flora and fauna (Akre 1980, Shanks & Chase 1981, Akre et al. 1981).

The Puyehue Volcano (Mapuche: puye hue, 'instead of puyes (fish) ´) is an active volcano, located in Southern Andean range, in the Los Ríos Region, Chile (2236m, S 40° 02´24"; W 70° 14´26") on the eastern edge of the Puyehue National Park. The Puyehue volcano forms a volcanic system oriented northwest-southeast volcanology known as volcanic complex Puyehue-Cordón Caulle (PCC). This volcanic complex, only the Puyehue and Cordón Caulle volcano have erupted during the Holocene, and of these only the Cordon Caulle has recorded historical eruptions beginning its last eruption on June 4, 2011 (Lara et al. 2006).

The eruption of the complex Puyehue-Cordón Caulle deposited large amounts of volcanic ash over Patagonia. This volcanic complex dispersed about 100 million metric tons of ash over 7.5 million hectares mainly in northern Patagonia [Argentina] (Gaitán et al. 2011). Several hundred million tons of volcanic tephra were dispersed over ~25000 km2 along a west-to-east gradient (Gaitán et al. 2011), which comprised a directional shift in ash-grain size and thickness of tephra deposits (i.e., a proxy for disturbance 'intensity', sensu Pickett &White 1985). Fine ash particles were dispersed several thousand kilometers by wind, while larger particles settle closer to the volcano (Ayris & Delmelle 2012). Lower ash particle size appeared in the east over the Atlantic Ocean, arriving South Africa, Australia, Tasmania and New Zealand (Environment Canada MSC 2011). The chemical analyses of the volcanic ash showed that is extremely abrasive (Informe UNCO-Neuquén 2011) and predominantly composed of volcanic glass shards (SiO_2) and alumina (Al_2O_3) (Buteler et al. 2011, Mogni et al. 2011), two substances with insecticidal properties (Shanks & Chase 1981, Subramayan & Roesli 2000).

The magnitude of PCC eruption was so important that affected distant places, mainly in Río Negro and Neuquén (Figure 1). In the Andean-patagonic forest and places close to the volcano the ash particles size were thicker, while in distant places ash particles were finer.

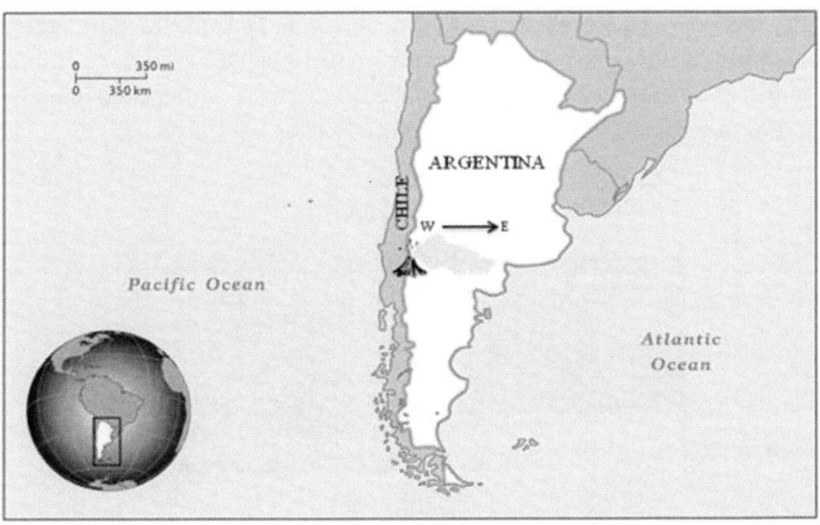

Figure 1. Map with the ash plume covering northern Patagonia (Provinces of Neuquén and Río Negro. Map courtesy National Geographic. National Geographic does not review or endorse content added to this map by others.

In Argentina, the Andean-Patagonian forest is characterized by a strong rainfall gradient rising East-West (Dimitri, 1972) and extends as a narrow strip lying over the mountain massif from northern Neuquén to Tierra del Fuego e Isla de los Estados. In the wetter areas of the west dominate the trees of the genus *Nothofagus*, and in the east are replaced by forests of "Ciprés de la Cordillera" (*Austrocedrus chilensis*). It is one of the latest global reserves of temperate forests with relatively little anthropogenic disturbance, with valuable flora and fauna diversity, and is even one of the best preserved biomes of Argentina (Primer Inventario Nacional de Bosques Nativos, 2005).

Impact of the Volcanic Ash in Insects

The mechanism of action of the volcanic ash is through the abrasion and adsorption of the epicuticular waxes phenomena, leading to insect's desiccation (Figure 2). Occlusion of spiracles, excessive salivation activity, cleanliness and the interruption of digestive activity by the accumulation of ash in the intestine are contributing factors (Wigglesworth 1944, Wille & Fuentes 1975, Edwards & Schwertz 1981, Stadler et al. 2010, Figure 3).

Volcanic ash often acts as inert dusts (inorganic dusts). Inert dusts exert their toxic action not by biochemical mechanisms (organic pesticides) but through physical phenomena such as abrasion, adsorption of cuticular hydrocarbons and desiccation (Subramanyam & Roesli 2000). One of the inert dusts used as an insecticide is diatomaceous earth, is composed mostly of silicon dioxide (SiO_2) (Ebeling 1971, Golob 1997).

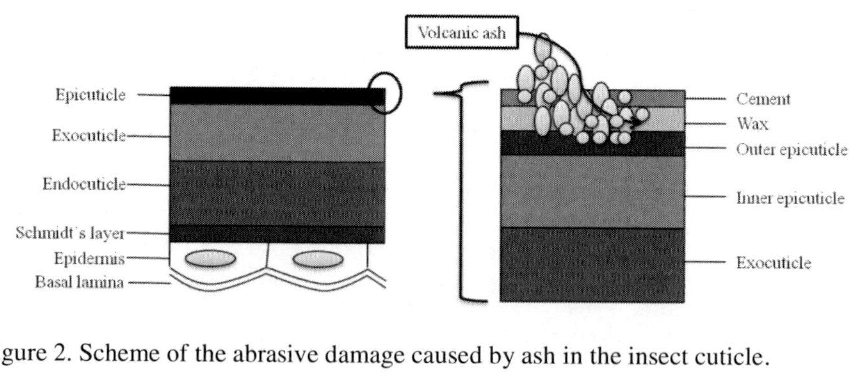

Figure 2. Scheme of the abrasive damage caused by ash in the insect cuticle.

These inert dusts are often used to control pests and are commercialized, for example, for the protection of stored grain due to its high efficacy and low toxicity to the environment (Ebeling 1971, Subramanyam & Roesli 2000). Insecticidal activity of the inorganic dusts, including volcanic ash, depends on the size of dust particles (e.g., thin or thick), form and structure (e.g., amorphous, non-circular, cylindrical, etc.), chemical composition and electrostatic of dust particles (Jia et al. 2005, Stadler et al. 2010).

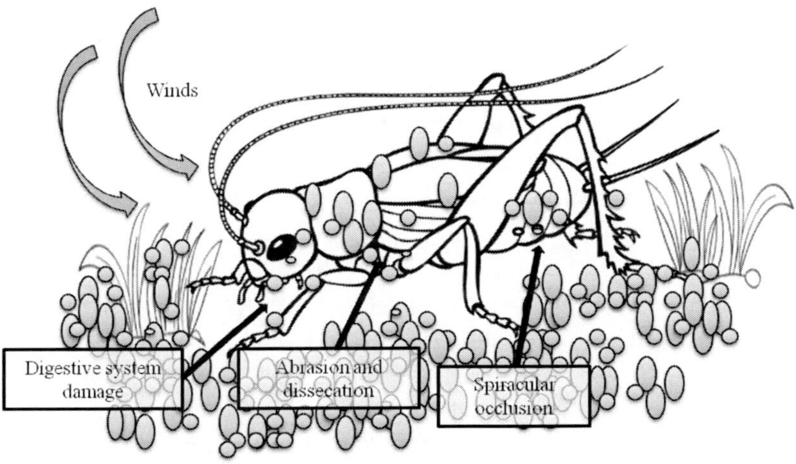

Figure 3. Damage caused in the insect body through different mechanisms.

All of these factors affect, directly or indirectly, the biological activity of the insects. For example, the finer particles tend to be more toxic than larger particles, with the same chemical composition (Paull & Lyons 2008, Buteler et al. 2011, Fernández-Arhex umpublished data). The shape and structure affects the kinetics of deposition, income and translocation of particles within the body of the organism (Jia et al. 2005).

Volcanic complex Puyehue-Cordón Caulle

A volcanic eruption could affect the habitat of arthropods, changing food sources, shelter, and microclimate conditions (del Moral & Grishin 1999, Ayris & Delmelle 2012). These changes may influence their behavior, survival, diversity and richness.

1. Ash from PCC Affects the Behavior of Insects?

Insects have the ability to search and chose the resources required for their development and reproduction. Searching behavior is an active movement by which insects search for resources, hosts or a particular food source, mates, and sites for shelter, oviposition or nesting (Bell 1990). The location and selection of these resources depend on the integration of three kinds of factors: (i) the biological characteristics and abilities of an insect, including locomotory patterns and perception of sensory information, (ii) external environmental factors determining the resources available and the risks inherent in their quest; and (iii) internal factors, such as deprivation or sexual receptivity, determining what an individual needs at a particular time (Bell 1990).

A volcanic eruption causes changes in the environment, Chaneton et al. (2014) argued that ash fall on distant forest canopies and soils may disrupt species interactions and ecosystem level processes like primary productivity and herbivory (Bishop et al. 2005, Marske et al. 2007). Thus herbivorous searching behavior could be affected.

There are few studies that analyze the real impact of ash on the behavior of insects; most studies are focused on survival, diversity and richness. The insect behavior, their elections, and preferences are a key factor for immediate and future insect success.

The work performed by Pietrantuono et al. (2014) studied the influences of PCC volcanic ash on the host plant preferences of *Sinopla perpunctatus* Signoret (Hemiptera: Acanthosomatidae) a native green stink bug from the Andean-Patagonian forest. This sucking insect has a preference scale of host plants of the genus *Nothofagus* and its ability to choose their host plant is not affected by the presence of ash. Due to their way of eating we may assume that access to food resource was not affected. Even though the volcanic ash could exert a negative effect on insects behavior this did not occur in the case of *S. perpunctatus* probably because of the tendency of this insect to be located on the underside of the leaves or between folds of the bark, which act as protective barriers (Dajoz 2001, Faúndez & Osorio 2010). This behavior may have decreased the exposure and contact with the ash, and its potentially abrasive effect on the insect's integument.

In the case of leaf-miner insects (i.e., insect larvae that feed on plant tissue from the inside of leaves) we may assume that the ashes only could affect the adult insects because the egg and larva are fully protected within the leaf epidermis. However, ash-covered foliage shows altered energy and water balances, which may cause premature leaf senescence (Seymour et al. 1984) affecting the continuity of development of the larva. In addition, after the leaf emergency, the larva must select a substrate for pupation (except for those that form the pupa inside the leaf). This substrate can be more or less suitable for larval development depending on soil properties and/ or the insect needs and preferences (Fye 1978). Physical and chemical soil properties (i.e., organic matter concentration, pH, electrical conductivity, field capacity, transparency, and porosity) determine the environment where an insect will or will not develop (Prudic et al. 2005, Martínez et al. 2008). Deposition of volcanic ash changes the characteristics of the substrate (Cremona et al. 2011).

In the work made by Pietrantuono et al. (unpublished), preference tests with the leaf miner *Notofenusa surosa* (Hymenoptera: Tenthredinidae) were performed. This is a native sawfly commonly present in the Andean-Patagonic forest that uses *Nothofagus obliqua* as main host plant. In this assay the habitat preferences for the development of the pupa were assessed by offering substrates from different sites, including the two types of grain ash (Figure 4).

The larva of *N.*, actively choose their pupation substrate. This sawfly is capable of discriminating between different concentrations of organic matter in the soil (Figure 5).

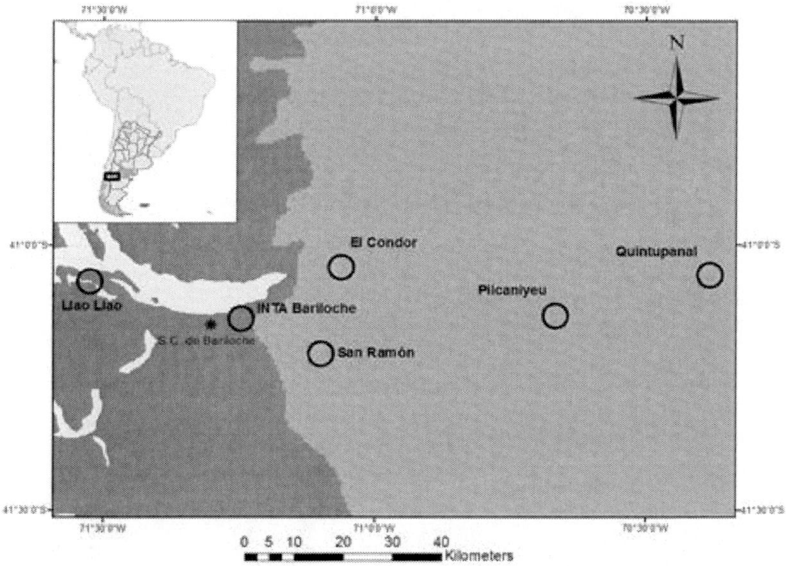

Figure 4. Sites of soil sampling at the Rio Negro province (Argentina). The sites are following a gradient of rainfall (West- East) and were affected by the volcanic eruption.

Thus volcanic ash which does not contain organic matter is avoided, causing repellant effect on the larva.

Noteworthy, phytophagous insects were not the only ones whose behavior was affected. Morales et al. (2014) found that foraging activity of bumble bees in patches of wild flowers decreased and overall in comparison to pre-eruption levels regarding behavioral changes, although a recent study confirms that flowers covered with PCC ash were less attractive and therefore less visited by honey bees (Martínez et al. 2013)

Elizalde (2014) established that volcanic ash produces behavioral several changes in insects reducing its mobility and feeding. Insects are affected due to loss of habitat and food resources (Bishop et al. 2005), and the physical impact of fine ashes on exoskeletons and feeding activity (Edwards & Schwartz 1981, Buteler et al. 2011). However, it is possible that behavioral change also be due to a decrease in the ability of resource perception or a change in the scale of preferences.

In summary behavioral responses seem to be related with life history traits, the type of development, habits, ways of feeding (Dale et al. 2005, Marske et al. 2007) and ultimately its ability to perception (Martínez et al. 2013, Pietrantuono et al. 2014).

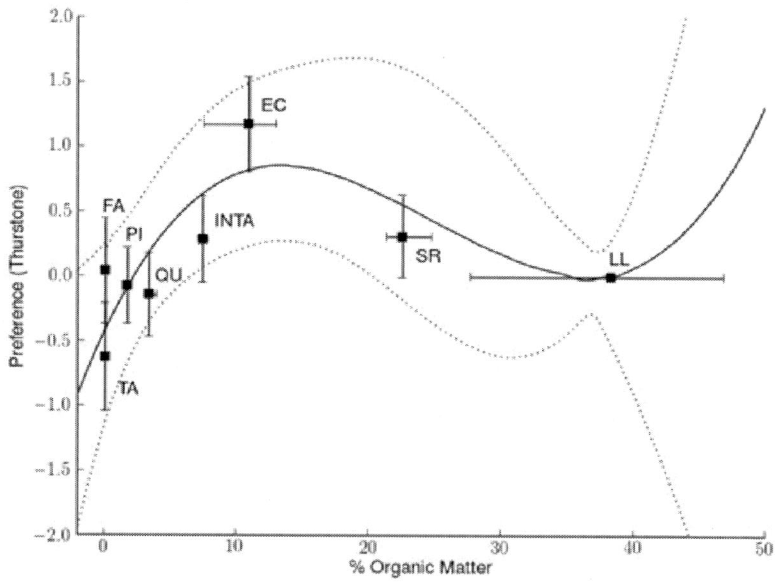

Figure 5. Preference curve as a function of organic matter. This function was calculated from the weighted average of model 1. The weight of each model in the calculation of the weighting curve is the percentage in the Table 2. The Y axes represent the Thurstone scale of attractiveness / preference. The X axis is the percentage of organic materials at each substrate (FA: Fine Ash, TA: Thick Ash, QU: Quintupanal, INTA EEA Bariloche: Instituto de Tecnología Agropecuaria, EC: El Cóndor, SR: San Ramón, LL: Llao-Llao). Negative values on the Y axes indicate a lower preference for the parameter.

2. Survival, Diversity and Richness

Natural disturbances are important components of ecosystem dynamics. Their ecological consequences are variable and depend on their nature, frequency and extent (Pickett & White 1985). Many authors predict climate change will have a number of effects on insects: survival; sweeping shifts in herbivory rates; altered distribution and outbreak frequency of key insect pests; and unpredictably altered relationships with natural enemies (Williams & Liebhold 1995, Fleming 1996, Coley 1998, Tenow et al. 1999). Considering this, it is relevant to study the dynamics of the insects that could be affected by natural disturbances such as volcanoes, to assess in what way were affected.

The ash plume of the PCC affects natural distribution of insects. In places close to the volcano the ash particles size were thicker, while in distant places ash particles were finer, comprising forests, shrub lands and steppes.

Some studies demonstrated the impact of the volcanic ash of PCC in some nordpatagonian species of insects. The analyses of the chemical composition of this volcanic ash showed that it is extremely abrasive and predominantly composed by *O*, *Si*, *Al*, *Fe*, *Na* and *K*. The bioassay results of two species of Coleoptera, *Oryzaephilus urinamensis* L. (Coleoptera: Silvanidae) and *Tribolium castaneum* (Herbst) (Coleoptera: Tenebrionidae), exposed continuously for seven days to the volcanic ash, indicated that fine grain sizes thoroughly adheres to body surfaces and are toxic, when mixed into the substrate at low concentrations (Buteler et al. 2011). Also, in honeybees (*Apis mellifera*) this volcanic ash reduces its survival, indicating that there is no mechanism to prevent ingestion of food contaminated with ash (Martínez et al. 2013). In the case of invasive wasp *Vespula* spp., their populations were severely affected by the ash deposition and plume, caused by this eruption. Populations of this wasp were completely devastated in areas where ash thickness was >3 cm (Masciocchi et al. 2013). In turn, the laboratory data showed that constant exposure to volcanic ash and diatomaceous earth (both high 75% and low 40% humidity) (Figure 6) induces mortality in adult grasshopper *Dichroplus vittigerum* (Blanchard) (Orthoptera: Acrididae).

Interestingly, the toxicity of both products was very similar. Laboratory results also showed that survival of *D. vittigerum* significantly decreased once exposed to the two ash granulometry sizes (fine <500 and medium =500 μm). In turn, for green locusts (*Burgilis* sp) survival was significantly reduced when exposed to fine grain size ashes. However, the eruption of this volcano caused little effects on ant community. Total ant abundance tended to be lower after the eruption, but species richness and composition were similar before and two seasons after the ash fall. This small impact could be due to a consequence of the timing of the eruption, ants' social nature, and ash thickness (Pirk 2014). On the other hand, Morales et al. (2014) studied the impact of the ash in the foraging behavior of bees. They evaluated the effect of the gradient of increasing ash layer thickness on wild bees, native (*Bombus dahlbomii*) and invasive (*B. terrestris* and *B. ruderatus*) bumble bees. They found, with the increase of ash deposition, a consistent and significant decrease in: the number of wild bees and total bee richness visiting raspberry flowers; the number of bumble bees (particularly *B. terrestris*) visiting wild flowers; and the proportion of triggered flowers of scotch broom. Thus, volcanic eruptions can exert a detrimental effect on bee fauna.

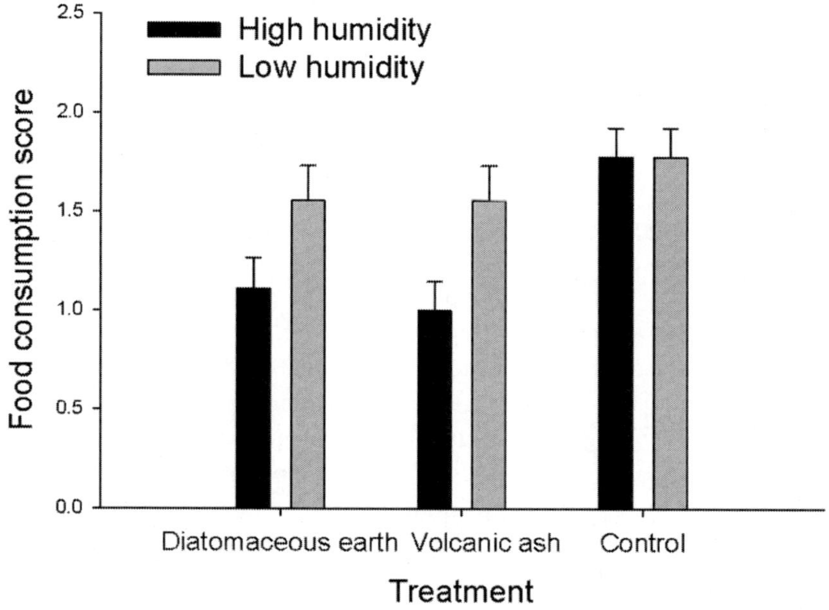

Figure 6. Food (fresh dandelion leaves) consumption scores of *Dichroplus vittigerum* adults during a 24 h dry dust toxicity bioassay in which each grasshopper was placed in a plastic dish with of 0.5 g of volcanic ash or diatomaceous earth and with 100 mm^2 of fresh leaves of dandelion (*Taraxacum officinale*). Control insects were placed in clean container with food. Each insect that consumed 50% or less of the leaf area, it received a score of 1, and each insect that consumed more than 50% of the leaf area received a score of 2. Bars topped with different lower case letters are significantly different.

DISCUSSION

Volcanic Ash Is Beneficial or Detrimental?

Volcanic ash has a greater or lesser detrimental effect on the state of insects. Whether causing a modification on behavior or a decreasing survival.

Miserendino et al. (2012), makes a list of the negative effects of the ash on terrestrial and aquatic insects:

a) Spiracular occlusion: probably not important in aquatic species since most aquatic species that breathe through their spiracles usually have them protected by different structures (hairs, elytra, etc.).
b) Excess of salivation: also not important in aquatic insects since water is not a limiting resource.
c) Interference with the digestive processes by the ingestion of the ash: this affects both terrestrial and aquatic species.
d) Abrasion of the mandibles and mouthparts: this can also affect both terrestrial and aquatic species (Wiederholm 1984, Edwards and Schwartz 1981, del Moral and Grishin, 1999, Collier 2002, Harrison et al. 2007, Marske et al. 2007).

We can establish that different taxa display different levels of susceptibility, indeed would be incorrect to state that the ash is always harmful. Even for phytophagous insects seem that there are two opposing approaches to the effect of the ash. Marske et al. (2007), argued that volcanic ash adversely affect the insect causing a lower herbivore pressure. Benefiting plant increasing rate and photosynthetic leaf area, as well canopy productivity (Schowalter 2000).

However, the rains, high humidity and dew, causing flue ash particles adhere to the leaf surface and interfere on photosynthesis, transpiration and respiration of plants, even years after the volcano eruption (Grosfeld & Puntieri 2011). Thus plants under stress which in turn makes them more susceptible to suffer attack by phytophagous and pathogens (Dajoz 2001, Varela & Weigandt 2009). Nevertheless, folivores that find refuge from ash fall might then exert a greater consumptive impact on stressed host plants (Schowalter 2000).

Chaneton et al. (2014) considered that the effects from ash fall varied with site distance to the crater (see also Dale et al. 2005). Foliar production dropped abruptly after the 2011 eruption in the wet forest near the PCC crater, but did not change in the dry forest farther away from the crater. In contrast, leaf damage by insects generally decreased with heavy ash fall, although the effect was most pronounced in the dry forest, which sustained the highest folivory rates. Thus, a major decline in folivory levels may have a large positive influence on annual foliage production. While the intensity of ash fall declined with distance to the crater, the relative impact on insect herbivory was greater.

We may assume that the ashes will have a long term effect on the insects' survival. The interaction between the time when the volcano erupts and insect taxon seems to be crucial in determining the outcome of insect populations affected by ash. In this case, the PCC erupted at the end of autumn, when temperatures in the area were low and not much insect activity. In the case of grasshoppers, their eggs were located underground, fully protected of ash effect; as a consequence the population from the area affected with the volcanic ash would be negatively influenced in the following seasons. In these seasons the nymphs and adults will emerge in an environment contaminated with ash, together with the prevailing conditions of wind and warm weather from the region, so that the volcanic ash will have a negative effect on insects due to its abrasive and desiccant action (Fernández- Arhex et al, 2013). In the case of ants, Pirk (2014) cited that their total abundance tended to be lower after the eruption, but species richness and composition were similar before and two seasons after the ash fall. The little effects on ant community are mainly a consequence of the timing of the eruption, ants' social nature, and ash thickness. When the eruption occurred, ant activity was reduced due to low temperatures. Also, the potential mortality of outside workers during the acute deposition phase does not risk colony survival since they represent a small percentage of it (Pirk 2014). But, not all social insects have the same advantages as ants. Contrary to ants, yellowjackets (*Vespula* spp.) populations were devastated in areas with volcanic ash. These wasps have annual colonies founded in the spring by overwintering queens. These queens hibernate in protected places, which were probably buried under the ash, killing them or complicating their emergence in spring. So, the timing of the eruption affected a crucial stage of these wasps' life cycle (Masciocchi et al. 2013, Pirk 2014).

Other impact of the PCC could be on bee fauna. Volcanic eruptions can exert a detrimental effect on bee fauna and concomitant on the plant-pollinator interactions, with a potential cascade effect on the pollination service to crops, the spread of invasive bumble bees, and the pollination success of invasive plants (Morales et al. 2014).

CONCLUSION

Effects of volcanic disturbance on insect communities may be complex, being dependent on species life-history traits (Schowalter 2000, Marske et al. 2007; Figure 7), trophic position (Parmenter et al. 2005), and timing of ashfall relative to insect phenology (Chaneton et al. 2014, Pirk et al. 2014). Moreover, climatic conditions, type (direct or indirect), duration of exposure, and amount of deposited volcanic ash are factors that may affect the welfare of insects.

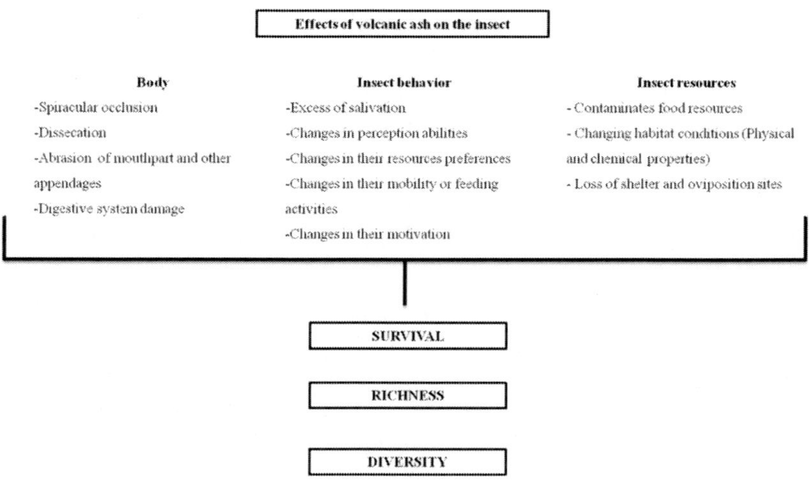

Figure 7. Table summarizes the effect of volcanic ash on insects.

The combination of all the above factors may induce a number of direct and/or indirect effects on individual:

- Direct effect: affects the insect in terms of physiology, survival, behavior, etc.
- Indirect effect: ash affects the environment of the insect, by causing destruction of the vegetation that insects use for food or habitat (Wille & Fuentes 1975, Buteler et al. 2011).

Not only we must take into account the time a volcano erupts, also we have to study the chemical composition of the volcanic ash and evaluate their potential toxicity. The toxicity of the volcanic ash of PCC has an insecticidal effect similar to that of diatomaceous earth (an inert dust with insecticidal properties). Suggesting that volcanic ash could be use as "natural insecticide". Therefore, this ash may be compared to the application of non-persistent and broad spectrum natural insecticide as well as it can be used in integrated pest management strategies. Further studies are needed to understand the effect of this volcanic ash on these insects population in the field. It is also necessary to evaluate the effectiveness of volcanic ash as an indoors insecticide such as in greenhouses.

REFERENCES

Akre RD, LD Hansen, HC Reed, LD Corpus. 1981. Effects of volcanic ash from Mt. St. Helens on ants and yellow jackets. Melanderia, 37: 1-19.

Akre, RD. 1980. *Effect of volcanic ash on insects*. Wash. State Univ. Conf. Aftermatch of St. Helens. July 8-9. pp. 14-15.

Ayris PM, P Delmelle. 2012. The immediate environmental effects of tephra emission. B Volcanol., 74:1905-1936.

Bell, W. J. 1990. Searching behavior patterns in insects. *Annu. Rev. Entomol.* 35: 447-467.

Bishop, JG; WF William; JD Schade & CM Crisafulli. 2005. Causes and consequences of herbivory on prairie lupine (*Lupinus lepidus*) in early primary succession. Pp. 151- 162 in: Dale, VH; FJ Swanson & CM Crisafulli (eds.).Ecological Responses to the 1980 Eruption of Mount St.Helens. Springer, New York.

Buteler M, T Stadler, GP López García, MS Lassa, D Trombotto Liaudat, P D'adamo, Fernández-Arhex V. 2011. Propiedades insecticidas de la ceniza del complejo volcánico Puyehue-Cordón Caulle y su posible impacto ambiental. *Rev. Soc. Entomol. Arg*., 70 (3-4):149-156.

Chaneton EJ, Mazía N, Garibaldi LA, Chaij J, Kitzberger T. 2014. Impact of volcanic ash deposition on foliar productivity and insect herbivory in northern Patagonia deciduous forests. *Ecol Aust* 24: 51-63

Coley, PD. 1998. Possible effects of climate change on plant/herbivore interactions in moist tropical forests. *Climatic Change,* 39: 455–72.

Collier, K; J Quinn & M Scarsbrook. 2002. Bouncing back: how fast can stream invertebrates recolonise? *Water & Atmosphere*, 10:9-11

Cremona MV, Ferrari J, López S. 2011. Las cenizas volcánicas y los suelas de la región. Presencia: Sitio Argentino de Producción Animal. 4pp.

Cremona V, J Ferrari, S López. 2011. Las cenizas volcánicas y los suelos de la región. Revista Presencia Nº 57: 8-11.

Dajoz, R. 2001. Entomología forestal. Los insectos y el bosque. Ediciones Mundi-Prensa, España 548 pp.

Dale, VH; FJ Swanson & CM Crisafulli. Eds. 2005. Ecological Responses to the 1980 Eruption of Mount St. Helens. Springer, New York.

Del Moral R, SY Grishin. 1999. Volcanic disturbances and ecosystem recovery. Chapter 5. In: L.R. Walker(ed) Ecosystems of disturbed ground. Elsevier. pp. 137–160.

Dimitri, M. 1972. La región de los bosques andino-patagónicos. Sinopsis general. Colección Científica Instituto Nacional de Tecnología Agropecuaria., 10.

Ebeling E. 1971. Sorptive dusts for pest control. *Annu. Rev. Entomol.*16: 123-158.

Edwards, J. S. & L. M. Schwartz. 1981. Mount St. Helens ash: a natural insecticide. *Can. J. Zool.* 59:714-715.

Elizalde, L. 2014. Volcanism and arthropods: a review. *Ecología Austral* 24:3-16

Environment Canada MSC. 2011. [Available on: http://all-geo.org /volcan01010/wp-content/uploads/2011/06/cordon_caulle_map_big.png (downloaded on 19/Agust/2014)]

Faúndez EI, Osorio GA. 2010. New data on the biology of Sinopla perpunctatus Signoret, 1864 (Hemiptera, Heteroptera: Acanthosomatidae). Bol. Biodivers. Chile 3: 24-31.

Fernández -Arhex, V; Buteler, M; Amadio, ME; Enriquez, A; Pietrantuono, AL; Stadler , T; Becker, G & O, Bruzzone . 2013. The effects of volcanic ash from Puyehue-Caulle range eruption on the survival of *Dichroplus vittigerum* (Orthoptera: Acrididae). *Fla. Entomol.*, 96:286-288.

Fleming, RA. 1996. A mechanistic perspective of possible influences of climate change on defoliating insects in North America's boreal forests. *Silva Fenn*, 30: 281–94.

Fye RE. 1978. Pupation preferences of Bollworms, Tobacco budworms and Beet armyworms and impact on mortality resulting from cultivation of irrigated cotton. *J Econ Entomol* 71: 570-572.

Gaitán JJ, F Raffo, JA Ayesa, F Umaña, DB Bran. 2011. Zonificación del área afectada por cenizas volcánicas. INTA EEA Bariloche "Dr. Greenville Morris", Ministerio de Agricultura, Ganadería y Pesca de la Nación. Bariloche. http://inta.gob.ar/documentos/zonificacion-del-area-afectada-por-cenizas-volcanicas-en-rio-negro-y-neuquen/ [Accesed 26 August 2013]

Golob P. 1997. Current status and future perspectives for inert dusts for control of stored product insects. J.Stored Prod. Res. 33: 69-79.

Grosfeld, J and JG, Puntieri. 2011. Puyehue – Cordón Caulle: algunos efectos de las cenizas volcánicas en la vegetación boscosa. *Patagonia Forestal* 2:11–12.

Harrison ET, Norris R, Wilkinson SN. The impact of fine sediment accumulation on benthic macroinvertebrates: implications for river management. In: Harrison Wilson AL, Dehaan RL,Watts RJ,Page KJ, Bowmer KH, Curtis A, editors. Proceedings of the 5th Australian Stream Management Conference. Australian rivers: making a difference. New SouthWales: Charles Sturt University, Thurgoona; 2007. p. 139–44

Informe De Los Laboratorios De La Facultad De Ingeniería, Departamentos De Geología Y Petróleo (Cimar-Cpem) Y Departamento De Química. 2011. Análisis y caracterización de cenizas procedentes del Complejo Volcánico Puyehue – Cordón Caulle depositadas en la ciudad de Neuquén y Alto Valle del Río Negro. Univ. Nac. Comahue, Neuquén. 6 pp.

Jia G, H Wang, L Yan, X Wang, R PeI, T Yan, Y Zhao, X Guo. 2005. Cytotoxicity of carbon nanomaterials: single-wall nanotube, multi-wall nanotube, and fullerene. *Environ. Sci. Technol.* 39: 1378-1383.

Lara LE, H Moreno, J A Naranjo, S Matthews, C Pérez De Arce. 2006. Magmatic Evolution of the Puyehue-Cordón Caulle Volcanic Complex (40° S), Southern Andean Volcanic Zone: From shield to unusual fissure volcanism. *Journal of Volcanology and Geothermal Research* (Elsevier) 157 (4): pp. 343–366. doi:10.1016/j.jvolgeores.2006.04.010.

Marske KA, Ivie MA, Hilton G M. 2007. Effects of volcanic ash on the forest canopy insects of Montserrat, West Indies. *Environ. Entomol.* 36(4): 817-25.

Martínez HE, Fuentes JP, Acevedo E. 2008. Carbono orgánico y propiedades del suelo. *J Soil Sci Plant Nutr* 8 (1):68-96

Martínez, AS; M Masciocchi; JM Villacide; G Huerta; L Daneri; A Bruchhausen; G Rozas & JC Corley. 2013. Ashes in the air: the effects of volcanic ash emissions on plant–pollinator relationships and possible consequences for apiculture. *Apidologie,* 44: 268-277.

Masciocchi, M; AJ Pereira; MV Lantschner & JC Corley.2013. Of volcanoes and insects: the impact of the Puyehue–Cordon Caulle ash fall on populations of invasive social wasps, *Vespula* spp. *Ecol. Res.,* 28:268-277.

Miserendino, ML; M Archangelsky; C Brand & LB Epele. 2012. Environmental changes and macroinvertebrate responses in Patagonian streams (Argentina) to ashfall from the Chaitén Volcano (May 2008). *Sci. Total Environ.*, 424:202-212.

Mogni L, C Cotaro, R Daga. 2011. Análisis preliminar cenizas volcánicas sistema Puyehue-Cordón Caulle – 04-06-11. http:// organismos.chubut.gov.ar/ambiente /files/ 2011/06/Informe-Cenizas-Puyehue1.CAB_.pdf.

Morales CL, A Saez, MP Arbetman, L Cavallero, MA Aizen. 2014. Detrimental effects of volcanic ash deposition on bee fauna and plant-pollinator interactions. *Ecología Austral* 24:42-50.

NASA. 2011. Available on: http://www.nasa.gov/topics/earth/features/ stratospheric-aerosols.html (downloaded on 19/Agust/2014)

Parmenter, RR; Risafulli, CMC; ORBE, NCK; Parsons, CLP ; Reutzian, MJK & JA Macm Ahon . 2005. Posteruption arthropod succession on the Mount St. Helens Volcano: the ground-dwelling beetle fauna (Coleoptera). Chapter 10. In: Dale, VH; FJ Swanson & CM Crisafulli (eds). Ecological Responses to the 1980 Eruption of Mount St. Helens. Springer-Verlag, pp. 139-150.

Paull J, K Lyons. 2008. Nanotechnology: the next challenge for organics. *J. Org. Syst.* 3(1): 3-22

Pickett, STA & PS White. 1985. *The ecology of natural disturbance and patch dynamics.* Academic Press, New York.

Pietrantuono A.L., Fernández-Arhex V. & Bruzzone O.A. 2014. First study of host-plant preferences of Sinopla perpunctatus (Hemiptera: Acanthosomatidae) a stink bug from Andean-patagonic forest. *Florida entomologist* 97(2):534-539.

Pirk, G. 2014. Did ash fall from Puyehue-Cordón Caulle volcanic complex affect ant abundance and richness in the Patagonian steppe? .*Ecología Austral* 24:23-30.

Primer Inventario Nacional De Bosques Nativos. 2005. Proyecto Bosques Nativos y Áreas Protegidas Préstamo BIRF 4085-AR.

Prudic KL, Oliver JC, Bowers MD. 2005. Soil nutrient effects in oviposition preference, larval performance and chemical defense of a specialist insect herbivore. *Oecologia* 143: 578-587.

Schowalter , TD. 2012. Insect responses to major landscape-level disturbance. *Annual Review of Entomology*, 57:1-20.

Seymour, VA; TM Hinckley; Y Morikawa & JF Franklin. 1983. Foliage damage in coniferous trees following volcanic ash fall from Mt. St. Helens. *Oecologia,* 59:339-343.

Shanks CH Jr, and DL Chase. 1981. Effect of volcanic ash on adult *Otiorhynchus* (Coleoptera: Curculionidae). *Melanderia,* 37, 63-66.

Sparks RSJ, MI Bursik, SN Carey, JS Gilbert, LS Glaze, H Sigurdsson, AW Woods. 1997.Volcanic Plumes. John Wiley & Sons, Chichester.

Stadler T, M Buteler, DK Weaver. 2010. Nanoinsecticidas: Nuevas perspectivas para el control de plagas. Rev. Soc. Entomol. Argentina, 69: (3-4): 149- 156.

Subramanyam B, and R Roesli. 2000. Inert dusts, pp. 321-379 In B. Subramanyam and D.W. Hagstrum [eds.], Alternatives to Pesticides in stored-product IMP. Kluwer Academic Publishers, Boston, Massachusetts.

Tenow, O; Nilssen, AC; Holmgren, B & F, Elverum. 1999. An insect (*Argyresthia retinella*, Lep., Yponomeutidae) outbreak in northern birch forests, released by climatic changes? J. Appl. Ecol., 36:111–122.

Varela, S. Y M, Weigandt. 2009. Estrés en árboles y su efecto sobre la susceptibilidad a invasión por insectos. Serie técnica: Manejo Integrado de Plagas N°8.

Wicderholm T. Responses of aquatic insects to environmental pollution. In: Resh VH, Rosenberg DM, editors. *The ecology of aquatic insects.* New York: Praeger; 1984. p. 508–57.

Wigglesworth VB. 1944. Action of inert dusts on insects. *Nature,* 153: 493-494.

Wille , A & G F Uentes . 1975. Efecto de la ceniza del Volcán: Irazú (Costa Rica) en algunos insectos. *Rev. Biol. Trop.* 3:165-175.

Williams, DW & M Liebhold. 1995. Herbivorous insects and global change: potential changes in the spatial distribution of forest defoliators. *J. Biogeogr., 22*: 665–71.

INDEX

A

acetone, 123
acid, 28
adsorption, 9, 144
aerosols, ix, x, 118, 119, 120, 121, 122, 123, 124, 126, 128, 130, 133, 135, 138, 139, 157
age, 25, 29, 46, 47, 51, 124
air temperature, 24
airports, 125
aldehydes, 123
algae, 3
amplitude, 32
anaerobic digesters, 5
architect, 42
Argentina, x, 117, 132, 139, 141, 143, 144, 147, 157, 158
aromatics, 123
arthropods, 145, 155
ASI, 134
atmosphere, vii, ix, x, 10, 49, 117, 118, 119, 120, 122, 123, 124, 125, 131, 142

B

bacteria, 3
barometric pressure, 24
barriers, 146
base, 8, 19, 28
beams, 44
behavioral change, 148
bioassay, 149, 150
biological activity, 145
boreal forest, 155
bromine, ix, 117, 121, 123

C

Cairo, 136
calibration, 51, 132
campaigns, 127, 128, 130, 132
canals, 44
carbon, 4, 156
carbon dioxide (CO_2), 4
Caribbean, viii, 23, 25, 26, 29, 30, 31
case studies, vii, 2, 10, 125, 141
chemical, vii, 1, 2, 5, 119, 120, 121, 140, 143, 145, 147, 149, 153, 157
chemicals, 4
Chile, x, 125, 139, 141, 142, 155
China, 122
chlorine, ix, 117, 121, 123, 133, 136
circulation, ix, 117, 119, 120, 121, 122, 134
cities, 2, 28, 41, 125
classes, 31, 32
classification, 16, 33
cleaning, 17, 19

climate, vii, 23, 24, 25, 34, 40, 47, 51, 119, 135, 149, 154, 155
climate change, vii, 135, 149, 154, 155
climatic factors, 40
CMC, 157
coal, 122, 125
community(ies), x, 142, 149, 152, 153
complexity, 25, 28
complications, 34
composition, x, 118, 119, 145, 149, 152, 153
compounds, 119, 123
condensation, 133
conductivity, 9
conifer, 51
conservation, 42
construction, 19, 44
consumption, 122, 150
convergence, 26
cooling, 24, 25, 48, 124
correlations, viii, ix, xi, 23, 24, 34, 45
cosmic ray flux, 24
Costa Rica, 158
cotton, 155
covering, 28, 44, 47, 48, 143
critical infrastructure, vii, 1
critical value, 45
crops, 152
crust, 25, 27, 34
crystals, 119
cultivation, 155
cuticle, 144
cycles, viii, 23, 24, 25, 29, 30, 31, 32, 34

D

damages, vii, 2, 3
data collection, 132
data set, 134
database, viii, 25, 39, 41, 42, 46, 135
decay, 25
deformation, 24, 28
deposition, x, 5, 133, 142, 145, 149, 150, 152, 154, 157
deposits, 25, 28, 44, 143
depth, 27, 119, 120, 128, 129, 131, 134
desiccation, 144
destruction, 121, 133, 153
detection, 36, 136
diffraction, 123
disequilibrium, ix
dispersion, 18, 136, 137
distribution, viii, 2, 8, 13, 14, 17, 18, 23, 31, 40, 124, 140, 149, 158
diversity, 144, 145, 146
DNA damage, 123
DOI, 133
drought, 50, 51
dusts, 144, 155, 156, 158

E

earthquakes, ix, xi, 2
ecology, 157, 158
ecosystem, xi, 142, 146, 149, 155
EEA, 141, 148, 155
El Niño, 119
electrical conductivity, 147
elytra, 151
emergency, 146
emission, 10, 18, 124, 125, 154
energy, 4, 49, 146
energy supply, 4
engineering, 20
environment, xi, 36, 51, 142, 145, 146, 147, 152, 153
environmental effects, vii, 154
environments, vii, 51, 142
epidermis, 146
equipment, 3, 4, 5, 17
Europe, viii, 10, 28, 40, 43, 48, 122, 136
European Commission, 19
evidence, 24, 31, 48, 49, 50, 121, 136
evolution, 27, 28, 34, 35, 36, 118
exposure, x, 142, 146, 149, 153
external environment, 146
extraction, 42

F

Fairbanks, 138
fauna, 150, 152, 157
fires, 42
fish, 142
flight, 125
floods, 2
flora and fauna, vii, x, 141, 142, 144
flowers, 148, 150
fluid, 6, 7, 36
food, 3, 4, 145, 146, 148, 149, 150, 153
force, 7, 34
forest fire, 124
formation, 5, 121, 135
formula, 14
fractures, 27
France, 2, 23
frequency distribution, 21, 31
friction, 7
fullerene, 156

G

genus, 144, 146
geometry, 123
global scale, viii, 39, 40, 124
global warming, 24, 36
governments, 42
grain size, vii, 142, 143, 149
granules, 8
grasslands, x, 142
gravity, 3, 4, 7, 27
grazing, 42
Greece, 25, 26, 29, 30, 31, 138
greenhouse gases, 24
greenhouses, 154
grids, 2
growth, viii, 4, 25, 28, 40, 41, 42, 45, 47, 48, 49
growth rings, 45

H

habitat, vii, x, 141, 142, 145, 147, 148, 153
halogen, 122
harmful effects, 123
Hawaii, 27
hazardous materials, 2
hazards, vii, 1, 2, 20, 21
haze, 138
heat transfer, 20
hemisphere, viii, 23
historical data, 35
Holocene, 28, 142
honey bees, 148
host, xi, 142, 146, 147, 151, 157
human health, vii, 2
humidity, 149, 151
hydrocarbons, 144
hydrogen, 119

I

Iceland, 2, 122, 137
image, 125, 127, 132
imagery, 125
impurities, 4
indirect effect, 153
individuals, xi, 142
industry, vii, 1, 2, 125
information technology, 40
ingestion, 149, 151
insecticide, 144, 154, 155
insects, x, 141, 145, 146, 147, 148, 149, 150, 151, 152, 153, 154, 155, 156, 158
integration, 146
integument, 146
intestine, 144
invertebrates, 154
islands, 25, 27, 29
isolation, 119
Italy, vii, 1, 2, 10, 11, 25, 28, 31, 35, 36, 139

J

Japan, 125

K

kinetics, 145

L

laminar, 7, 18
landscape, 157
larva, 146, 147
larval development, 146
lead, xi, 3, 34, 124, 142
liberation, 27
lidar, 136
life cycle, 152
light, 18, 124
localization, 35
logistics, 132
low temperatures, 152

M

magnitude, ix, xi, 143
management, 19, 154, 156
mantle, 27, 29, 37
mapping, 3
marine environment, 140
mass, 8, 20, 24, 25
materials, 3, 9, 148
measurements, 8, 9, 14, 16, 46, 120, 122, 131, 132, 136, 137, 138
media, 140
median, 32
Mediterranean, viii, 23, 24, 35, 36, 37, 138
melting, 36
methodology, 5, 6, 8, 12, 13, 19
microclimate, 145
microorganisms, 3, 128
migration, viii, ix, 24, 34
Miocene, 27, 29
models, ix, 117, 121
Moderate Resolution Imaging Spectroradiometer, 125
modifications, ix
MODIS, 125, 127, 132, 139
Montreal Protocol, 122
mortality, 149, 152, 155
Moscow, 138
motivation, x, 141

N

nanomaterials, 156
nanometer, vii, 142
nanotube, 156
NATO, 134
natural disturbance, 149, 157
natural enemies, 149
natural hazards, 124
negative effects, 151
New Zealand, 143
nitrates, 3
nitrogen, 9, 119, 123
North America, 27, 155
nucleation, 133, 136
nutrients, xi, 142, 157

O

occlusion, 151
oil, 2
Oklahoma, 120, 134
operations, 17, 19
optical properties, x, 118, 124
organic matter, 4, 147, 148
organism, 145
oscillation, 119
oxidation, 120
oxygen, 119
ozone, ix, x, 117, 118, 119, 120, 121, 122, 123, 126, 129, 130, 133, 134, 135, 136, 138
ozone layer, x, 118, 119, 120, 122, 126, 134

P

Pacific, 24, 25, 50
PAN, 123
parallel, 35
particle mass, 136
pastures, x, 142
pathogens, 151
pathways, 27
permeability, 7, 8, 16
Peru, viii, 39, 40, 48, 50, 51
pests, x, 142, 144, 149
pH, 147
phosphates, 3
photosynthesis, 49, 151
physical phenomena, 144
physical properties, 20
physiology, 153
plants, vii, xi, 2, 5, 48, 142, 146, 151, 152
Poland, 138
polar, 119, 121, 133, 135, 136
pollen, 128
pollination, 152
pollutants, 3
pollution, 125, 139, 158
population, 152, 154
porosity, 7, 14, 18, 147
positive relationship, xi
precipitation, 120, 126
probability, 31, 47, 121
probe, 129
protection, 144
pupa, 146, 147

R

race, 44
radiation, x, 118, 119, 123, 124, 128, 129, 138, 139, 140
radius, 26, 45, 123
rainfall, xi, 144, 147
reactions, 120, 121
reconstruction, 44, 46
recovery, x, 122, 142, 155
regionalization, 50
reproduction, 4, 145
reserves, 144
resources, 145, 148
respiration, 151
response, ix, 26, 34, 118, 120, 122, 135, 136
restoration, 43
rheology, 34
rings, viii, 40, 41, 45, 46, 48, 49, 50, 51
risk management, 19
risks, 2, 19, 21, 146, 152

S

scatter, 123
scattering, x, 118, 123, 124, 140
scope, 10
Scots pine, 42
sea level, 24, 25, 34, 36
seasonality, 24
sedimentation, 4
sediment(s), 21, 24, 25, 156
senescence, 146
sensitivity, 14, 18
sewage, 3, 4, 5, 6, 18
shape, 18, 19, 145
shelter, 145, 146
shrubs, 127
Siberia, 50
signals, 24, 134
silicon, 144
silver, 43
simulations, 121, 134, 135, 138
SiO2, 143, 144
software, 46, 47
solar activity, 24
sorption, 9, 14, 18
South Africa, 143
South America, 140
Spain, viii, 35, 39, 41, 42, 48, 49, 50, 51
species, x, 127, 141, 146, 149, 151, 152, 153
species richness, 149, 152
specific surface, 6, 7, 8, 9, 14, 15, 18
spin, 25

standard deviation, 47, 128, 129, 130
state, 34, 42, 151
stereomicroscope, 46
stress, ix, 24, 25, 34, 151
structure, 25, 37, 44, 145
substrate, 146, 147, 148, 149
succession, 154, 157
sulfate, 119, 121, 124
sulfur, ix, 117, 120, 122, 123, 139
sulfur dioxide, 120, 123, 139
sulfuric acid, 120
Sun, vii, x, 23, 24, 25, 26, 29, 31, 32, 34, 118, 123, 140
sunspots, 26
surface area, 7, 8, 14, 15
survival, x, 141, 145, 146, 149, 151, 152, 153, 155
synchronization, 47

T

tanks, 3, 4
taxa, 151
techniques, 40
technology, 4, 20, 44
temperature, 50, 120, 121, 136
Tibet, 137
tides, 24
time series, 51
toxicity, 145, 149, 150, 153
traits, 148, 153
translocation, 145
transmission, 138, 140
transparency, 147
transpiration, 151
transport, vii, 2
transportation, 2, 132
treatment, 2, 3, 4, 5, 10, 11, 20
tropical forests, 154
turbulent flows, 6
Turkey, 19

U

UK, 19, 20, 35, 36, 121
UNESCO, 42
United Nations, 132, 133
urban, 10, 12, 124, 139
urbanization, 10
USA, 36, 37, 50, 51
USDA, 139
UV, x, 24, 118, 119, 123, 124, 125, 126, 132, 137, 138, 139, 140
UV radiation, x, 118, 123, 124, 140

V

variations, 24, 25, 31, 119, 129, 133, 138
vegetation, 153
velocity, 6, 7, 12
viscosity, 6, 7
vitamin D, 132
vulnerability, 2, 19

W

Washington, 19, 36
wastewater, vii, 2, 3, 5, 6, 12, 16, 17, 21
water, xi, 2, 3, 4, 9, 10, 18, 24, 124, 142, 146, 151
water quality, 4
wavelengths, 123, 125, 129, 132
West Indies, 156
wood, viii, 39, 42, 44, 46, 49